Rheumatology Nursing

For Churchill Livingstone

Senior commissioning editor: Alex Mathieson
Project manager: Valerie Burgess
Design direction: Judith Wright
Project controller: Pat Miller
Illustrator: Robert Britton
Copy editor: Carolyn Holleyman
Indexer: Tarrant Ranger Indexing Agency
Sales promotion manager: Hilary Brown

Rheumatology Nursing

A Creative Approach

Edited by

Jackie Hill MPhil RGN FRCN

Lecturer and Rheumatology Nurse Practitioner,
Clinical Pharmacology Unit (Rheumatism Research),
University of Leeds, Chapel Allerton Hospital, Leeds, West Yorkshire, UK

Foreword by

Vicky Stephenson RGN FRCN

Chair of Congress,
Royal College of Nursing of the UK 1995–1998

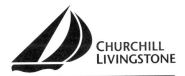

CHURCHILL
LIVINGSTONE

EDINBURGH LONDON NEW YORK PHILADELPHIA SYDNEY TORONTO 1998

CHURCHILL LIVINGSTONE
An imprint of Harcourt Brace and Company Limited

Churchill Livingstone, Robert Stevenson House,
1–3 Baxter's Place, Leith Walk, Edinburgh,
EH1 3AF, UK.

First published 1998

ISBN 0 443 05792 3

British Library Cataloguing in Publication Data
A catalogue record for this book is available from the British
Library.

Library of Congress Cataloging in Publication Data
A catalog record for this book is available from the Library
of Congress.

Note
Medical knowledge is constantly changing. As new
information becomes available, changes in treatment,
procedures, equipment and the use of drugs become
necessary. The editors, contributors and the publishers have,
as far as it is possible, taken care to ensure that the
information given in this text is accurate and up-to-date.
However, readers are strongly advised to confirm that the
information, especially with regard to drug usage, complies
with the latest legislation and standards of practice.

The
publisher's
policy is to use
**paper manufactured
from sustainable forests**

Produced by Addison Wesley Longman China Limited, Hong Kong
EPC/01

Catherine Sturdy RGN FAETC
Rheumatology Clinical Nurse Specialist, Friarage
Hospital, Northallerton, UK
4. *Assessing rheumatic patients*
14. *Surgical interventions*

Angela Vale BSc RGN
Sister, Rheumatology Ward, Devonshire Royal
Hospital, Buxton, UK
6. *Body image and sexuality*

Christine E. White RGN
Rheumatology Nurse Specialist, Pinderfields and
Pontefract Hospital Trust, Wakefield, West
Yorkshire, UK
9. *Fatigue and sleep*

Contents

Contributors

Valerie Arthur SRN
Rheumatology Nurse Specialist, University Hospital
Birmingham NHS Trust, Birmingham, UK
2. The rheumatic conditions – an overview

Jane Billington RGN LicAc MMAcC MIFA
Hospital Macmillan Nurse, Withington Hospital,
Manchester, UK
13. Complementary therapeutic interventions

Jill Byrne MSc RN SCM
Nurse Clinician/Ward Manager, Rheumatology
Unit, St Helens and Knowsley Hospitals Trust,
St Helens, Merseyside, UK
10. Skin and nutrition
12. Medication in rheumatic disease

Anne Cawthorne RGN OND DipN BSc RNT CertCouns
MISPA
Lecturer Practitioner, Neil Cliffe Cancer Care Centre;
Honorary Tutor, Manchester University, UK
13. Complementary therapeutic interventions

Lynne Dargie RGN NDNCert CPT
District Nurse and Community Practice Teacher,
Sonning Common Health Centre, Reading, UK
16. Seamless care

Jane Douglas BSc DPSN RGN
Rheumatology Nurse Specialist, Freeman Hospital,
Newcastle Upon Tyne, UK
3. Immunology and investigative techniques
10. Skin and nutrition

Jackie Hill MPhil RGN FRCN
Lecturer and Rheumatology Nurse Practitioner,
Clinical Pharmacology Unit (Rheumatism Research),
University of Leeds, Chapel Allerton Hospital,
Leeds, West Yorkshire, UK
6. Body image and sexuality
8. Pain and stiffness
15. Patient education

Juliet Prady RGN
Senior Sister, Head Injury Rehabilitation Unit,
Devonshire Royal Hospital, Buxton, Derbyshire,
UK.
6. Body image and sexuality

Jane Proctor RGN
Practice Nurse, Sonning Common Health Centre,
Reading, UK
16. Seamless care

Sarah Ryan BSc MSc RGN
Clinical Nurse Specialist Rheumatology,
Staffordshire Rheumatology Centre, Haywood
Hospital, Stoke on Trent, UK
1. The essence of rheumatology nursing
5. Psychological aspects
7. The social implications of rheumatic disease

Joan Stamp RGN
Clinical Nurse Specialist and Manager in
Department of Rheumatology, South Cleveland
Hospital, Middlesborough, UK
11. The team approach to mobility and self care

Foreword

Prior to 1980, there was no distinct body of rheumatology nursing knowledge in the UK. Hundreds of nurses were involved in caring for patients with rheumatic diseases but they were practising in comparative nursing isolation and there was little opportunity for them to come together to share their skills and expertise. There was still less opportunity for them to be involved in nursing research or to define a body of rheumatology nursing knowledge. Many of the contemporary textbooks focused upon diagnosis rather than the nursing response to the many complex problems presented by patients.

The Royal College of Nursing Rheumatology Nursing Forum (RNF) held its inaugural meeting in Manchester in 1981 with 96 registered nurses present. The membership today is greater than 2000. During its formative years, the RNF concentrated upon the professional development of its members – gradually, nursing journals featured articles by rheumatology nurses, and textbooks written by nurses began to appear.

The authors of this book are highly knowledgeable practising rheumatology nurses and they are members of the RNF. In this research-based text, they have focused upon therapeutic nursing responses to the many complex problems of patients with a rheumatic disease, and their families. In addition to the science, the art and caring components of good rheumatology nursing shine out.

Such is the prevalence of the rheumatic diseases, that all nurses, regardless of their field of practice, will regularly encounter such patients. This text will be invaluable to them, as well as to those for whom rheumatology nursing is a chosen career.

As founder members of the RNF, we view this book as an exciting development for rheumatology nursing, for patient care and for the RNF, which is now recognised world-wide as a body of expert nursing knowledge. It is with pride that we salute our successors who are realising the hopes we shared 17 years ago.

1998   Vicky Stephenson

Preface

Musculoskeletal diseases are the most common causes of disability in developed countries throughout the world. In the United Kingdom, a significant rheumatic disease affects one in seven of the population and is responsible for one third of all the severe disabilities. Rheumatic disease affects people from all walks of life and of all ages, from babies to the very elderly. They are so widespread and so common that it is inevitable that all nurses, no matter which health setting they work in, will at some time provide care for rheumatic patients. This makes it essential that all nurses have sufficient knowledge of rheumatology nursing to allow them to deliver high quality care. Historically this knowledge has been difficult to acquire, as there is a paucity of textbooks specifically about rheumatology nursing. Therefore, the aim of this book is to fill this gap. It is written by fourteen experienced nurses who work in the field of rheumatology and are active members of the Royal College of Nursing Rheumatology Nursing Forum. Many are renowned experts in their chosen topics, and all are keen to share their knowledge.

The book is intended primarily for nurses working at post-basic level, but it will also be a useful resource for pre-registered nurses. It is also intended to accommodate continuing nurse education, and this is emphasised by the inclusion of aims and intended learning outcomes at the beginning of each chapter, and action points for practice at the end.

The book aims to enhance all aspects of nursing practice and will be particularly helpful to nurses working in the fields of rheumatology, orthopaedic surgery, in general practice and in the community. It will also prove useful to nurses caring for patients on elderly care or general medical and surgical wards, as rheumatic disease is often a secondary diagnosis. One area that has not been included is the care of the child with rheumatic disease. This is a specialist subject that warrants a book in its own right, and as such is outside the scope of this textbook.

The essence of rheumatology nursing is the 'Three E's': educating, empowering and enabling our patients. This requires the nurse to work in partnership with the patient and his or her carers, and to adopt a holistic approach to care.

The book is in three sections. The first sets the scene and comprises three chapters. Chapter one discusses the underlying principles of rheumatology nursing and focuses on the benefits of adopting a therapeutic rather than a purely supportive approach to care delivery. The next two chapters are devoted to the diseases, their diagnosis and their effect on the immune system.

The second section of the book is structured on The Royal College of Nursing Rheumatology Nursing Forum Problem Model. Its eight chapters address the patient's problems and include effective interventions that help relieve symptoms such as pain and stiffness, fatigue and sleep disturbance and the psychological and social effects. The effects of rheumatic diseases on the skin are explored and also included is a discussion of the relationship between skin integrity and nutrition, and a summary of the effectiveness of dietary supplementation on the rheumatic diseases. Pain, disability and changes in body image can have a profound effect on both sexual function and pregnancy and this is explored in detail. One chapter is devoted to assessing the rheumatic patient and the section is completed by a description of the multidisciplinary team approach to mobility and self care.

The final section of the book focuses on therapeutic interventions including medications, complementary therapies and caring for the patient undergoing surgical interventions. Teaching patients about their disease and its treatments is the foundation upon which successful management programmes are built, and no book on caring for the rheumatology patient would be complete without a chapter on patient education. Various approaches to patient teaching are discussed and methods of assessing and writing educational material are described. The final chapter is devoted to care in the community and is written by a community and a district nurse.

Rheumatology as a speciality has often been described as one of the Cinderella services; it is not seen as a glamorous, emotive or technical branch of nursing. However, to those of us who work in it and love it, nursing the patient with rheumatic disease is a truly demanding yet satisfying experience. Although essential, our nurturing nursing skills alone will not provide the quality of service that our patients deserve. The aim of providing a high quality rheumatology nursing service will be achieved only through great depth and breadth of knowledge; this book represents one step on the road to realising that aim.

I would like to thank all my fellow 'scribes' who have contributed blood, sweat and tears to make the dream a reality; Alex Mathieson and Pat Miller at Churchill Livingstone for their guidance and unbelievable forbearance; and all the nurses and patients who have shared their knowledge and experience with me over the years. Finally, I have to give my love and thanks to my husband Geoff whose belief in me and my work has kept me going when I thought it impossible to continue.

1997   Jackie Hill

Setting the scene

Section one provides an overview of the rheumatic diseases, the effect they can have on the immune system and the different investigations used to diagnose and assess the diseases. The central role of the nurse in caring for patients is discussed and the benefits of adopting a therapeutic rather than exclusively supportive framework is advocated. The expanding role of the nurse within the speciality is explored and the benefit of nurse-led clinics and wards is described.

1

The essence of rheumatology nursing

Sarah Ryan

The aim of this chapter is to provide an understanding of the important contribution that therapeutic nursing can make to a patient living with a chronic rheumatological condition. After reading this chapter the reader should be able to:

- **Describe the key elements of nursing and explain why they are important to a patient with a rheumatological condition**
- **Discuss the skills and qualities required for the nurse to enter into a therapeutic relationship**
- **Describe the difference between supportive and therapeutic nursing and provide examples to illustrate this**
- **Discuss the actual and potential barriers to therapeutic practice**
- **Explain the advantages of having a shared philosophy of care within the clinical area.**

WHAT IS NURSING?

The role of the nurse appears to be all encompassing. The nurse is the only member of the health care team that provides a continuity of care 24 hours a day, 7 days a week. During this time she will not only be attending to the patient's physical, psychological, social and spiritual well-being, she will also be responding to:

- Requests from relatives
- Supervising the work of colleagues
- Accommodating the needs of the organisation.

The complexity and multifaceted nature of nursing makes it difficult to define. However, for the future of nursing, there is one mandate that remains central to our vision and to which nurses must remain committed, and that is:

All nursing care stems from patient-focused need.

and

All nursing development must be dedicated to providing holistic care for patients and their families.

Indeed the professional code of conduct (UKCC 1992) reinforces these values by highlighting the legal requirement for nurses to act always in the best interests of patients. This must remain the foundation stone of all nursing practice.

Definitions of nursing

The most widely known definition of nursing is that of Henderson (1966) who states that 'the unique function of the nurse is to assist the individual sick or well in the performance of those activities contributing to health or its recovery (or to a peaceful death) that he would perform unaided if he had the necessary strength, will or knowledge, and to do this in such a way as to help him gain independence as rapidly as possible'. Although this definition is not new, it contains the elements relevant to today's health care with its emphasis on empowerment, rehabilitation, education and where ever possible, enabling the patient to actively participate in self care activities. When nursing a patient with a chronic rheumatic illness, these objectives are relevant, but the goal of a complete reinstatement of health is not realistic. The patient will require the services of the nurse who will facilitate positive coping mechanisms and adaptation to develop by the actions of:

- Guiding
- Supporting
- Empowering.

Health and illness are not static but dynamic entities, fluctuating in response to many internal and external influences. The role that the nurse assumes will be governed by the patient's perceived need at any particular time. For instance, following a diagnosis of rheumatoid arthritis (RA), a patient's primary nursing need may be for information, but as the condition progresses, an increased emphasis on practical advice may be appropriate.

Bower (1972) views nursing as the 'application of knowledge to promote and maintain maximum health, comfort and care'. To fulfil these criteria, nurses must be knowledgeable practitioners who are leaders

within the clinical environment and who ensure that there are mechanisms in place that encourage and support ongoing personal and professional development. Once the nurse has acquired the necessary knowledge herself, she can safely provide patients with information that allows them to give informed consent on all aspects of their treatment.

Nursing is a practice-based profession, but this does not mean that because we use our hands we cannot use our minds as well (Clarke 1994). If nurses are to act in the best interests of patients providing informed answers, they need to be participating actively in, or be aware of, appropriate research. Research groups and practice networks can provide channels through which to share ideas and increase understanding with colleagues working in the same area of rheumatology.

Caring

Caring is one of the most important values of the nursing profession. Although often referred to as a basic requirement there is nothing basic about high quality nursing care. The term 'basic care' has been used and interpreted incorrectly to the detriment of the profession. Nursing requires a combination of:

- Knowledge
- Understanding
- Expertise.

Identifying and meeting the needs of patients who are unable to care fully for themselves involves having regard for people as individuals and being concerned about what happens to them (Malin & Teasdale 1991). The process of 'caring' comprises elements of both action and emotion. However, in practice the action element frequently dominates, as the nurse concentrates her energies on the patient's physical needs (Macleod-Clark 1983, May 1991, Henderson 1994). This can result in a neglect of the emotional needs that have been shown to be the predominating factor influencing the experience of 'good' or 'bad' care as perceived by patients (Smith 1992).

An over-emphasis on the physical manifestation of RA such as synovitis of the small joints, without consideration of the effects the condition has on the individual's lifestyle, will not provide comprehensive care and may well be harmful. If no one has explored the emotional impact of chronic illness with the patient, they may find themselves bewildered, and unsure of where to turn for help and advice. It is common for patients with a chronic condition to experience a plethora of emotions (Krueger 1984) including:

- Shock
- Anger
- Grief
- Depression.

It is essential that the nurse has the necessary support and education to provide the emotional elements of care, otherwise it will not be holistic, meaningful or relevant to the patient.

The elements of nursing

The key elements or functions of nursing can be seen in Box 1.1. The main link between the elements is the nature of the relationship between the nurse and the patient. This interaction is important, and should start at the preliminary encounter and continue through all subsequent activities.

To do this, the nurse must make time for the patient and show empathy towards their problems; intimacy and reciprocity are essential ingredients of the nurse/patient relationship (Muetzel 1988).

Box 1.1 Nursing functions (Wilson Barnett 1984)

- Understanding illness and treatment from the patient's viewpoint
- Providing continuous psychological care during illness and critical events
- Helping people cope with illness or potential health problems
- Providing comfort
- Coordinating treatment and other events affecting the patient.

Once problems have been identified, a plan of care will be formulated which incorporates nursing functions that meet identified needs. Chronic conditions have a global impact on the patient's life; living with a rheumatological illness will affect not only the individual but also their family and significant others (Ryan 1996). The social implications of rheumatological illness are discussed in Chapter 7.

As well as a sound knowledge base, the nurse will require the ability to understand exactly what physical disability means to each individual (Powell 1991). For instance, a mother with active inflammation in her hands may be prevented from lifting her child, causing feelings of guilt and anxiety. She must be allowed to express her feelings and be given support and advice about practical measures such as lying on the bed to cuddle her child. For others, inflammatory changes in the hands may affect their ability to work, causing depression and poor self esteem. Counselling will be required to support the individual through this life crisis, but until the nurse is able to appreciate and understand the impact of illness from the patient's perspective, they will not be able to offer care from a humanistic viewpoint.

Essentially, nursing is a social activity. The nurse will need to possess good communication skills and a level of understanding and knowledge about the complex nature of rheumatological illness to be able to offer a complete care package.

THE PHILOSOPHY OF NURSING

A philosophy of practice is essential. It should provide a clear outline of what nurses perceive to be important and central to their practice. This ensures a continuity of approach and can unify the team and ensure that care is practised from a shared understanding with an identified purpose. If nurses working within a clinical area do not share a common purpose, disunity and fragmentation of care can occur. To be meaningful, the philosophy should be derived from those working in both primary and secondary care. Each clinical area will need a team to determine and develop the beliefs that shape present practice. A philosophy imposed by the wider organisation without the necessary consultation with the team will probably fail in its objective. A rheumatology philosophy of care can be divided into four interlinked and complementary areas (see Fig. 1.1). Underpinning each area is the patient as the central focus of care delivery.

Beliefs relating to health

Health is the state in which the individual has adapted to physical, psychological and/or social imbalances and who is able to cope with their arthritis in a positive

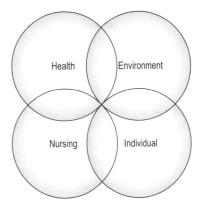

Figure 1.1 The rheumatology philosophy of care.

and constructive manner. In the context of rheumatological conditions, health does not mean the removal of all symptoms as this would be an unrealistic outcome and an unfair burden to place on patients. Health and illness are not static entities, many rheumatological conditions are characterised by flares and remissions and the patient will require advice, support, guidance, motivation and education to deal with problems presented by each new phase of their illness.

Beliefs relating to the environment

The hospital

The hospital environment is alien to most people and can cause anxiety and loss of confidence. To counter this, a person needs to believe that they can influence care management (Tones 1991) even if the belief is illusory, and participate actively at all levels. Neglect of the patient's individual concerns and perceptions can lead to isolation and the adoption of poor coping mechanisms. Nursing must create a positive atmosphere that will address both internal and external issues. If the orientation of the ward is committed to task delivery with little emphasis on interpersonal communication, the patient will be unable to explore their emotions to the detriment of their health and acceptance of their condition.

The clinical environment and the nursing staff within it should advocate a supportive welcoming approach, and encourage the patient to:

• Ask questions
• Learn about their disease
• Share personal issues.

A necessary prerequisite is that the nursing resources can meet this need and that high quality care is provided by an adequate number of qualified nurses. Assessment of the external environment, possibly by the occupational therapist, is essential to promote conditions that encourage independence and self care.

The community

As resources are increasingly diverted to the community, a person with arthritis may have reduced access to the specialist multidisciplinary hospital team. It is therefore necessary that nursing expertise moves in to the community. A community rheumatology nurse can act as the interface between primary and secondary care. The rheumatology nurse can liaise with practice nurses and other community workers to promote a greater understanding of the needs of the patients and to ensure continuity of care. Practice nurses are now conducting assessment clinics (Dargie & Proctor 1994) and monitoring second line disease-modifying drugs. It is important that primary care is supported by the secondary care service, and that community nursing staff have easy access to their hospital colleagues. In this way, the patient can be given ready access to which ever service best matches their need. Aspects of seamless care are discussed in Chapter 16.

Beliefs related to the individual patient

The beliefs of how the rheumatology nurse views the patient is essential to underpin care provision.

1. The individual is a person with an ongoing health-related problem. The individual should not be depowered, but encouraged to share their own valuable knowledge store which is essential to their care.

2. The individual will bring their own lay beliefs and life experience to all situations. These are usually consistent over time and pertinent to the individual concerned (Donovan 1991). They need to be shared with the nurse, as they will influence the success and acceptance of care management. For instance, if a patient believes that exercise damages the joints, this needs discussing so that the patient can incorporate new information into their existing knowledge. In this instance advice will be required on the type and amount of exercise needed and the anticipated outcome, enabling the patient to make an informed choice and contribute to the decision making process.

3. Patient autonomy should be the overriding principle that guides nursing practice. Paternalism is based on the principle of beneficence, i.e. the professional knows best, and is frequently used to justify actions such as forcing treatment on the individual for the individual's supposed 'good'. Use of the principle of autonomy to guide nursing decision making will remove the passivity and dependency implicit in paternalism. A heavy reliance on professional beneficence can unintentionally remove the rights or abilities of patients to participate in their own care. Non compliance with therapies is common in patients with RA. Estimates range from 28% to 78% (Bradley 1989, Jette 1982). Liang (1989) describes non compliance as the ultimate experience of independence. If patients are non compliant, this action may indicate that the management plan was not in accordance with the patient's wishes, beliefs or tolerance.

4. The individual has the right to be an active rather than passive recipient of care if they wish. However, to

assume that all patients wish to be empowered is not adopting an individualised approach. Research by Waterworth & Luker (1990) showed that some patients were 'reluctant collaborators in care'. They wished to leave decision-making to the nurse, regarding their own involvement as neglect of care. By carrying out an individual assessment, the nurse will recognise the patient's perceived needs and plan care accordingly. Some patients may prefer a partial involvement rather than a full contributing and participating role. This should be respected and reflected in care management. It will take time for patients to learn about their condition, and reliance on the nurse at a time of crisis, may be necessary for adaptation. As the therapeutic relationship develops, the patient may feel more able to contribute to care decisions. Nevertheless, the emergence of a new stressor such as a reduction in mobility may return the patients to a heightened state of dependency.

5. The patient is not an isolated being but lives as part of a social network. Any decisions concerning their care should incorporate the needs, values and expectations of these significant others. The individual has many social and occupational roles and the effects of illness must be addressed in a holistic manner.

6. The individual's values, perceptions and expectations will be central to care planning and the success of care interventions.

Beliefs relating to nursing

1. The nurse will assist the individual to achieve a state of adaptation by identifying the area of need and providing care from the patient's frame of reference.

2. The nurse will enter into a therapeutic relationship with the patient and provide both an action and emotional component to care incorporating the areas identified in the RCN Rheumatology Nursing Forum Patient Problem Model (see Fig. 1.2).

3. The nurse will empower, educate and support the patient and their families throughout all care episodes.

4. Nursing must be dynamic in nature and provide care that has meaning and relevance for the individual concerned. The nurse will strive to be a knowledgeable practitioner and use research-based findings to underpin practice.

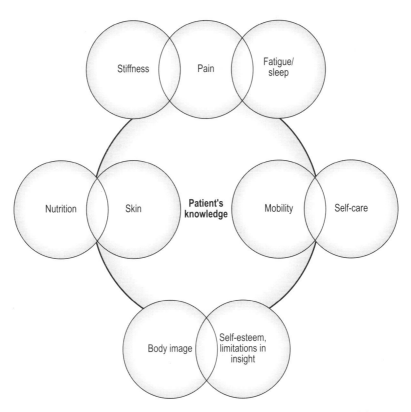

Figure 1.2 The RCN Rheumatology Nursing Forum Patient Problem Model (with permission from the RCN).

5. Nursing must have leaders with vision; providing support mechanisms to enable nurses to nurture and develop, allowing them to participate in their identified role.

EMPOWERMENT

The concept of empowerment is central to the provision of patient-focused care. Tones (1991) defines empowerment as the 'process whereby an individual or community of individuals acquire power', i.e. the capacity to control other people and resources. An empowerment approach to health recognises the rights of individuals and communities to identify their own health needs, to make their own health choices and to take action to achieve them (Wallestein & Bernstein 1988). This is a rather Utopian viewpoint, as the ability to make health choices necessitates active participation in the nurse/patient relationship and equality of access to the possible intervention which may not always be possible. For example, a young mother with RA may not be able to attend a pain management programme because of her inability to use public transport. However, there is some merit in Wallestein's contribution, as it challenges the traditional view of the passive patient, placing the patient (in this definition) in a more active role. Empowerment necessitates a relinquishing of the power held by the health care professional or a sharing of power on a more equal basis.

Empowerment is a complicated subject, so much so that some authors (Gibson 1991) have found it easier to define it by the consequences of its absence namely:

• Powerlessness
• Helplessness
• Hopelessness
• Alienation.

The combination of an internal locus of control and a belief in powerful other can be of benefit (Wallston 1995). For instance, the patient may respect the information offered by the nurse, but will judge its relevance against what is meaningful to them. If the nurse recommends an increase in exercise, they will experiment and balance the perceived benefits against time that could be spent on other activities. A person who believes only in powerful others, will preclude individual judgement and prevent an individual assessment of whether the situation is within their personal control.

Empowerment comprises three elements:

1. Responsibility

2. Accountability
3. Risk taking.

Responsibility can be allocated to a person, but unless the person accepts the responsibility they are powerless to act. It may also be the case that an individual is willing to take responsibility, but social and political constraints may prevent this. Tones (1991) states that acceptance of responsibility will be determined by the extent to which an individual possesses competence, skills and/or the belief they are capable of controlling central aspects of their lives and overcoming environmental barriers.

The process of empowerment

Keiffer (1984) conceptualises empowerment as a four stage process.

1. Era of entry

This is a developmental stage whereby patient participation is exploratory and authority and power is demystified.

2. Era of advancement

The patient and nurse spend time gaining an understanding of each other's perspectives and prioritise the interventions required to minimise the stressor that is affecting the patient. This can be a very interactive stage when mutually agreed objectives can be formed. The nurse should not seek to impose the goals of the multidisciplinary team, but employ an holistic approach to the effects that a rheumatological illness has on social and psychological functioning. For example, it should not be assumed that an increase in pain is attributed entirely to active synovitis. It may be related to a family or social problem, and unless this is acknowledged and addressed, the pain will continue.

3. Era of incorporation

In this phase activities are focused on confronting and contending with the 'permanence and painfulness of structural or institutional barriers to self determination' (Gibson 1991). Empowerment entails a process of helping the patient to develop a critical awareness of the root cause of the problem in an addition to a readiness to act on that awareness. This may require the sharing of new knowledge and information.

4. Era of commitment

This is a stage whereby the patient can integrate

new personal knowledge and skills into reality. As rheumatic diseases are not static conditions, the patient will require regular evaluations as their condition progresses or their perceptions change. The patient may have reverted to the era of advancement if this occurs.

Power

The balance of power in the relationship between nurse and patient is unequal. There is usually an expectation by the nurse and an acceptance by the patient that the nurse will be in control. Nurses are considered to have the right to give directions and orders, make rules and prescribe treatment (Roth 1984). Nurses are not independent professionals, but are subject to constraints both from nurse managers and medical hierarchies (Alm 1991, Chavasse 1992). Weaver & Wilson (1994) believe that these influences have led to an overwhelming emphasis on:

- Illness rather than health
- Tasks rather than personal relationships
- Accountability rather than autonomy.

Rather than striving to redress this situation, the nurse has become a translator of what is going to be done (Flemming 1992). Nurses need to work towards demystifying power by encouraging and valuing the patient's contributions and perceptions. It is only by working in partnership to achieve mutually identifiable goals that the patient will start to acquire the knowledge and skills necessary to begin the process of adapting to living with a chronic rheumatological illness.

Increasing patient knowledge

A principal goal of patient education should be to encourage and to enable patients to become as self-sufficient as possible (Weaver & Wilson 1994). Patient education should allow open sharing of information including questions and concerns, and encourage providers and consumers of health care to learn from each other (Hill 1997a, Fahrenfort 1987).

Lorig & Holman (1989) have developed an arthritis self management programme that has been successful at altering self efficacy beliefs and improving physical and psychological functioning. Research has shown that attending education groups leads to a reduction in pain, an increase in self reported behaviour and improvement in self esteem (Geoppinger et al 1987, Lindroth et al 1989, Lorig et al 1987). A meta-analysis of 15 patient education studies showed patient educa-

tion programmes to be comparable with the effects of non-steroidal anti-inflammatory drugs (Mullen et al 1987).

Patient education is an essential component of care as patients cannot be expected to take an active part in care management unless they have the relevant knowledge and skills to do so (Hill 1995). The importance of patient education is discussed in Chapter 15.

THERAPEUTIC NURSING

Therapeutic nursing has been defined as 'that practice where the nurse has made a positive difference to a patient or client's health state, and where he or she is aware of how and why this positive health difference has occurred' (Powell 1991). Four main areas (Box 1.2) in which nursing can be seen to be therapeutic have been highlighted by MacMahon & Pearson (1991). Therapeutic nursing should not be confused with simply offering support to the patient. Levine (1973) makes this distinction:

Nursing which is supportive in nature seeks to prevent further deterioration.

Whereas:

Therapeutic nursing promotes adaptation and contributes to the restoration of well-being.

Box 1.2   Areas of therapeutic nursing

- Nurse/patient relationship
- Conventional nursing interventions, e.g. pressure area care
- Unconventional nursing interventions, e.g. practices taken from therapies
- Patient teaching.

RA is an incurable condition, but the goal of well-being remains realistic. Supportive nursing has a role to play as many of the interventions, both medical and nursing, are to limit the potential for further deformity and disability. An example is disease-modifying drug therapy, such as methotrexate or gold injections. However, to adopt an exclusively supportive approach would be detrimental to the patient, as it does not allow them to participate in the control of their management. Control is retained by the nurse, stifling any attempt by the patient to take an active part in their care.

Some nurses do not wish to develop a therapeutic relationship with patients (Salvage 1990) and others do not value working with patients whose conditions are not amenable to cure (Nolan 1995). The UKCC code of conduct (1992) emphasises that nurses should act in such a way as to safeguard the well-being and interests of patients. If nurses do not seek to adopt a therapeutic role, they are probably falling short of fulfilling this fundamental aspect of nursing care.

In order to improve the patient's well-being, the nurse must incorporate the following skills:

- Teacher
- Guide
- Motivator
- Supporter.

The satisfaction obtained when the patient and the nurse grow together, will help to remove some of the negative perceptions that nurses sometimes acquire when caring for patients with long-term needs.

The nurse/patient relationship

The nurse/patient relationship should be viewed as an exciting challenge which brings benefits to both. There are critics of what has been termed a 'new nursing approach' (Melia 1987, Salvage 1990). These commentators draw attention to material and structural barriers such as the reduction in the number of qualified nurses and a philosophy of care still dominated by task. Indeed Salvage (1990) questions whether patients desire a close relationship if their immediate concern is likely to be relief from pain and discomfort. This may be relevant to patients experiencing acute illness, but in chronic conditions it takes time and close cooperation to cope with pain that cannot be alleviated. This is where individual patient assessment is so important. It should be remembered that some patients may not perceive benefits from developing a relationship and so long as the patient is aware of how to renew or establish contact should a problem occur, this view must be respected.

Patient perceptions

Some patients with RA have a negative concept of the future that persists even after their condition is in remission (Hewlett 1994). The nurse should identify and address any problems perceived by the patient in the initial assessment. If the patient is convinced that the future means a wheelchair existence, it is not helpful to be told that only 5% of people with RA require a wheelchair. The issue should be discussed and the care plan should incorporate therapies that the patient can use to minimise disability occurring. This could include:

- Advice on exercise
- Joint protection
- Pacing activities
- Encouraging expression of feeling
- Discussion with significant others
- Explanation on the role of drug therapy.

The concept of shared care, with the patient taking responsibility for their condition with support and guidance of a named nurse offers the best way forward. A patient who believes they can influence their condition will report fewer physical problems and enhanced well-being (Newman 1993).

Adopting an holistic/humanistic approach to care requires a change from the supportive role of 'doing' for the patient to a therapeutic approach which necessitates enabling the patient to feel in control (see Ch. 5). For instance, if the patient's main problem is that of pain the nurse can have a therapeutic input by establishing, in conjunction with the patient, the pattern, type and severity of the discomfort, whether or not it is related to activity and the apprehensions and anxieties associated with it. This is a two-way process, first achieving clarification of the problems from the patient's perspective and then working in partnership to minimise the stressor. By the use of empathy, respect and trust the nurse enables the patient to believe in her decisions.

It is also essential to encourage those who have value in the patient's life to participate in care management. For example, rest is an important part of the treatment for a patient with a systemic condition such as RA in which both physical and emotional fatigue can occur. If the family is unaware of this, pressure may be placed on the patient to abandon resting. This can be avoided if the family learns the role of rest in the management of the condition. If there is an absence of shared understanding within the family, the patient may try to disguise their limitations resulting in increased symptoms and a reduced quality of life.

Patient participation

Brownlea (1987) defines participation being involved with the:

- Decision-making process
- Delivery of a service
- Evaluation of a service
- Being one of a number of people consulted over an issue or matter.

Five classifications of possible patient participation have been developed by Klein (1974).

1. Information

Information is given to the patient who receives it passively. This is not beneficial for patients with a chronic illness because for care to be meaningful and relevant, the patient must participate in its planning. If the patient does not believe or understand the management programme they may not comply. This is a very paternalistic approach that serves no one's interest.

2. Consultation

The patient may be consulted and the information received may be acted upon. However, power is held solely by the professional who makes all the decisions. If the patient has not been properly consulted and involved, the health professional cannot be sure that they have understood the nature of the problem.

3. Negotiation

Here equality exists and both parties' viewpoints negotiate the treatment programme.

4. Participation

Patients' values are taken into account and underpin the decision-making process.

5. Veto participation

The patient holds the right not to comply with treatment. This decision should always be made from a stance of full knowledge and not out of ignorance or non-disclosure.

For a profession that has interpersonal relationships at its heart, treating patients as genuine participants should be the norm. However, the term participation can only be used correctly when the nurse is aware of the physical, psychological, emotional and social meaning of the illness. Conversely, the patient who is genuinely participating will be aware of the nurse as a person with a host of other demands and concerns. Participation involves a common understanding of the stock of knowledge which constitutes each other's experiences. It would be a mistake for nurses to assume that they intuitively know what it is like to live with a rheumatic illness. Patients have different problems arising from the physical and psychological demands of illness. Nurses will need to invest the time required to know each individual and their specific problems if therapeutic care is to materialise.

Encouraging the patient and their relatives to complete an assessment of their problems and health care needs may yield a very different result to that of the nursing assessment (Sanders 1995). This participation may well provide a useful starting point for a partnership to develop.

BARRIERS TO THERAPEUTIC PRACTICE

The view of nursing

Some nursing activities, such as assisting a patient to bath, are often considered to be basic or menial where in fact they are essential to a patient's well-being. Technical skills are associated with greater status and are therefore deemed to be more important than basic care skills. Therapeutic nursing will include technical skills, but at its core is the realisation of the value of expressive skills (Wright 1991) which include the ability to:

- Be with the patient
- Provide comfort
- Provide education
- Provide the emotional element of care.

Within the framework of therapeutic practice, no act of care having relevance to the patient can be described as menial. Indeed high technology skills without the addition of high touch skills have little meaning for the patient concerned (Wright 1991). The importance of these expressive skills must be emphasised and should therefore be taught at both basic and post basic level. A nurse engaged in therapeutic practice will relate to the patient as an individual, adopting a combination of skills that are perceived to be beneficial and solve the patient's problems. Nursing should not be embarrassed by this caring element, but strongly endorse it as the component that the patient directly relates to the success of their nursing care (Smith 1992). The challenge to nurses is to combine both technical and comprehensive skills into a 'healing whole' which serves the patient (Wright 1991).

Emotional involvement

It has been suggested that nurses do not want to develop the relationship required to nurse patients with a chronic or indeed an acute illness. A study of communication between nurses and patients on a surgical ward found that nurses in close relationships concentrated on medical treatment rather than emotional need (Macleod-Clarke 1983). To some nurses, working with patients with ongoing needs offers little job satisfaction because they are unable to sustain a sense of therapeutic optimism (Evers 1991, Reed & Bond 1991, Reed & Watson 1994). It is possible that rather than working in partnership with the patient to establish shared objectives, nurses set themselves unrealistic care objectives from their own frame of reference. Establishing and being committed to a relationship is demanding, as it is necessary to give of oneself to develop the trust needed for partnerships to grow. To encourage this depth of involvement or 'emotional labour' (Smith 1992) a nurse needs to work within a supportive framework with an assigned supervisor to assist with personal and professional development. The profession must incorporate this objective within the mandatory establishment of clinical supervision in order to develop autonomy and self esteem (Platt-Kock 1986). Wright (1986) has stated that all nurses need the opportunity to:

- Share feelings
- Express views
- Raise questions relating to practice in a structured fashion.

Work environment

The culture in which nurses work does not encourage them to spend time talking to patients (Beeb 1987, Melia 1987), but time is essential if a relationship is to develop. There is still emphasis on achieving tasks rather than engaging in therapeutic interventions, and a growth of support workers at the expense of qualified nurses. If these trends continue, it is questionable whether it will remain possible for a relationship to develop on anything but a superficial level.

In some hospitals, the outpatient department may be the only environment where the patient with a chronic disease is cared for, and so all newly diagnosed patients should be referred to a rheumatology nurse to begin the process of therapeutic care. A realistic personal profile of care should be established which could be used by other key workers, such as the physiotherapist or practice nurse, so maintaining the continuity of care between the secondary and primary health care sections. Care profiling and planning needs to be dynamic, otherwise it will raise expectations and then cause dissatisfaction if identified needs are not met (Altschul 1983). Therapeutic nursing requires a non-hierarchical method of care delivery that enables nurses to be involved in the decision-making process and places them in a position where they can develop a partnership with the patient. The philosophy of the

work environment is of vital importance because if the nursing team is not committed to developing a relationship, a relationship will not occur. The belief that therapeutic practice is of mutual benefit will only become reality if it is actively fostered and reinforced by the organisation which delivers care. A routinised and ritualistic approach will not serve the needs of the patients.

INNOVATIONS IN NURSING

Nursing development units

If nurses are to practise therapeutic nursing, the environment in which they practise, whether in primary or secondary care, needs to be supportive and conducive to their needs. The work of existing nursing development units has shown that the development of nursing is firmly linked to the development of the nurses (Bamber et al 1989, Salvage 1989). An investment in nurses in both time and money is essential for personal and professional development. The main features of a practice development unit are cited in Box 1.3.

Box 1.3 Features of a Nursing Development Unit

- Philosophy – one team of nurses responsible to one ward manager throughout 24 hours to ensure continuity and consistency of care delivery
- Dedicated time for education and development
- Team building – all members actively involved in decision-making
- Focus on communication skills, assertiveness, self awareness, research skills and complimentary therapies
- Therapeutic relationship with patients
- A knowledge of nursing and its value
- The nurse as a charge agent, implementing research based practice
- Disseminate excellence in practice
- Patient is central to all care activities.

The majority of nursing development units are within inpatient areas, but with the reduction in the number of specialised rheumatology beds, the majority of patients with a rheumatological disorder will be nursed as outpatients. It is therefore important to adapt the characteristics listed in Box 1.3 to the clinical areas where patients are nursed. One of the central aspects of a nursing development unit is that all 'practice initiatives are driven by patients' needs in order to develop a more flexible and responsive service' (D Dobbs, personal communication, 1996). Achieving nursing development status and altering practices of care is a demanding process requiring great commitment from all involved. However this provides a rewarding environment which allows nurses to function in a system of care delivery that encourages the essence of nursing and the creation of a therapeutic partnership between nurse and patient.

Clinical supervision

Patients with chronic rheumatic diseases have a multitude of needs that require a therapeutic understanding prior to care planning. If the nurse is to undertake this emotional aspect of care, her own personal and professional needs must be catered for. The clinical area should incorporate a framework that encourages nurses to become involved in clinical supervision that will provide the necessary:

- Guidance
- Support
- Learning.

Supervision encourages the development of reflective learning; the process of creating and clarifying the meaning of experience (present or past) in terms of self in relation to self, and in terms of self in relation to the world. The outcome of the process is a changed conceptual perspective (Boyd & Fales 1983).

Clinical supervision provides nurses with the opportunity of focusing on their practice and the effect nursing has on both a personal and professional level. This type of learning offers the nurse the opportunity to:

1. Develop a problem-solving approach to nursing situations
2. Learn from practice
3. Transfer the knowledge to other situations.

It also provides the opportunity to share personal feelings about a particular nursing situation, and assess whether that situation has provoked 'positive' or 'negative' feelings. It is essential to provide this level of support so that nurses can undertake both the physical and emotional care components of nursing which are essential when caring for patients where ongoing care is required. The main objectives of clinical supervision are stated in Box 1.4.

Supervision can take place in an individual or group setting. However, group supervision enhances a collective approach to care and enables reflection on practice that affects the team as a whole. Each clinical area will adopt a model that best suits the need of the population involved. The essential element is that a framework exists and is intertwined with practice.

Box 1.4   Objectives of clinical supervision

- Emotional support
- Learning and developing nursing practice
- Increased self awareness and self evaluation
- Individual and collective growth
- Reflection on practice
- Accountability
- Safe and quality-governed patient care.

Nursing research

Pearson (1991) believes that the creation of a nursing focused environment will ensure that:

- Nursing is recognised as therapy in its own right
- Foster the development of knowledge
- Provide a milieu for research and development.

It is widely accepted that to provide effective care, nursing needs to underpin its practice with research. Historically there has been an over-emphasis on the need for scientific-based quantitative methodology, but the essence of nursing is sophisticated and complex and this approach is not always appropriate. Nursing should use the research methodology that best suits the objective. This requires being open to a combination of approaches. For instance, Ryan (1996) used a phenomenological qualitative approach to elicit the patients' perceptions of living with RA. This produced a wealth of illustrative data that highlighted five main areas that patients felt had enormous effects on their lives. These were:

- Self esteem
- Role alteration
- Frustration at limitations
- Negative perceptions of the future
- Dissatisfaction with their medical care provision.

Using this methodology enabled exploration of the patient's view, which must be taken into account if care delivery is to be meaningful and relevant to their individual needs. A qualitative methodology that seeks to arrive at discovery and meaning will help to expand the care base within rheumatology nursing. It will also enable exploration of how nursing as a therapy can be most beneficial.

A study based on interviews with families where one of the adults had RA found that many men felt frustrated when they could no longer continue in their employment (Le Gallez 1993). Nurses can now be made more aware of this problem and seek to address it by engaging the services of the disability employment adviser or by providing counselling support themselves. This will enable the individual concerned and if necessary their family, to work through their feelings of anger and grief. The consequences of not working will affect the individual's self esteem and confidence and may also involve family members in role alteration. Working with an individual at this stage is essential to prevent the negative mechanisms of depression and isolation occurring.

One of the main objectives of qualitative research is to provide a description of the patient's experience. This can influence care delivery by increasing our understanding of the wide-ranging implications of chronic illness. The creation and recognition of nursing development units may be a more viable way of securing clinical nursing research at a local level and reduce the barriers that presently exist between theory and practice.

Nursing beds

Nursing beds have traditionally catered for patients in rehabilitation or in a non-acute phase of their illness. These patients continue to need intensive nursing but have significantly less need of intensive medical care (Pearson 1988). There are many reasons why a patient with a chronic rheumatological condition would benefit from admission to a nursing bed, cared for by nurses with both an understanding and knowledge of the implications of living with rheumatic illnesses (Box 1.5).

Box 1.5   The benefits of rheumatology nursing beds

- The need to acquire understanding about the condition
- To learn coping and self management strategies, e.g. pacing activities
- To acquire the knowledge, skills and confidence to regain and retain the maximum level of independence through guidance and learning
- The encourage the expression of feelings/emotions
- To help adjust to the stressors of the illness (e.g. physical, psychological and social consequences)
- To provide help for those who are dependent in their self care activities
- Reassessment of self care needs and individual care profiling
- To adapt a multidisciplinary approach to care
- The need to receive comfort and support and to develop the motivation to adjust to the demands of illness.

A study on the effectiveness of nursing beds concluded that patients reported increased satisfaction with their care compared with those nursed in a tradi-

tional setting, and there were financial savings from lower readmission rates (Pearson 1988).

Nurse-led clinics

The nursing role is essentially expressive in nature (Hill 1992), consisting of a combination of skills such as:

- Caring
- Helping
- Supporting
- Teaching
- Comforting
- Guiding.

Rheumatology nurses have been conducting their own clinics and using these skills to educate and support patients for a number of years (Hill 1985, Hill 1986). This makes excellent use of the knowledge and communication skills that nurses possess. Nurse-led clinics enable nurses to take an holistic approach to care using the framework of the Rheumatology Nursing Forum Patient Problem Model (see Fig. 1.2), which incorporates the physical, psychological, social, spiritual and sexual needs of the patient. The activities undertaken in a nurse-led clinic are stated in Box 1.6.

Box 1.6   The activities undertaken in the nurse-led clinic

- Assessing the progress of the disease
- Monitoring the progress of the disease
- Identifying patient-focused problems and providing a plan of care
- Assessing the patient's acceptance and knowledge of the disease
- Providing education to patients and their families
- Acting as an expert source of referral to other members of the multidisciplinary team
- Conducting research.

It is essential that the role of the nurse working within this sphere remains firmly rooted in patient need and that all role expansion focuses on the patients' care. Otherwise there is a danger that the nurse could be viewed as a medical assistant instead of being at the forefront of developing their own profession in the interests of their patient group (Bird et al 1985). Nursing requires strong leadership. It would be a tragedy if nursing were to be subsumed and lose its identity in a medically-orientated alliance. The nursing profession needs to be clear as to what constitutes nursing and the necessity for both an action and emotional element in nursing practice.

The value of a clinic run on true nursing principles was demonstrated by Hill et al (1994). This study was an evaluation of the effectiveness, safety and acceptability of a nurse practitioner in a rheumatology outpatient clinic. It consisted of a single blind parallel group study, in which 70 patients with RA were randomly allocated to either the nurse practitioner or consultant's care. One of the most noticeable aspects of the research was the marked difference in the referral patterns of the two practitioners. The rheumatology nurse practitioner made more use of the other members of the multidisciplinary team such as the occupational therapist and physiotherapist. This study also reinforced the view that one of the primary roles of the nurse working with patients with rheumatology conditions is that of educator. Education is required to increase the patient's cognitive understanding and to impart knowledge of self management techniques such as exercise regimes. The knowledge shared with patients was well received and there was a greater improvement in knowledge and satisfaction with care than in the control group. Education takes time and this was reflected in the fact that the nurse practitioner saw fewer patients than the consultant over the study period. However, the patients in the nursing cohort showed reductions in pain and depression compared with those patients in the consultant's group. The nurse was shown to be a safe practitioner who was able to initiate and interpret clinical and laboratory data. These results are encouraging and demonstrate the effective and safe contribution the nurse can make to the care of rheumatology patients with a diversity of needs.

THE FUTURE OF RHEUMATOLOGY NURSING

The scope of professional practice (UKCC 1992) has presented the profession with the opportunity to shape its own future by developing and utilising specialist skills and knowledge in areas where it will best meet the needs of the patient. It reinforces the need for nurses to remain receptive to the requirements of patients and to provide care that meets the identified needs. It also emphasises professional accountability and places decisions regarding the boundaries of practice in the hands of the nursing profession. This should provide the opportunity and framework for nurses to look at their practice and develop a strategy for improving the quality of care offered.

Within the field of rheumatology, nursing must continue to be dynamic and make an active difference to care management. With the reduction in patient facilities, the majority of patients are nursed entirely as outpatients, so further increasing the need for nursing time. Nurses must develop convincing arguments for more resources to be channelled into nurse-led clinics.

Nurses with a holistic ideology and good communication/education skills are best suited to engage in a therapeutic relationship. However, in the process of expanding skills they must not lose the essence of nursing, nor should they delegate inappropriately to unqualified colleagues. If nurses accept new aspects of care they may risk ignoring others. For example the administration of intra-articular injections should be viewed as part of a complete package of care rather than as an isolated intervention. The nurse has reviewed the patient in clinic and been able to address physical, psychological and social nursing requirements. During the consultation, she has diagnosed a knee effusion that requires aspiration and injection. If the nurse is not competent to undertake this procedure, the therapeutic relationship will have to be interrupted whilst the procedure is carried out by another health professional. A nurse proficient in this procedure would have been able to offer a complete package of care. On the other hand, a nurse conducting an injection clinic involving no other assessment, would not be providing holistic care and this could be considered an inappropriate use of the nurse's skills. Some nurses have questioned the value of saving doctors' time at the expense of nursing time. They suggest that role development could lead to the fragmentation of care, with patients receiving 'second class doctoring from professional nurses and second class nursing from those individuals who take on the nursing functions' (Dodds 1991). This scenario is perhaps a little extreme but it serves to remind nurses that new roles must not be to the detriment or neglect of others. Role development must centre around the needs of the patient and not the needs of other health care professionals. The code of conduct emphasises the need for all members of the health care team to work together, and this is essential in the area of rheumatology, where the multidimensional needs of the patients require services from many different but allied disciplines. Communication is vital for the rheumatology team to work together, as they must share a vision of the future provision of rheumatology services and the roles of team members.

Education for patients

Phelan et al (1992) examined the responsibilities and work areas that rheumatology nurse specialists considered to be part of their role. Nearly all respondents (96%) stated that the counselling and education of patient and staff were the most important areas of their work. Nurses should remain pro-active in this area and develop it further. To enable patients and their families to develop the positive coping mechanisms needed to live with incurable chronic conditions will take:

- Time
- Understanding
- Intimacy
- Reciprocity.

It is essential that as nurses develop new skills, patient education is not neglected but remains the foundation of patient-centred care.

Role development

Nurses should not be afraid of role expansion; indeed if it enhances patient care it should be fostered. It has already been a time of great development within the profession; nurse practitioners and specialists are increasing in numbers (Castledine 1991) and nurse prescribing has become law. Many nurses are developing their role and carrying out extended activities (Hill 1997b) such as:

- Administration of intra-articular joint injections
- Musculoskeletal examinations
- Clerking of patients on admission to the ward.

All these areas of care have traditionally been the province of the medical staff. By learning new skills the nurse can offer a more complete package of care that will strengthen the therapeutic partnership providing she retains the expressive elements of nursing.

Nursing is a growing profession and change should be welcomed. Nurses may have come to believe that 'real nursing' is that which is associated with acute scientific medical interventions (Wright 1995). Clearly, some nurses would be competent to carry out such interventions given the correct training and education, but role development must be part of a wider care initiative that combines the emotional care element of nursing with technical interventions. Well-educated nurses who are able to make clear decisions about what should or should not be within the remit of the profession are needed to underpin role development. Leaders involved in clinical practice are needed to take the profession forward. Nursing must set its own agenda and find its political voice, using the framework provided within the scope of professional practice. The potential exists to create a multitude of nursing roles that form the basis of genuine clinical

career structures based on developing knowledge and skills in patient care rather than on a managerial hierarchy (Wright 1991).

Nursing as therapy

Caring is not exclusive to nursing, but it does lie at the core of nursing philosophy. More research is required to provide a description and exploration of the value of nursing and its therapeutic role. Much of the current research has been conducted on the impact/value of the nurse/patient relationship in the acute care setting. Thomas et al (1996) showed that patients who were able to identify one nurse in charge of their care, reported more positive experiences of nursing and rated their satisfaction with nursing highly. This applied to all types of wards practising a variety of modes of care delivery.

Education for nurses

Although there are increasing numbers of specialist posts within rheumatology and other disciplines of nursing, there is often a shortage of experienced nurses. Early authors viewed the nurse specialist as an 'expert direct care provider who serves as a model of expertise representing advanced or newly developing practice' (Peplau 1965). More recent authors (Beecroft & Papenhausen 1988) have expanded this definition to include the role of:

- Educator
- Coordinator
- Researcher
- Practitioner.

At present there is no clear structural career pathway for nurses specialising in rheumatology and there is a shortage of academic courses to provide the knowledge base required. The nursing profession needs to move to an all-graduate status, so that academic knowledge can match practice-based skills and the academic status of rheumatology nursing would be enhanced by the introduction of a Chair of Rheumatology Nursing (Hill 1997b).

Nursing may be a practice-based profession, but knowledge is still essential to guide decision-making in practice and education must be a constant feature of professional development. The United Kingdom Central Council (UKCC) is making inroads into this area, with evidence of post qualification, education and practice development becoming a mandatory requirement. However, the profession must not accept the requirements of the UKCC as a maximum standard, but rather as a minimum standard providing a springboard to further educational development.

In addition the profession requires a pre-registration framework that ensures nursing students acquire a wide experience of both acute and chronic illness. This should include gaining an understanding of the needs of patients with a rheumatological condition. This would help to prevent patients with ongoing needs being viewed as 'unpopular patients' due to a lack of understanding of the condition and what its influence on lifestyle is really like. Only by involving nurses at their training stage can they begin to develop an appreciation of the needs of these patients and the therapeutic difference the application of nursing skills can make. This would entice more students to consider specialising in rheumatology nursing on completion of their training.

As patient care continues to move from a secondary to primary setting nurses must look at the education facilities for both colleagues and patients within the community. Dargie & Procter (1993) highlighted the success of running an arthritis clinic from a general practitioner surgery. This topic is expanded in Chapter 16. Networks of communication are needed between hospital-based and community-based nurses. This would allow working relationships to be established and foster an understanding of the problems encountered in either setting. This in turn would lead to the development of shared care protocols ensuring that in whatever setting the patient is cared for, there will be consistency of practice.

The future of nursing is both exciting and challenging. It is incumbent upon nurses to ensure that they are able to practise therapeutic nursing within a therapeutic environment, which is after all the essence of nursing.

Action points for practice

- Review the philosophy of care in your clinical area. Does it encourage therapeutic practice?
- In clinical supervision groups reflect on the emotional element of nursing and the additional organisational mechanisms required to underpin this practice.
- Conduct a small research project on the organisation of care within your clinical area. Is it fulfilling patients' needs?
- Discuss the components needed to develop the nurse/patient relationships and compile a standard for practice.

REFERENCES

Alm T G 1991 Power in nursing. Journal of Advanced Nursing 16(5): 503

Altschul A T 1983 The consumer's voice nursing implications. Journal of Advanced Nursing 8: 175–183

Bamber T, Johnson M L, Purdy E, Wright S 1989 The Tameside experience. Nursing Standard 22(3):26

Beeb R 1987 Care to talk? Nursing Times 83(37): 40–41

Beecroft P C, Papenhausen J L 1988 What is a specialist? Clinical Nurse Specialist 2(3): 109–112

Bird H A, LeGallez P, Hill J 1985 Combined care of the rheumatic patient. Springer-Verlag, Berlin, ch10, p258

Bower F L 1972 The process of planning nursing care. Mosby, St Louis

Boyd E M, Fales A W 1983 Reflective learning: key to learning from experience. Journal for Humanistic Psychology 23(2): 99–117

Bradley T 1989 Patient control of treatment is essential. Arthritis Care and Research 13(3): 163–166

Brownlea A 1987 Participation: myths realities and prognosis. Social Science and Medicine 25(6): 605–614

Castledine G 1991 The advanced nurse practitioner. Nursing Standard 5(44): 33–36

Chavasse J 1992 New dimensions of empowerment in nursing and challenges. Journal of Advanced Nursing 17: 1–2

Clarke J 1994 Graduate status for nurses. Does this create an elitist profession? Annual Celebrity Lecture, N. Ireland

Dargie L, Proctor J 1994 Setting up an arthritis clinic. Community Outlook 4(7): 14–17

Dargie L, Proctor J 1993 Arthritis health promotion. Practice Nurse 6: 144–148

Dodds F 1991 First class nurses or second class doctors. British Journal of Theatre Nursing 1(9): 6–8

Donovan J 1991 Patient education and the consultation: the importance of lay beliefs. Annals of Rheumatic Diseases 50: 418–421

Evers H K 1991 Care of the elderly sick in the United Kingdom. In: Redfern S J (ed). Nursing elderly people, 2nd edn. Churchill Livingstone, Edinburgh, 417–436

Fahrenfort M 1987 Patient emancipation by health education: an impossible goal? Patient Education and Counselling 10: 25–37

Flemming V 1992 Client education: a futuristic outlook. Journal of Advanced Nursing 17: 158–163

Geoppinger J M, Arther M W, Brunk S E, Reidesit S 1987 The effectiveness of community-based arthritis self care programmes. Arthritis Rheumatism 30: S194 (suppl)

Gibson C 1991 A concept analysis of empowerment. Journal of Advanced Nursing 16: 354–361

Henderson V 1966 The nature of nursing. Collier-MacMillan, London

Henderson A 1994 Power and knowledge in nursing practice. Journal of Advanced Nursing 20: 935–939

Hewlett S 1994 Patients' views on changing disability. Nursing Standard 8(31): 25–29

Hill J 1985 Nursing clinics for arthritics. Nursing Times 81: 33–34

Hill J 1986 Patient evaluation of a rheumatology nursing clinic. Nursing Times 82: 42–43

Hill J 1992 A nurse practitioner rheumatology clinic. Nursing Standard 7(11): 35–37

Hill J 1995 Patient education in rheumatic disease. Nursing Standard 9(25): 25–28

Hill J 1997a A practical guide to patient education and information giving. Ballière's Clinical Rheumatology 11(1): 109–127

Hill J 1997b The expanding role of the nurse in rheumatology. British Journal of Nursing 36(4): 410–412

Hill J, Bird H, Lawton C, Harmer R, Wright V 1994 An evaluation of the effectiveness, safety and acceptability of a nurse practitioner in a rheumatology outpatient clinic. British Journal of Rheumatology 33: 283–288

Jette A 1982 Improving patient co-operation with arthritis treatment regimes. Arthritis and Rheumatism 25: 447–453

Keiffer C 1984 Citizen empowerment: a developmental perspective. Prevention in Human Services 3: 9–36

Klein R 1974 Notes towards a theory of patient involvement. Canadian Public Health Association, O'Hawa, Canada

Krueger D W 1984 Rehabilitation psychology. Aspin, Maryland

Le Gallez P 1993 Rheumatoid arthritis: effects on the family. Nursing Standard 7(39): 30–33

Levine M E 1973 Introduction to clinical nursing, 2nd edn. F A Davis, Philadelphia

Liang M 1989 Compliance and quality of life: confessions of a difficult patient. Arthritis Care and Research 2: 571–574

Lindroth Y, Bauman A, Barnes C, Brookes P M, McCrede M 1989 A controlled evaluation of arthritis education. British Journal of Rheumatology 28: 7–12

Lorig K, Gonzaler V, Konkol L 1987 Arthritis patient education: a review of the literature. Patient Education and Counselling 10: 207–252

Lorig K, Holman H R 1989 Long term outcomes of an arthritis self management study: effects of reinforcement efforts. Social Science Medicine 29: 221–224

Macleod-Clark E W 1983 Nurse-patient communication – analysis of conversation from surgical works. In: Wilson-Barnett J (ed). Nursing research. Ten studies in patient care. John Wiley, Winchester

MacMahon R, Pearson A (eds) 1991 Nursing as therapy. Chapham Hall, London

Malin N, Teasdale K 1991 Caring versus empowerment. Considerations for nursing practice. Journal of Advanced Nursing 16: 657–662

May C 1991 Affective neutrality and involvement in nurse-patient relationships: perceptions of appropriate behaviours among nurses in acute medical and surgical wards. Journal of Advanced Nursing 16: 552–558

Melia K M 1987 Learning and working: the occupational socialisation of nurses. Tavistock Publications, London

Muetzel P 1988 Therapeutic nursing. In : Pearson A (ed) Primary nursing. Nursing in the Burford and Oxford nursing development units. Croom Helm, Beckenham

Mullen P D, Biddle A K, Laville E A, Lorig K 1987 Efficacy of psycho-educational interventions on pain depression and disability with arthritis – a meta-analysis. Journal of Rheumatology 14(15): 33–39

Newman S 1993 Coping with rheumatoid arthritis. Annals of the Rheumatic Diseases 52: 553–554

Nolan M, Nolan J 1995 Responding to the challenge of chronic illness. British Journal of Nursing 4(3): 145–147

Pearson A 1988 Primary nursing. Nursing in the Burford and Oxford nursing development units. Croom Helm, London.

Pearson A 1991 Taking up the challenge, the future for therapeutic nursing. In: McMahon R, Pearson A. Nursing as therapy. Chapman and Hall, London

Peplau H 1965 Specialisation in professional nursing. Nursing Science 3(8): 268–287

Phelan M J I, Byrne J, Campell A, Lynch M P A 1992 Profile of the rheumatology nurse specialist in the United Kingdom. British Journal of Rheumatology 31(12): 858–859

Platt-Kock L M 1986 Clinical supervision for psychiatric nurses. Journal of Psychiatric Nursing 26(1): 7–15

Powell J 1991 Reflection and the evaluation of experience pre-requests for therapeutic practice. In : MacMahon R, Pearson A (eds) Nursing as Therapy, Chapman Hall, London

Reed J, Bond S 1991 Nurse assessment of elderly patients in hospital. Internal Journal of Nursing Studies 28(1): 55–64

Reed J, Watson D 1994 The impact of the medical model on nursing practice. Internal Journal of Nursing Studies 31(1): 57–66

Roth J 1984 Staff in male bargaining tactics in long term treatment institutions. Sociology of Health and Illness 6(2): 111–131

Ryan S 1996 Living with rheumatoid arthritis: a phenomenological exploration. Nursing Standard 10(41): 45–47

Salvage J 1989 Shifting Boundaries Nursing Times 85(10): 24

Salvage J 1990 The theory and practice of the 'new nursing'. Nursing Times 86(4): 42–44

Sanders P 1995 Encouraging patients to take part in their own care. Nursing Times 91(9): 42–43

Smith P 1992 The emotional labour of nursing. Macmillan, Worcester

Thomas L, Bone D, McCole E, Priest J 1996 The impact of primary nursing on patient satisfaction. Nursing Times 92(22): 36–38

Tones K 1991 Health promotion, empowerment and the psychology of control. Journal of the Institute of Health Education 29(1): 17–25

United Kingdom Central Council for nursing midwifery 1992 Code of conduct. UKCC, London

United Kingdom Central Council for Nursing Midwifery 1992 Scope of professional practice. UKCC, London

Wallerstein N, Bernstein E 1988 Empowerment education. Frere's ideas adapted to health education. Health Education Quarterly 4: 379–394

Wallston K 1995 Adaptation coping and perceived control in persons with rheumatoid arthritis. Rheumatology in Europe 2: 291–304 (suppl). Eular Publication

Waterworth S, Luker K 1990 Reluctant collaborators: do patients want to be involved in decisions concerning care. Journal of Advanced Nursing 15: 971–976

Weaver S, Wilson J 1994 Moving towards patient empowerment. Nursing and Health Care 15(9): 481–483

Wilson-Barnett J 1984 Key functions in nursing: the fourth Winifred Raphael memorial lecture. Royal College of Nursing, London

Wright S 1986 Building and using a model for nursing. Edward Arnold, London

Wright S 1991 Facilitating therapeutic nursing and independent practice. In: MacMahon R Pearson A (eds) Nursing as therapy. Chapman Hall, London

FURTHER READING

Ashworth P, Longmate M, Marnstone P 1992 Patient
    participation, its meaning and significance in the context
    of nursing. Journal of Advanced Nursing 17: 1430–1439

2

The rheumatic conditions – an overview

Valerie Arthur

The aim of this chapter is to provide a description of the anatomy and physiology of the musculoskeletal system, and provide a general overview of the diseases that relate to this system. After reading this chapter you should be able to:

- Describe the structures that make up the musculoskeletal system
- Describe the anatomy and physiology of the musculoskeletal system in relation to the rheumatic diseases
- Discuss the current thinking on the aetiology and pathology of the common rheumatic diseases
- Differentiate between inflammatory, non-inflammatory and soft tissue rheumatological conditions
- Describe the extra-articular manifestations of the rheumatic diseases
- Show evidence of the management of the various rheumatic diseases and the implications for nursing care
- Describe the problems that arise from these diseases and how they may affect patients and their families.

THE IMPACT OF RHEUMATIC DISEASE

The rheumatic or musculoskeletal diseases are many and complex and although they have been the subjects of research for several decades there still remains much to be learnt about them (Symmons & Bankhead 1994). Musculoskeletal diseases cause some of the greatest suffering and disability experienced by mankind and place a great social and economic burden on patients, their families and society at large. They account for 18.7% of all consultations in general practice and it has been predicted that as the elderly population increases so will the incidence of these complaints (Badley 1991). Although rheumatic disease can affect any age group, from babies to the very elderly, the greatest incidence in the UK is in females over the age of 65 years (Symmons et al 1994). With an ever-increasing elderly population of which the greater proportion will be women, the full impact of the consequences of these diseases has yet to be felt by health professionals, health authorities and society at large.

The nurse has an integral role to play in the care of patients with rheumatic disease, as the one member of the multidisciplinary team with whom the patient is likely to have the most contact (Arthur 1994). The reduction of junior doctors' hours and the advent of nurse-led clinics has increased the nursing component of care (Hill 1992, Hill 1997). As the role of the nurse is extended, the nursing care of these patients will expand even further. In order to practise at such a level, the nurse specialising in rheumatology must have a sound knowledge of rheumatic diseases and the anatomy and physiology of the systems and organs relating to the musculoskeletal system. This knowledge is essential for the correct assessment and planning of the nursing interventions necessary for the holistic care of patients with rheumatic disease.

THE HISTORY OF RHEUMATIC DISEASE

Evidence of rheumatic disease has been found in mummies and skeletons from ancient Egypt and since that time literature and art have provided further evidence of man's suffering from these diseases down the centuries (Buchanan & Dequeker 1994). During the 19th century clinical observations, descriptions and drawings made by physicians such as Adams and Charcot increased the body of knowledge (Dieppe & Klippel 1994). However, the individual rheumatic diseases were not comprehensively catalogued or classified until the beginning of this century. The advent of radiology led to sub-classification and since then the specialities of molecular biology, immunology and bacteriology have produced further differentiations (Buchanan & Dequeker 1994). Today it is accepted that there are around 200 different types of rheumatic disease (Symmons & Bankhead 1994).

The latter part of this century has seen increased research into the aetiology, epidemiology and pathology of these diseases, not only in the search for a cure,

but also to improve our understanding of this varied and complicated speciality. Despite this, the cause of the majority of the rheumatic diseases and their cure remains one of the great enigmas of medical science. As we embark into the twenty first century it is to be hoped that this situation will be resolved. Until a solution is found, nursing care in common with the care given by all members of the multidisciplinary team, will remain important in enabling patients to cope with the distressingly painful and disabling effects of many of these diseases.

ANATOMY AND PHYSIOLOGY OF THE MUSCULOSKELETAL SYSTEM

This section comprises:

- Components of the musculoskeletal system
- Structures and functions of these components
- Specific joints most commonly affected by rheumatic disease
- Physical structure and common disorders of these joints.

Components of the musculoskeletal system

The musculoskeletal system consists of:

1. Bones
2. Skeletal muscle
3. Connective tissue
4. Joints.

All these structures function as separate units within an overall interdependent system that allows a complex range of movement.

Structure and functions of the components of the musculoskeletal system

1. Bones

The skeleton is made up of various bones. Its functions are to:

- Provide a framework to support the body
- Protect organs
- Store minerals
- Produce blood cells.

There are around 200 different bones in the body which are held together by cartilage and ligaments and it is this complex structure, the skeleton, which supports the body (Fig. 2.1).

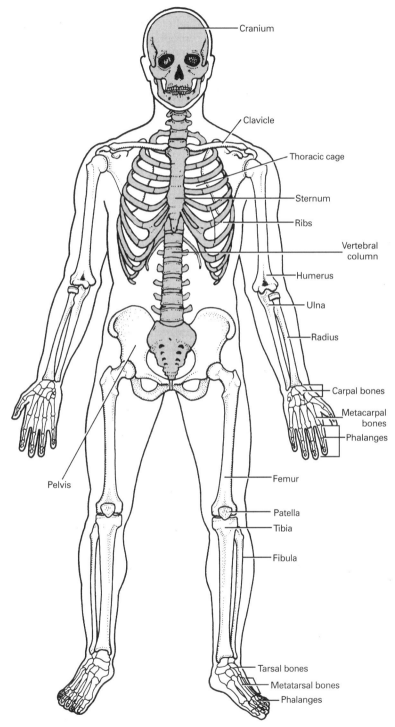

Figure 2.1   The skeleton. Anterior view (adapted from Wilson and Waugh 1996, with permission).

The brain, heart, lungs and spinal cord are protected by the bony structures of the cranium, rib cage and vertebral spine. The pelvis and the muscles of the abdomen protect the vital abdominal organs.

Calcium is stored within the bones of the skeleton and is vital for bone formation, blood coagulation, nerve production and cardiac and skeletal muscle contraction. The musculoskeletal system contains 97% of the total bodily contents of calcium salts.

As well as storing calcium, the bones contain marrow that produces vital blood cells.

Structure of bone

Bone is the hardest tissue in the body and is made up of collagen fibres which consist of crystals of hydroxy-apatites formed from phosphates of calcium. It is living tissue nourished by a system of blood and lymphatic vessels.

Box 2.1 Composition of bone	
Osteoblasts	deposit collagen fibres to form the matrix of the bone
Osteocytes	form the calcified matrix of the bone
Osteoclasts	reabsorb bone by phagocytic action

Osteoblasts secrete collagen and become osteocytes once calcium deposition has occurred. Osteocytes form the matrix or framework of bone and are connected to each other by a network of channels. Bone is reabsorbed by the phagocytic action of the osteoclasts. There are two different types of bone:

- Compact
- Trabecular.

The mature skeleton contains 80% compact bone and 20% trabecular bone.

Compact or dense bone is hard and white and makes up the shafts of the long bones and the surface of flat bones. Microscopic investigation reveals concentric plates of bone (lamella) interspersed by a system of Haversian canals. These provide access for blood and lymphatic vessels which nourish the osteocytes.

Trabecular or cancellous bone is spongy in appearance and is surrounded by compact bone. The strut-like arrangement of the cells can be seen under a microscope. This formation increases the strength of the bone. Haversian canals are also present in trabecular bone to supply the necessary nutrients.

Red bone marrow is a pulpy tissue found in the central cavity of the shaft of long bones and in the cancellous bone of the flat and irregular bones. The vertebrae, sternum, ribs, clavicles, scapulae, cranial bones and proximal ends of the femoral and humeral bones of adults all contain red bone marrow. Erythrocytes are produced in the red bone marrow. A good dietary intake of vitamin B_{12}, folic acid and iron is necessary for this process.

Bones are covered by a tough, vasculitic outer covering known as the *periosteum*. In addition to blood supplied from the periosteum and the Haversian canals, long bones receive blood from an artery which enters the shaft through the nutrient foramen.

Foetal bone

Foetal bones are outlined as fibrous or cartilaginous tissue. As the foetus develops, calcification of the bone occurs as calcium salts are deposited into the cartilage and osteoblasts lay down bone to replace the cartilage.

During childhood this process occurs mainly at the centres of ossification which enable the bone to grow. The centres of ossification are situated in the extremities of long bones and in the centre of bones. Each extremity or epiphysis of a long bone is separated from the shaft (diaphysis) by the epiphyseal line which is made of a layer of cartilage. Once adulthood is reached this layer becomes calcified and the epiphysis and diaphysis become fused and there is no further growth of the bone. Growth in the circumference of a bone occurs when osteoblasts lay down new bone under the periosteum which is the tough fibrous covering of the bone.

Requirements for bone formation

Bone formation and reabsorption is a continuous process which requires an adequate intake of calcium and vitamin D. This process, known as bone turnover, is especially high during childhood, when an adequate dietary intake of calcium is necessary for the development of strong bones.

The growth of bones is affected by:

- Pituitary growth hormone
- Sex hormones (oestrogens and androgens)
- Thyroid hormone.

Bones contain calcium salts. These are present in greater quantities in adults than in the bones of children which tend to be more elastic with a loose matrix. If trauma occurs, it may result in a 'greenstick' or partial fracture, instead of a complete break as would normally occur in mature, dense bones. In a freshly healed fracture, the bone matrix is less dense than normal.

Hormonal influence

Loss of bone density occurs as hormone levels decrease, in for example menopausal women, resulting in osteoporosis, a condition where the bones become less strong and are liable to fracture.

Specific bones

Bones come in all shapes and sizes depending on the size and function of the muscles which are attached to them.

Long bones (Fig. 2.2). Long bones consist of a shaft (diaphysis) with two extremities (epiphysis). The limbs are a made up of typical long bones such as the femur, tibia, fibula, humerus, ulna and radius. In mature bones the central shaft is made of compact bone which has a central channel filled with bone marrow. The extremities are made up of cancellous bone containing red bone marrow and are covered with a thin layer of compact bone.

Short bones. Short bones consist of cancellous bone covered by a layer of compact bone. They are box-like in shape, such as the carpus of the wrist and tarsus of the ankle.

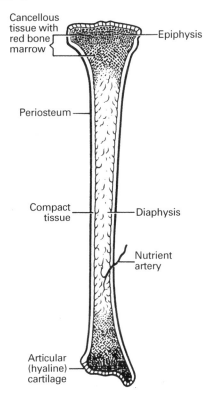

Figure 2.2 A mature long bone — a longitudinal section (from Wilson and Waugh 1996, with permission).

Flat bones. Flat bones are composed of a layer of cancellous bone between two layers of compact bone. Examples are the scapula, innominate bone and cranial bones.

Irregular bones. Irregular bones are formed from cancellous bone covered by an outer layer of compact bone. Examples are the vertebrae and facial bones.

Sesamoid bone. Sesamoid bones develop in the tendons of specific joints such as the sesamoid bone of the thumb. The most important sesamoid bone is the patella.

2. Skeletal muscles

Skeletal muscles:

- Provide force and power for the body to work
- Produce movement by working with other muscles.

Physical structure

Skeletal muscles are also known as striated or voluntary muscle and are made up of bundles of muscle fibres called fasciculi. The individual muscle fibres consist of thin filaments of contractile proteins that are covered by the sarcolemma. The endomysium is the fibrous tissue found in the spaces between the individual fibres. These lie parallel to each other and are grouped into fasciculi and covered by perimysium. The groups of fasciculi are in turn covered by a tough fibrous sheath or epymisium that covers the muscle itself (Fig. 2.3).

Nutrition

Skeletal muscles are amply supplied by blood vessels and capillaries which provide the oxygen, calcium, chemical nutrients necessary for action and remove the waste materials incurred by such action.

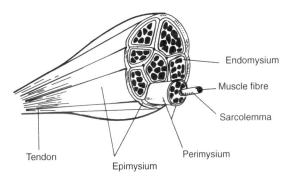

Figure 2.3 Composition of skeletal muscle (from Wilson and Waugh 1996, with permission).

Types of muscle (Box 2.2)

> **Box 2.2** The titles of many muscles reflect their characteristics. For example:
>
> | | |
> | --- | --- |
> | Triceps (three heads) | formation |
> | Flexor carpi ulnaris | movement |
> | Sternomastoid | attachment |
> | Occipitalis | position |
> | Deltoid | shape |

The action of muscles

Striated muscle is supplied with motor nerves that enable it to contract in one direction. When action occurs the muscle fully contracts (shortens and thickens), and this is known as an isotonic state. They may also be stimulated to contract by electrical shock.

The upright posture of the body is maintained by muscle tone which provides the necessary amount of force to counteract the effects of gravity. Muscle tone means that the length of muscle does not change but that the muscle remains tense in an isometric state. This partial contraction of the muscle is absent during sleep or periods of unconsciousness.

Movement

Movement of the joints is produced by voluntary contraction of one or a group of muscles which pull the bones together.

Muscles are grouped in pairs, one muscle being the agonist or prime mover, and its partner being the antagonist. For example, the main agonist in the upper arm is the biceps, and the antagonist is the triceps. When the biceps contracts the triceps relaxes. Large muscles are often composed of several muscles. For example the quadriceps extensor is made up of four different muscles, the rectus femoris, vastus medialis, vastus lateralis and vastus intermedius.

Synergistic muscle groups act together to provide complicated actions at the wrists, shoulders, ankles and hips. They work as a group to perform one action that no one of them could perform alone. This synchronised action is called synergism.

Skeletal muscles are capable of a wide variety of movements (Box 2.3). They range from powerful complicated actions as in the quadriceps, to the small, slight movements produced by the muscles of facial expression.

3. Connective tissue

The functions of connective tissue are to:

> **Box 2.3** Movement of muscles
>
> | | |
> | --- | --- |
> | Flexors | bend limbs |
> | Extensors | straighten limbs |
> | Adductors | move limb from midline |
> | Abductors | move limb towards midline |
> | Rotators | rotate a limb |
> | Pronators | turn palm downwards |
> | Supinators | turn palm upwards |
> | Plantarflexors | pull the foot up |
> | Dorsiflexors | push the foot down |
> | Levators | raise part of the body |
> | Depressors | lower part of the body |

- Attach bone to bone
- Attach muscle to bone
- Provide a point of anchorage for the action of muscles and bones
- Help to stabilise joints.

Tendons

Groups of muscles are attached to each other and surrounding tissue by tendons and fascia. Tendons are the connective tissue extensions of the perimysium and epimysium. They are strong, fibrous, inelastic cords which attach the muscle extremities to the bone at points of insertion or entheses.

A flat expansion of tendonous tissue is known as an aponeurosis. For example, the lumbar fascia is an aponeurosis which attaches the latissimus dorsi muscle to the vertebral column. Where tendons pass under ligaments or through bony tunnels, as in the wrist and ankle, they are enclosed in a synovial membrane sheath that reduces friction and enables the tendons to glide smoothly.

Ligaments

Ligaments resemble tendons and are strong bundles of connective tissue attached from one bone to another bone around a joint. They are thickened and enlarged around many of the synovial joints and thus increase the strength of the joint capsule. They act as restraints and ensure that the joint movement is within an acceptable plane and range.

4. Joints

The functions of joints are to:

- Stabilise the skeleton
- Permit a range of movement.

Physical structure

Joints are where two or more bones meet. There are three different types of joint:

1. *Fixed joints*, such as the squamous sutures of the skull that interlock with each other. Whilst the brain is developing and growing these joints expand. As a child grows older they become fixed and immovable and so protect the soft tissue of the brain.

2. *Fibrocartilaginous joints* are slightly moveable. Examples are the symphysis pubis, the costosternal joints and the vertebral bodies. In the case of the symphysis pubis the action of a hormone, relaxin, makes the joint more flexible and thus permits enlargement of the birth canal.

3. *The diarthroses or synovial joints* (see Fig. 2.4). Synovial joints are the most common types of joint in the body. They are of particular interest in rheumatology as they are the joints most commonly affected by inflammatory joint diseases such as rheumatoid arthritis (RA).

Synovial joints are freely moveable and are surrounded by a joint capsule lined with synovium. This lining, also called the synovial membrane, covers all the intra articular surfaces except the cartilage itself. It produces synovial fluid which lubricates the joint and feeds the cells of the articular cartilage.

The ends of the bones are covered and cushioned by hyaline cartilage. The joint capsule is made of fibrous tissue and strengthened by ligaments. It surrounds the whole joint and thus holds the bones together.

Cartilage

There are two types of cartilage:

• Hyaline
• Fibrocartilage.

Hyaline (articular) cartilage is a resilient structure that forms a firm cushion between the articulating or moveable surfaces of bone. It is not supplied with blood but gains all its necessary nutrients from the vasculature of surrounding tissues. These nutrients are carried to the cartilage by the synovial fluid which also removes the byproducts of metabolic activity within the cartilage.

Fibrocartilage has a definite matrix, is fibrous and compact. It is found at non-articulating joints such as the sternocostal, symphysis pubis and also between the intervertebral discs of the vertebrae.

Bursae

Bursae can be found close to joints where the skin moves directly over the bone. They are small synovial sacs acting as cushions to help relieve the pressure and friction over joints such as the knee, hip and ankle.

Movement of the joint

Movement of the joint is produced by the action of muscles and tendons and stabilised within a plane by ligaments. The different types of synovial joint permit a wide range and variety of movement (Box 2.4).

Types of synovial joints

• Uniaxial – (hinge) joints are capable of flexion and extension as in the elbow and interphalangeal joints.
• Polyaxial – (ball and socket) joints can extend, abduct, adduct, rotate and circumduct as in the hips and shoulders.
• Ellipsoid joints – permit flexion, extension, abduction and adduction but cannot rotate and combine the other movements to permit circumduction as in the wrist.
• Saddle joints – flex, extend, circumduct and rotate as in the carpometacarpal joint of the thumb.
• Plane joints – glide one across another as in the metatarsal joints.

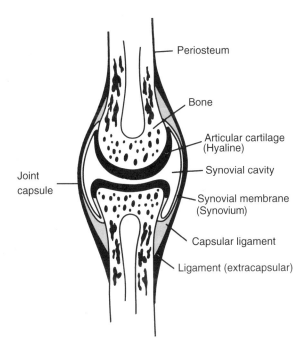

Periosteum

Bone

Articular cartilage (Hyaline)

Synovial cavity

Synovial membrane (Synovium)

Capsular ligament

Ligament (extracapsular)

Joint capsule

Figure 2.4 Synovial joint (adapted from Wilson and Waugh 1996, with permission).

Box 2.4	Planes of movement
Flexion	bending a joint
Extension	straightening a joint
Abduction	moving from the median or mid-line
Adduction	moving towards the median or mid-line
Circumduction	flexion, adduction, extension and abduction in sequence or in reverse order
Rotation	movement around the long axis of a bone
Pronation	rotation of the hand to face palm downwards
Supination	rotation of the hand to face palm upwards
Opposition	bringing the tip of the thumb to the tips of the fingers
Dorsiflexion	pulling the foot up towards the leg
Plantar flexion	pointing the foot down towards the ground
Inversion	pointing the sole of the foot inwards
Eversion	pointing the sole of the foot outwards

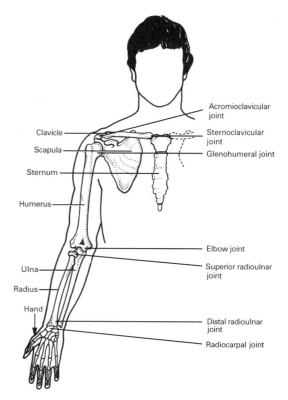

Figure 2.5 Shoulder girdle and upper limb (adapted from Wilson and Waugh 1996, with permission).

- Bicondylar joints – flex, extend and slightly rotate as in the knee and temperomandibular joints.
- Pivot joint – only rotate, an example is the atlas vertebra.
- Compound joints – are capable of several movements which involve more than two bones articulating with each other, for example the elbow.

Joints commonly affected by rheumatic disease

The joints or groups of joints most commonly affected by rheumatic disease are the:

1. Shoulder girdle.
2. Elbow.
3. Wrist and hand.
4. Pelvic girdle.
5. Knee.
6. Ankle and foot.
7. Vertebral column.
8. Jaw.

1. The shoulder girdle

The shoulder girdle (Fig. 2.5) is made up of the humerus, clavicle and scapula, which together provide a framework for the variety of movement found at this joint. Movement is synchronised and therefore dependent on the joints, ligaments and muscles working in harmony. Failure of any of these structures results in restricted or deficient movement.

The four joints of the shoulder girdle are:

- Glenohumeral
- Acromioclavicular
- Sternoclavicular
- Scapulothoracic.

The *glenohumeral* is multiaxial and the principal joint of the structure. The head of the humerus articulates within the glenoid fossa of the scapula, the diameter and depth of which is increased by a ring of fibrocartilage called the glenoid labrum. Free movement at this joint is allowed by the lax joint capsule which is strengthened by the glenohumeral, transverse humeral and coracoacromial ligaments. The long head of the biceps muscle inserts into the capsule and stabilises the joint.

Further stability is given by the rotator cuff which provides a band around the anterior, superior and posterior aspects of the glenohumeral joint and thereby stabilises the head of the humerus within the glenoid fossa. The muscles that form the rotator cuff are the supraspinatus, infraspinatus, subscapularis, and teres major.

The *acromioclavicular joint* is a plane joint formed by the distal end of the clavicle and the acromion process of the scapula. It is surrounded by a joint capsule which is strengthened above by the acromioclavicular ligament. A fibrous pad permits some movement at this joint. It is stabilised by the coraclavicular ligaments that hold the scapula and clavicle together during movement.

The *sternoclavicular* joint is a saddle joint formed between the medial end of the clavicle and the manubrium sterni. This joint contains an intra articular fibrous disc and is strengthened by anterior and posterior ligaments. The clavicle rotates during abduction and elevation of the shoulder.

The *scapulothoracic* joint is formed by the scapula articulating with the thoracic cage. The rotator cuff muscles, deltoid and trapezius insert around this articulation. Normal movement of the shoulder is dependent upon this joint.

The wide range of movement at the shoulder girdle depends upon the joints, muscles, tendons and ligaments working together (Box 2.5).

> **Box 2.5** Range of movement at the shoulder
>
> *Movements*: Flexion, extension, abduction, adduction, rotation and circumduction.
> *Muscles*: Deltoid, teres major, latissimus dorsi, trapezius, pectoralis major, subscapularis, teres minor, infraspinatus, supraspinatus and coracobrachialis.

Common disorders of the shoulder are:

- Synovitis
- Capsulitis (frozen shoulder)
- Dislocation
- Rotator cuff tears
- Tendinitis
- Bicipital tendinitis
- Subacromial bursitis
- Osteoarthritis.

2. The elbow joint

The elbow joint is a compound hinge joint formed by the articulation between the distal end of the humerus and the proximal ends of the ulna and radius. The radial and ulnar collateral ligaments provide support for the elbow and prevent varus or vagus instability.

The *superior radioulnar* joint is a fibrocartilaginous, uniaxial, pivotal joint at the articulation of the proximal ends of the radius and ulna. The joint capsule of the elbow joint also surrounds this joint. Several bursae can be found around the joint, the main one being the olecranon bursa.

The elbow muscles and their movements are listed in Box 2.6.

> **Box 2.6** Muscles responsible for the range of movement at the elbow
>
> | | |
> |---|---|
> | *Biceps, brachialis, flexor carpi ulnaris* | flexion |
> | *Triceps* | extension |
> | *Pronator teres* | pronation |
> | *Supinator* | supination |

Common disorders of the elbow are:

- Synovitis
- Lateral epicondylitis (tennis elbow)
- Medial epicondylitis (golfer's elbow)
- Olecranon bursitis
- Entrapment neuropathy
- Referred pain often from cervical or shoulder problems.

3. The wrist and hand

The wrist and hand (Fig. 2.6) form a complex structure, which together with the bones of the forearm permit complete manual dexterity. The range of movement is

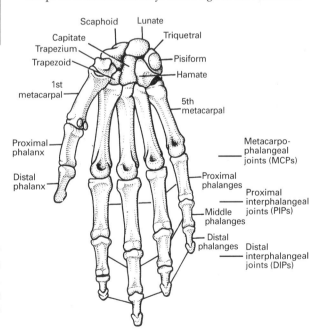

Figure 2.6 The bones and joints of the wrist, hand and fingers — anterior aspect (adapted from Wilson and Waugh 1996, with permission).

varied (see Box 2.7) and is essential for all the complex movements necessary for self-care. Any problems within this structure will directly affect independent living.

The bones which make up the wrist are the distal ends of the radius and ulna and the eight carpal bones: trapezoid, trapezium, scaphoid, lunate hamate, pisiform, triquetrum, and capitate. This structure provides a stable, strong support for the hand and its many functions.

The wrist is made up of the following joints:

* Radiocarpal
* Distal radioulnar
* Intercarpal.

The *radiocarpal* joint of the wrist is an ellipsoid, compound joint between the distal end of the radius and the scaphoid, lunate and triquetrum. The radiocarpal and collateral ligaments strengthen the joint capsule.

The *distal radioulnar* joint is a pivot joint. The radius is attached to the ulna by an articular disc, which permits rotation of the ulna head around the radius thereby pronating and supinating the hand.

The *intercarpal joints* are fibrocartilaginous, uniaxial, pivotal joints joined together by strong ligaments. One of the ligaments is the transverse carpal ligament (flexor retinaculum) on the volar aspect of the wrist. This forms the roof of the carpal tunnel by connecting the four bony prominences of the pisiform, hamate, scaphoid and trapezium. The flexor retinaculum prevents the flexor tendons from bowing out. Where tendons cross the wrist they are enclosed in tenosynovial sheaths. The flexor pollicis longus tendon sheath, the common flexor tendon sheath and the median nerve pass through the carpal tunnel to the hand. The ulnar nerve, artery and vein cross over the flexor retinaculum.

The extensor tendons are also enclosed in tendon sheaths and pass through fibro-osseous tunnels beneath the extensor retinaculum. This ligament binds deeply with the radius on the dorsum of the wrist and holds the extensor tendons to the wrist.

The *anatomic snuffbox* is the depression formed on the dorsum of the wrist by the extensor and abductor tendons of the thumb.

The *carpometacarpal* joints (CMCs) are formed between the trapezium, trapezoid, capitate and hamate bones and the proximal ends of the metacarpal bones. They are capable of flexion and extension and are classed as ellipsoid joints with the exception of the thumb which is a saddle joint. This articulation between the distal end of the trapezium and the proximal end of the first metacarpal is capable of abduction, adduction and rotation as well as extension and flexion.

The *metacarpophalangeal* joints (MCPs) or knuckles are hinge joints capable of flexion and extension. They are formed by the articulation of the distal ends of the metacarpal bones with the proximal ends of the phalanges.

The *proximal* and *distal interphalangeal* joints (PIPs and DIPs) are hinge joints which permit flexion and extension of the fingers. Fibrous tenosynovial sheaths enclose the flexor tendons of the fingers.

Common disorders of the wrist and hand are:

* Synovitis
* Carpal tunnel syndrome
* Trigger finger
* De Quervain's tenosynovitis
* Dupuytren's contracture
* Raynaud's phenomenon.

4. The pelvic girdle

The pelvic girdle (Fig. 2.7) is composed of the innominate bone and the sacrum. There are three joints in the pelvis. They are the:

* Hip joint
* Sacroiliac joint
* Symphysis pubis.

The *hip* is a multiaxial (ball and socket) joint. It is extremely strong, stable and capable of a variety of complex movements (see Box 2.8). The head of the

---

Box 2.7 Muscles responsible for the range of movement at the wrist

Flexor carpi radialis, flexor carpi ulnaris	flexion
Extensor carpi radialis, extensor carpi ulnaris	extension
Flexor carpi radialis, extensor carpi radialis	abduction
Flexor carpi ulnaris, extensor carpi ulnaris	adduction

Box 2.8 Muscles responsible for the range of movement at the hip

Iliopsoas, sartorius	flexion
Gluteus maximus, hamstrings	extension
Gluteus medius, gluteus minimus	abduction
Adductors longus, brevis and magnus	adduction
Gluteus medius, gluteus minimus	rotation (lateral)
Obturator, quadratus femoris	rotation (medial)

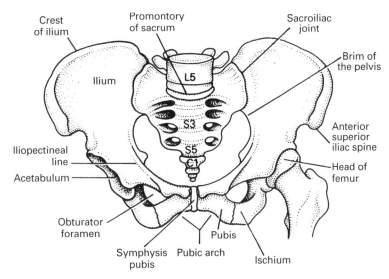

Figure 2.7 The pelvic girdle (from Wilson and Waugh 1996, with permission).

femur articulates within the acetabulum of the innominate bone. The acetabulum is strengthened and made deeper by a ring of fibrocartilage. The stability of the joint is maintained by three large ligaments; the iliofemoral, the pubofemoral and the ischiofemoral. The trochanteric bursa is the most important of the bursae found around the hip joint.

The *sacroiliac joint* is a synovial joint with limited movement. It holds the sacrum firmly between the two ilium bones and thereby anchors the vertebral column to the lower limbs. The strong sacroiliac, sacroprial and sacrotubal ligaments help to stabilise and strengthen this joint and enable it to take some of the stress that occurs during the gait cycle.

The *symphysis pubis* is a fibrocartilaginous joint which holds the two pubic bones together. There is little or no movement at this joint except during late pregnancy and childbirth. Then hormonal changes alter the structure to allow more flexibility and permit enlargement of the birth canal.

Common disorders of the pelvic girdle are:

- Trochanteric bursitis
- Synovitis
- Avascular necrosis
- Congenital dislocation of the hip
- Sacroiliitis.

5. The knee

The knee (Fig. 2.8) is a compound joint and is the largest joint in the body. It is supported by strong thigh muscles (see Box 2.9), which help to maintain its stability. Several ligaments strengthen the joint capsule. The patellar ligament supports the patella and the anterior part of the capsule. The anterior and lateral collateral ligaments, the anterior and posterior cruciate ligaments and the transverse ligament all increase the strength of the joint capsule. They are also vital in maintaining the strength and stability of the knee and in preventing valgus and varus deformities. Within the knee the semilunar cartilages or menisci help to deepen the articular surfaces at the proximal end of the tibia. Anteriorly the patella moves at the front of the knee between the lateral and medial condyles of the femur. There are many bursae around the knee, the main one being the prepatellar bursa.

Box 2.9 Muscles responsible for the range of movement at the knee	
Quadriceps	extension
Hamstrings, gastrocnemius, sartorius and gracilis	flexion
Medial hamstrings, popliteus, sartorius and gracilis	rotation (medial)
Biceps femoris	rotation (lateral)

Common disorders of the knee are:

- Synovitis
- Bursitis
- Tendinitis
- Prepatellar bursitis (housemaid's knee)
- Patellar bursitis (jumper's knee)

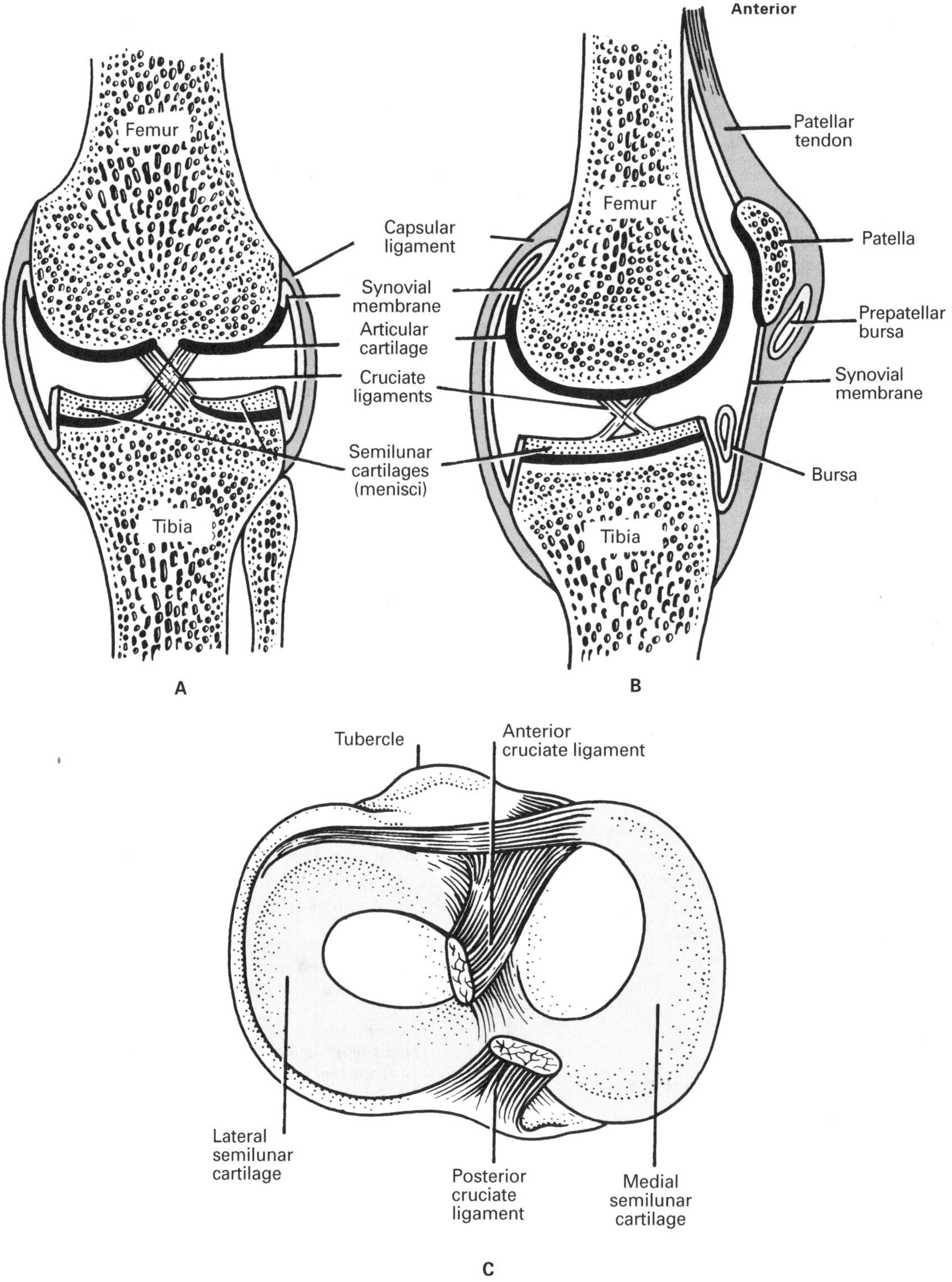

Figure 2.8 The knee. (A) Anterior view. (B) Lateral view. (C) Superior surface of the tibia showing the semilunar cartilages and cruciate ligaments (adapted from Wilson and Waugh 1996, with permission).

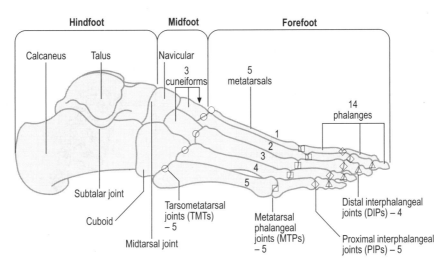

Figure 2.9 Bones and joints of the foot — lateral view (adapted from Wilson and Waugh 1996, with permission).

- Popliteal cysts
- Synovial chondromatosis
- Chondromalacia patellae
- Meniscal lesions
- Ligamentous injuries.

6. The ankle and foot

The ankle and foot (Fig. 2.9, Box 2.10), are composed of many bones and several joints. The foot is divided into the hind-, mid- and forefoot.

The *ankle*, also known as the *talocrural joint*, is a compound hinge joint. The distal ends of the tibia and fibula articulate with the talus and form the ankle joint. The hindfoot consists of the calcaneus and talus.

The talus also articulates inferiorly with the calcaneus at the subtalar joint and distally with the navicular bone at the midtarsal or talonavicular joint.

The distal tibiofibular joint is a fibrous joint that holds the distal ends of the tibia and fibula firmly together. Ligamentous bands strengthen the joint capsule medially and laterally.

Tenosynovial sheaths cover the tendons that run through this area. The extensor retinaculum, on the anterior aspect of the ankle is divided into two parts; the superior and inferior retinaculi. This strong ligament anchors the extensor tendons to the ankle and prevents them from bowing out. Medially, the flexor tendons are strapped down by the flexor retinaculum and the peroneal tendon is held down by the superior and inferior retinucli. Posteriorly, the Achilles tendon inserts into the calcaneus. Numerous bursae can be found in the ankle especially around the Achilles tendon.

Box 2.10 Muscles responsible for the range of movement at the ankle

Soleus, gastrocnemius	plantar flexion
Anterior tibialis,	dorsiflexion
extensor digitorum longus	
Peroneus longus, peroneus brevis,	eversion
extensor digitorum longus	
Tibialis anterior, tibialis posterior,	inversion
gastrocnemius	

Common disorders of the ankle are:

- Sprains
- Achilles tendinitis
- Achilles tendon rupture
- Achilles bursitis
- Plantar fasciitis
- Abduction sprains of the medial ligament
- Capsular ligament tears (sprained ankle)
- Calcaneal spur (policeman's heel).

The *midfoot* is composed of the navicular, cuboid and the three cuneiform bones. It articulates with the hindfoot at the midtarsal joint and with the forefoot at the tarsometatarsal joints.

The midtarsal or transverse tarsal joint is the articulation of the talus with the navicular (talonavicular) and the calcaneus with the cuboid (calneocuboid). These are fibrous plane joints.

The *forefoot* is made up of the metatarsals and phalanges. The proximal ends of the metatarsals articulate with the distal ends of the three cuneiform bones and the cuboid at the tarsometatarsal joints.

The metatarsophalangeal joints (MTPs) are the articulations of the distal ends of the metatarsal bones with the proximal ends of the phalanges. These are ellipsoid joints and are surrounded by a joint capsule which is strengthened by collateral ligaments and the plantar aponeurosis. Small bursae lie between the metatarsal heads, which are held together by the transverse metatarsal ligament. An aponeurosis of the extensor tendons covers the dorsum of the foot.

Extension, flexion, abduction and adduction of the toes is achieved by the intrinsic muscles of the foot.

The proximal interphalangeal (PIPs) and distal interphalangeal (DIPs) joints are hinge joints capable of flexing and extending the toes.

The arches of the foot are formed by an arrangement of the bones, ligaments and muscles. Each foot has four arches; two transverse and two longitudinal which act as shock absorbers during weight bearing.

Common disorders of the mid and forefoot are:

- Metatarsalgia
- Metatarsal stress fractures
- Hallux valgus (bunion)
- Hallux rigidus (hammer toe)
- Pes planus (flat foot)
- Pes cavus (claw foot).

7. The vertebral column

The vertebral column (Fig. 2.10) forms a framework which supports the rest of the body and also encloses the spinal cord. It is constructed of several different types of bones or vertebrae, some of which are fused together. The vertebrae (Box 2.11) are separated by discs of fibrocartilage and attached to each other by strong ligaments and muscles, thus combining

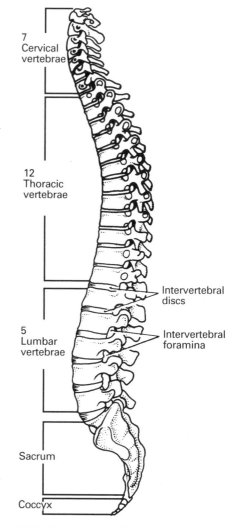

Figure 2.10 The vertebral column, lateral view (from Wilson and Waugh 1996, with permission).

strength with a degree of flexibility. The spinal column is constructed and curved to permit walking in an upright posture. At birth the infant has two spinal curves. These primary curves are in the thoracic and sacral regions. The secondary spinal curves develop in the cervical and lumbar regions as an upright stance is assumed.

Although the vertebrae are of different shapes and sizes, with the exception of the atlas (the first cervical vertebra), they all have the features shown in Box 2.12.

All vertebrae are separated by intervertebral discs of fibrocartilage which are made up of a central ring-like structure called the annulus fibrosis surrounding the nucleus pulposus. The bodies of the vertebrae are held

---

Box 2.11	The types of vertebrae			

There are 33 vertebrae:

7 cervical	Moveable	Convex forwards	Lordotic
12 thoracic	Moveable	Convex backwards	Kyphotic
5 lumbar	Moveable	Convex forwards	Lordotic
5 sacral	Fused (sacrum)	Concave forwards	Kyphotic
4 coccygeal	Fused (coccyx)	Concave forwards	

In the figure labels:
7 Cervical vertebrae
12 Thoracic vertebrae
5 Lumbar vertebrae
Sacrum
Coccyx
Intervertebral discs
Intervertebral foramina

Box 2.12 Features possessed by all vertebrae		
1 Spinous process Vertebral arch Body	2 Transverse processes Pedicles Laminae	4 Articular processes

together by anterior and posterior longitudinal ligaments. The spinous processes are held together by the supraspinous ligaments. Spinal nerves pass from the spinal cord through the intervertebral foramen, a space between individual vertebrae.

Of the seven *cervical vertebrae* of the neck, the lower five are similar in shape (Fig. 2.11). However, the upper two, the atlas and the axis (Fig. 2.12), are different because they are specially adapted to carry the head and enable it to move in many directions. The atlas has no spinous process and no body. It supports the cranium at the atlanto-occipital joint and permits nodding of the head and lateral flexion of the neck. The axis has a peg, the odontoid process or dens, around which the atlas rotates at the atlanto-axial joint to enable movement of the head.

Common disorders of the cervical region are:

- Atlanto-axial subluxation
- Stenosis
- Torticollis
- Spondylitis
- Whiplash injury
- Osteoarthritis.

The 12 *thoracic vertebrae* have facets for the attachment of the heads of the ribs. This arrangement permits the expansion and contraction of the rib cage and therefore the lungs.

Common disorders of the thoracic region are:

- Osteoporosis
- Costochondritis
- Ankylosing spondylitis
- Osteoarthritis.

The five *lumbar vertebrae* are the largest and strongest (Fig. 2.13). Their design enables them to carry the weight of the body and control its movements on the pelvis in the upright position.

Common disorders of the lumbar region are:

- Sciatica
- Prolapsed intervertebral disc
- Low back pain

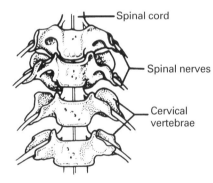

Figure 2.11   The lower cervical vertebrae separated to show the spinal cord and spinal nerves emerging through the intervertebral foramina (from Wilson and Waugh 1996, with permission).

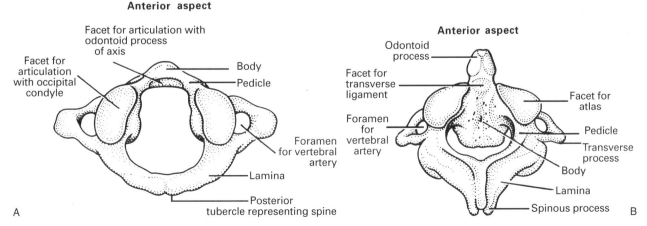

Figure 2.12   Upper cervical vertebrae — (A) atlas and (B) axis (both viewed from above) (from Wilson and Waugh 1996, with permission).

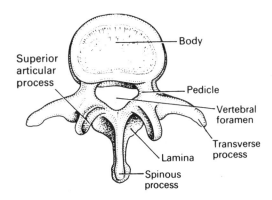

Figure 2.13 Lumbar vertebra (viewed from above) (from Wilson and Waugh 1996, with permission).

- Spinal stenosis
- Ankylosing spondylitis
- Osteoarthritis.

The five *sacral vertebrae* are fused together to form the sacrum which makes up the posterior aspect of the pelvis. The sacrum is fused to the ilium at the sacroiliac joint. This strong structure enables the body to maintain an upright position and to take the stress of walking and running. It provides posterior protection for the abdominal organs. Females have a larger sacrum than males to allow for a larger pelvic cavity necessary for child bearing.

Common disorders of the sacral region

- Low back pain.
- Sacroiliitis

The *coccyx* is a triangular structure, formed by the fusion of the four coccygeal vertebrae, the base of which articulates with the apex of the sacrum above.

The muscles and ligaments of the vertebral column facilitate the range of movement in the back (Box 2.13). These structures also support the vertebrae and thus the maintenance of an upright posture (Fig. 2.14).

Box 2.13	Range of movement of the spine
• *Cervical*	flexion (bending forwards) extension (bending backwards) rotation of the head, lateral movement (bending from side to side)
• *Thoracic*	lateral movement (bending from side to side)
• *Lumbar*	flexion (bending forwards) extension (bending backwards)
• *Whole vertebral column*	rotation and twisting

8. Jaw (temperomandibular joint)

The temperomandibular joint (TMJ) is formed between the condyle of the mandible (lower jaw) and the fossa of the temporal bone. It is the only articulating joint of the skull. It is lined by fibrous connective tissue rather than the normal hyaline cartilage and menisciaa help to extend the range of movement (Box 2.14). The joint itself is divided into two parts, the upper part enabling flexion and extension of the joint and the lower a gliding movement to permit lateral and protrusive movement of the lower jaw. It is the only joint in the body, which works with a partner, for example both TMJs work as a pair and enable the mouth to be opened.

Box 2.14	Muscles responsible for the range of movement of the jaw
Temporal, masseter	chewing
Buccinator	chewing and sucking
Pterygoid	closes the mouth

Common disorder of the jaw

- Synovitis.

THE COMMON RHEUMATIC DISEASES

The term rheumatic diseases is used to describe the many conditions that affect the musculoskeletal system. They can affect the bones, joints, soft tissues and muscles. There are around 200 such diseases (Symmons & Bankhead 1994). The gamut of conditions ranges from the milder soft tissue rheumatism such as tennis elbow, to inflammation of joint linings, as in rheumatoid arthritis (RA), and damage to the surface of the joints, as in osteoarthritis (OA).

Many of the rheumatic diseases relate to each other and in some instances have overlapping signs and symptoms. The management of patients with rheumatic disease likewise has many common features whatever the disease. However, the course of each patient's disease will be different and therefore each patient must be treated as an individual with an individual plan of care. The common rheumatic diseases are shown in Box 2.15.

INFLAMMATORY JOINT DISEASE
Rheumatoid arthritis (RA)

RA is a chronic inflammatory disease, mainly

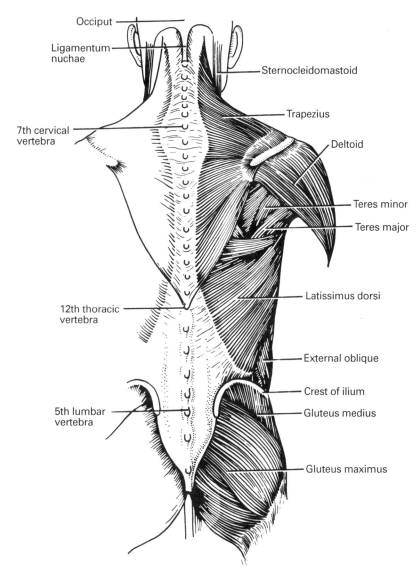

Figure 2.14 The main muscles of the back (from Wilson and Waugh 1996, with permission).

affecting the peripheral joints. It is characterised by exacerbation and remission of disease activity. Affected joints exhibit synovitis which is associated with pain, heat, stiffness, swelling and eventual joint destruction. The disease is systemic and may involve the organs.

Epidemiology

RA is found globally, although it appears to be less prevalent amongst oriental populations. It attacks all age groups and three times more women than men are affected (Lawrence 1994).

Aetiology

The aetiology is unknown but various factors such as infections, stress and trauma appear to act as a trigger in people with a genetic disposition. The body is unable to switch off the initial response to the disease and it becomes chronic. Although new criteria for the classification of RA were developed by the

---

> **Box 2.15** The common rheumatic diseases
>
> 1. *Inflammatory joint diseases*
>   Rheumatoid arthritis
>   Felty's syndrome
>   Juvenile chronic arthritis
> 2. *Spondyloarthropathies*
>   Psoriatic arthropathy
>   Ankylosing spondylitis
>   Reiter's syndrome
>   Behçet's syndrome
> 3. *Crystal deposition diseases*
>   Gout
>   Pyrophosphate arthropathy
> 4. *Joint failure*
>   Osteoarthritis
> 5. *Metabolic bone disease*
>   Osteoporosis
> 6. *Connective tissue diseases*
>   Systemic lupus erythematosus
>   Scleroderma
>   Polymyositis
>   Dermatomyositis
> 7. *Non-articular conditions*
>   Polymyalgia rheumatica
>   Giant cell arteritis
>   Raynaud's phenomenon
>   Sjögren's syndrome
> 8. *Soft tissue rheumatism*
>   Fibromyalgia
>   Carpal tunnel syndrome
>   Tennis and golfer's elbow

American Rheumatism Association in 1987 (Arnet et al 1988), many subsets exist.

Pathology

The synovial lining of the joint capsule becomes inflamed and congested with T lymphocytes, B cells, macrophages and plasma cells (Firestein 1994). This lining gradually thickens and forms a pannus that invades the articular cartilage causing erosion of the cartilage and bone visible on X-ray.

Increased disease activity produces an elevated erythrocyte sedimentation rate (ESR), positive rheumatoid factor (RF+) and an elevated C-reactive protein (CRP). The platelet count may also be raised and anaemia can be present. Some patients have a normal ESR and CRP with a negative rheumatoid factor (see Ch. 3). This type of disease is classed as seronegative RA and is usually less aggressive.

Presentation

The most common age of onset is the fourth and fifth decades. Symmetrical swelling, pain and tenderness of the peripheral joints of the hands and feet are usually the predominant features. As the disease progresses, other joints such as the shoulders, elbows, wrists, hips, knees and ankles are affected. Eventually, damage and destruction cause the joints to become unstable and subluxation can occur. RA is a systemic disease that also causes general malaise, fatigue and depression.

Clinical features

- Pain and swelling of the affected joints
- Early morning stiffness is an indicator of disease activity and can vary from minutes to hours
- Inactivity stiffness occurs after periods of rest
- Loss of mobility.

Specific problems may be:

- Hand problems can arise even in early RA (Fig. 2.15). Later problems include ulnar deviation (Fig. 2.16), Boutonnière (Fig. 2.17) and swan neck (Fig. 2.18) deformities. All cause loss of function. Tenosynovitis results in loss of flexion, triggering of the fingers and tendon rupture.
- Metatarsalgia, tendinitis of the plantar fascia and Achilles tendon cause pain and restrict mobility.
- Knee effusions can result in Baker's cysts which may be misdiagnosed as venous thrombosis.
- Bursitis of the greater trochanter, olecranon and knee can occur.
- Temperomandibular involvement can limit opening of the mouth.
- Cervical spine involvement causes pain and neuro-

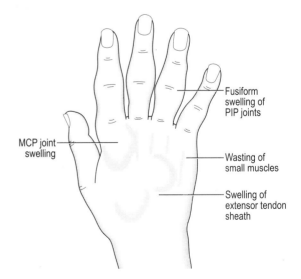

Figure 2.15 Hand problems in early RA (adapted from Dieppe et al 1985, with permission).

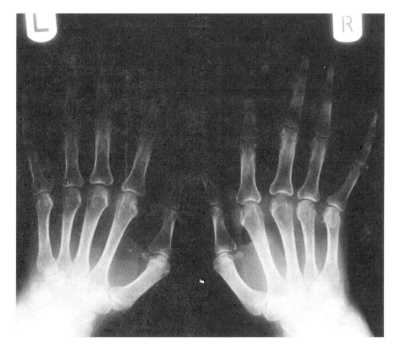

Figure 2.16   X-ray of hands showing ulnar deviation and erosions in the MCPs and PIPs in RA (with permission from the University Hospital Birmingham NHS Trust).

logical symptoms in the arms and hands. Atloaxial subluxation results in paralysis or even death.

Extra-articular features which may be present:

- Anaemia which normally resolves as the disease remits
- Muscular wasting around inflamed joints
- Entrapment neuropathies such as median nerve involvement (carpal tunnel syndrome)
- Rheumatoid nodules on the elbows, occiput, sacrum, scapulae, Achilles tendon, lungs and myocardium
- Sjögren's syndrome (dry eyes and mouth)
- Lymphadenopathy resulting in diffuse pitting oedema of the ankles
- Osteoporosis causing fractures of the spine, hip and wrist
- Pericarditis, pericardial effusions and amyloidosis
- Hepatomegaly caused by amyloid deposits
- Fibrosing alveolitis and pleural effusions
- Felty's syndrome causing splenomegaly
- Vasculitis causing nail fold infarcts and leg ulcers.

Management

Daily living activities are greatly restricted by disease

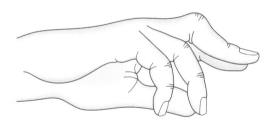

Figure 2.17   Boutonnière deformity (adapted from Dieppe et al 1985, with permission).

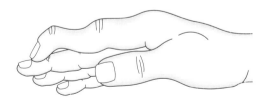

Figure 2.18   Swan neck deformity (adapted from Dieppe et al 1985, with permission).

activity. Assessment of the problems, a plan of care and subsequent implementation and evaluation are important to enable the patient to lead as normal a life as possible within their own capabilities.

Therapy may include:

- Analgesia
- Non-steroidal anti-inflammatory drugs (NSAIDs) to relieve pain, swelling and stiffness
- Second line drug therapy to induce disease remission.

Referral to members of the multidisciplinary team for:

- Education and information
- Joint protection
- Rest and relaxation
- Physiotherapy
- Advice about a healthy diet
- Special shoes, wrist and ankle supports, collars.

Surgical intervention may be helpful for some patients (see Ch. 14). Joint replacement of the hips, knees and shoulders may be indicated to give some measure of mobility, function and relief from pain. Other surgical procedures such as excision of metatarsal heads may also be undertaken to relieve pain and improve function. Cosmetic surgery is sometimes undertaken for deformities of the hand.

Felty's syndrome

Felty's syndrome occurs in 1% of the rheumatoid population (Campion & Maddison 1986) and is characterised by splenomegaly, leucopaenia and chronic arthritis.

Aetiology

Little is known of the aetiology of this syndrome except that it affects both sexes equally, although men seem to develop the syndrome earlier in their rheumatoid disease. Morbidity and mortality are high and infection often leads to death.

Pathology

The production of neutrophils is decreased and the bone marrow reserve is suppressed. Raised levels of IgM, IgG and ANA are present in the blood serum (see Ch. 3).

Presentation

Patients with long standing, seropositive, nodular, deforming rheumatoid arthritis may develop Felty's syndrome (Matteson et al 1994). Changes in the joints are usually mild with little clinical or radiological evidence. Splenomegaly, neutropenia and vasculitis may be present and weight loss is common. Frequent infections of the skin, lungs and kidneys occur but are not necessarily related to the neutropenia (Dieppe et al 1985a). Liver involvement occurs in 65% of patients (Matteson et al 1994).

Clinical features

- Hyperpigmentation may occur on the shins
- Chronic leg ulcers are more common than in rheumatoid arthritis
- Raynaud's phenomenon and Sjögren's syndrome may be present.

Management

The problems are similar to those associated with rheumatoid arthritis and should be managed in a similar fashion. Spontaneous remission of the neutropenia occurs in some cases.

Therapy may include:

- Second line drug therapy to suppress the rheumatoid disease (see Ch. 12). This should induce neutrophilia and reduce the likelihood of infection.
- Splenectomy is sometimes undertaken but it is a controversial intervention. The benefit derived from the increase in neutrophils induced by the removal of the spleen, the site of neutrophil destruction, has to be balanced against the risks of operation and infection.

Juvenile chronic arthritis

Juvenile chronic arthritis (JCA) is defined as an inflammatory arthritis which presents before the sixteenth birthday.

Epidemiology

George Frederick Still first described juvenile chronic arthritis 100 years ago and for many years it was known as Still's disease. Since then three subsets have been identified:

- Pauciarticular
- Polyarticular
- Systemic onset.

Aetiology

The aetiology of this disease is unknown although viral infections such as rubella, mumps and parvo virus are thought to trigger juvenile chronic arthritis in children with a genetic predisposition (Leak 1991).

Pathology

The pathology is similar to that of RA but repair of damaged joints can occur during disease remission. Growth problems such as retardation and shortened limbs result from overgrowth (caused by hyperaemia around the joint), premature fusion of the epiphyses and the use of corticorsteroids.

Presentation

Symptoms are difficult to elicit especially with very young children but joint effusions, limitation of movement, pain and tenderness are typical (White 1994).

Pauciarticular:

- Most common subset accounting for about 60% of cases
- Majority of cases in the under fives
- Girls affected more than boys at a ratio of 4:1
- Affects four or less joints, usually the knees, ankles, wrists and elbows
- Asymmetrical pattern.

    Further subsets within this group:

- Females under 2 years of age
- Asymptomatic with uveitis
- ANA positive
- Boys over the age of nine
- Enthesitis of the knees, ankles and hips
- Later development of sacroiliitis
- Children with a family history of psoriasis
- Asymmetrical, destructive, peripheral arthritis
- Dactylitis.

Polyarticular:

- Approximately 20% of cases
- Five or more joints affected within the first six months of the disease.

    Further subsets within this group:

1. Rheumatoid positive (RF+):

- Predominately affects females between 12 and 16 years
- Symmetrical involvement of the peripheral joints of the hands
- Flexor tenosynovitis
- Nodules, vasculitis, carpal tunnel, cervical myelopathy and Sjögren's syndrome.

2. Rheumatoid negative (RF–):

- Low grade fevers
- Symmetrical involvement of the hands, knees, wrists and ankles
- Hepatosplenomegaly.

Systemic onset:

- Approximately 20% of cases
- Occurs throughout childhood
- Affects boys and girls equally
- Fever and rash on the trunk and thighs
- Lymphadenopathy and hepatosplenomegaly
- Arthritis of the wrists, knees, ankles, cervical spine, hips, temperomandibular joints and hands.

Management

Early referral to the multidisciplinary team is essential so that they can support the family and treat problems as they arise. In addition to the usual team members a paediatrician, orthopaedic surgeon and ophthalmologist should be involved. The prognosis is usually good but is dependent on the number and size of joints affected and the severity of extra-articular involvement.

Therapy may include:

- Aspirin to control fever
- Non-steroidal anti-inflammatory drugs; usually ibuprofen, naproxen, diclofenac, tolmetin and piroxicam in liquid or suppository form
- Low dose methotrexate is well tolerated and effectively induces remission
- Corticosteroids although these can lead to growth retardation – myocarditis always requires the use of long-term steroids
- Joint injections performed under a light general anaesthetic
- Physiotherapy
- Splinting of affected joints
- Hydrotherapy
- Surgery to release soft tissues around the knees and hips and prevent flexion contractures.

THE SPONDYLOARTHROPATHIES

The rheumatological conditions grouped under this heading share many similarities such as peripheral arthropathy, seronegative rheumatoid factor, positive HLA B27, sacroiliitis evident on X-ray examination and a genetic predisposition (Dieppe et al 1985b).

Psoriatic arthritis

Psoriatic arthritis is a chronic peripheral, polyarthritis similar to RA and is associated with a previous, ongoing psoriasis. It may progress to a severe form of psoriatic arthritis known as arthritis mutilans.

Epidemiology

A familial history of psoriasis is common. Males and females are affected equally.

Pathology

Blood tests show a normal ESR and negative rheumatoid factor. HLA B27 is positive especially in those patients with sacroiliitis and spondylitis. X-ray examinations reveal erosions of the joints, sclerosis of joint margins, cysts and ankylosis. Arthritis mutilans produces more severe changes such as the destruction of the ends of the distal bones making them impact and causing the fingers to 'telescope'.

Presentation

The usual age of onset is between 20–50 years. Some patients have associated asymptomatic sacroiliitis and spondylitis. Psoriasis will be present in 75% of patients and one third will have some eye involvement (Wright & Helliwell 1992, Helliwell & Wright 1994).

Clinical features

- Inflammation of the DIPS and PIPs, dactylitis (sausage finger)
- Hot, swollen and painful feet
- Enthesitis – Achilles tendon and plantar fascia
- Psoriasis – extensor surfaces of the knees, elbows and scalp
- Onycholysis (nail pitting).

Management

Patients with psoriatic arthritis experience similar problems to those with rheumatoid arthritis and management varies according their needs. Counselling should be considered because in addition to unsightly skin lesions the difficulties of coping with arthritis can have a tremendous psychological impact (Espinoza & Cuellar 1994).

Ankylosing spondylitis

Ankylosing spondylitis affects the axial skeleton. Initially, the sacroiliac joints are involved followed by the vertebral column (Rai & Struthers 1994). In chronic progressive disease the vertebral column may fuse resulting in the characteristic bent spine. Ankylosing spondylitis can occur in association with other diseases such as Reiter's syndrome, psoriasis, ulcerative colitis or Crohn's disease.

Epidemiology

Approximately three times more males are affected than females. There is considerable variation in the incidence of ankylosing spondylitis, both geographically, and between racial groups.

Pathology

Blood tests show an elevated ESR and CRP and a negative rheumatoid factor. The majority of patients are HLA B27 positive. Radiological examination eventually shows calcification of the spinal longitudinal ligaments, squaring of the vertebrae (bamboo spine), spinal osteoporosis and the characteristic blurring of the sacroiliac joints.

Presentation

The average age of onset is 26 years (Khan 1994). It starts in an insidious fashion with pain and stiffness in the lumbosacral region. Peripheral arthritis may be present but is uncommon and does not persist. Sleep disturbance due to pain and stiffness in the spine causes fatigue. Remissions and exacerbation of disease activity occur early in the disease, but eventually the spine stiffens and body posture changes as thoracic kyphosis develops and lumbar lordosis is lost. Cervical ankylosis with kyphosis leads to the loss of forward gaze (Fig. 2.19). The majority of patients are able to remain in work and lead a normal life. However, those who develop hip and neck problems may become severely disabled.

Clinical features

- Fatigue
- Low backache initially severe and later becoming dull
- Pain and stiffness particularly in the lower back after periods of inactivity but improved by exercise
- Unilateral or bilateral pain in the sacroiliac and gluteal regions
- Sciatica type pain radiating from the buttock into the leg
- Enthesopathy – costosternal, manubriosternal, Achilles tendinitis and plantar faciitis.

As the disease progresses there may be:

- Restriction of spinal movement caused by ankylosis of the vertebrae
- Restricted range of movement in the hips and shoulders
- Flexion fractures of the hips

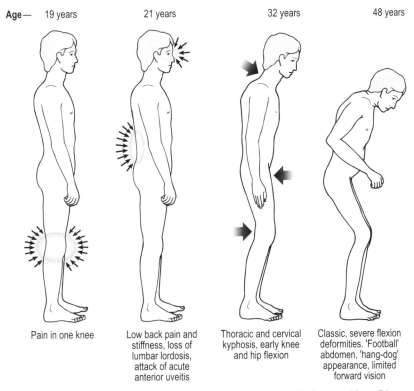

Figure 2.19 Classic progression of severe ankylosing spondylitis (adapted from Dieppe et al 1985, with permission).

- Stiff neck resulting in torticollis
- Reduced chest expansion caused by fusion of the ribs to the transverse processes of the vertebrae.

Extra-articular features:

- Iritis, conjunctivitis and uveitis
- Pulmonary fibrosis and aortic incompetence in severe cases.

Management

Education is vital in order that patients and their families understand the value of daily exercises and prone lying which will ensure that spinal fusion is restricted and a straight spine is maintained. Regular physiotherapy and hydrotherapy are essential to maintain movement of the spine and hips.

Therapy may include:

- Non-steroidal anti-inflammatory drugs to relieve pain and stiffness
- Phenylbutazone, methotrexate and cyclosporin are also used.

Psychological support is important for this group of patients who often experience anxiety, depression and problems with lack of self-worth and altered body image. Patients should be encouraged to join support groups such as the National Ankylosing Spondylitis Society which is known as NASS.

Reiter's syndrome and reactive arthritis

Reiter's syndrome is the triad of:

1. Arthritis
2. Urethritis
3. Conjunctivitis.

It usually occurs as a result of a reaction to a genital or gastrointestinal tract infection (Dieppe et al 1985c, Keat 1986).

Epidemiology

Hans Reiter, a military doctor with the German Army first described this syndrome. Reiter's syndrome is also termed a reactive arthritis, because the initial infection whether genital or gastrointestinal, causes a reaction elsewhere in the body. In one third of patients no infectious cause is found. Men and women are affected equally (Toivanen 1994).

Aetiology

A reactive arthritis which has been caused through sexual contact is termed SARA (sexually acquired reactive arthritis). Chlamydia trachomatis and gonococcal organisms are thought to be responsible. Shigella, salmonella, campylobacter and yersinia are the organisms associated with a reactive arthritis contracted through the gastrointestinal tract. The majorities of patients (65–96%), are HLA B27 positive and often develop a more chronic type of disease (Toivanen 1994).

Pathology

Blood tests reveal a negative rheumatoid factor and elevated ESR and CRP. Radiological examination shows osteopenia around the joints, calcaneal and plantar spurs and bilateral sacroiliitis.

Presentation

The peak age of onset is 16–35 years and it follows sexual contact or sometimes an attack of dysentery. A typical presentation is that of a young man with an acute, asymmetrical oligoarthritis affecting either the knees, ankles or feet. The affected joints are often severely inflamed with erythema, tenderness and large effusions. The lower limbs may be involved one at a time over several weeks. The elbows, wrists and fingers are occasionally affected. Sacroiliitis and spondylitis occur in the one third of those with recurrent disease. Symptoms may recur over a few years but they eventually resolve.

Clinical features

- Fever
- Synovitis of the knee or ankle
- Dactylitis or 'sausage toe'
- Plantar faciitis and Achilles tendinitis
- Conjunctivitis may be bilateral but it usually resolves
- Urethral discharge may be mild, non purulent and is often missed
- Circinate balinitis and vulvitis
- Cystitis
- Keratoderma blenorrhagica – these skin lesions resemble pustular psoriasis and may appear on the palms of the hands and soles of the feet of patients with SARA

- Onycholysis (nail pitting)
- Ulcers on the tongue, palate, buccal mucosa and lips.

Management

Treatment should be symptomatic. Musculoskeletal symptoms may persist for several months and then resolve. Counselling and advice may be necessary especially where there is a worry about future sexual activity. In the case of SARA, sexual contacts should be traced so that they can be treated.

Therapy may include:

- Non-steroidal anti-inflammatory drugs
- Tetracycline to treat urethritis
- Second line drugs such as sulphasalazine and methotrexate for persistent disease
- Splinting or bed rest of the affected joints
- Aspiration and steroid injection of joint effusions
- Physiotherapy to regain muscle power and tone
- Local steroid injections to relieve pain caused by enthesopathies of the feet and ankles.

Behçet's syndrome

Behçet's syndrome is a systemic vasculitis associated with oral and genital ulceration and inflammatory eye disease.

Epidemiology

Behçet's syndrome is prevalent in Turkey, Iran, China, Japan and around the Mediterranean but relatively unknown in Northern Europe and the Americas. Its distribution has suggested some link with the silk route from Europe to the Far East (Yazici 1994). Both sexes are affected equally although the disease tends to be worse in males.

This syndrome was originally described as a triad of oral and genital ulcers and inflammatory eye disease. However, neurological, gastrointestinal and vasculitic clinical features are now recognised as part of the syndrome.

Aetiology

The aetiology remains unknown although streptococcal infections are thought to play a part and it has been suggested from Japan that there is a possible link with exposure to toxic chemicals (Barnes 1991).

Pathology

Necrotising vasculitis is found in the vessels of skin,

vulva, retina and brain. Blood tests may show a raised ESR, mild to moderate anaemia and hyperglobulin-aemia.

Presentation

The peak age of onset is the third decade. The first symptom is usually recurring oral ulcers that are often very deep and cause scars. Genital ulcers occur in the majority of patients. They start as painful nodules in the groin, perineum, vulva and vagina of females and on the scrotum of males. Monoarticular or oligo-articular inflammatory arthritis affects 45% of patients (Barnes 1991). Skin lesions such as erythema nodosum and acneiform nodules are typical features. Vasculitis occurs in a small number of patients and often leads to severe problems. The eyes can be affected and in some cases blindness may ensue. Gastrointestinal and neurological involvement may also occur.

Clinical features

- Oral ulcers – buccal mucosa, lips, tongue and pharynx
- Genital ulcers occur in both sexes
- Eye involvement – iritis is easily treated, posterior uveitis may lead to blindness
- Inflammatory arthritis of the knees, ankles, wrists and elbows may be chronic or episodic
- Subcutaneous nodules and vasculitis similar to erythema nodosum may appear on the legs and feet
- Acne type pustules similar to those seen during adolescence
- Vascular symptoms – superficial thrombophlebitis, deep venous and arterial thromboses, aneurysms and occlusion of major vessel
- Central nervous system involvement – confused states and meningitis
- Colonic ulcers – pain, diarrhoea and haemorrhage
- Pathogenic reaction may occur when the skin is hypersensitive to simple trauma; for example a needle prick causing a papule to form over the site of the injury.

Management

The aim of therapy is to treat symptoms and the ophthalmologist and dermatologist will need to be involved.

Therapy may include:

- Non-steroidal anti-inflammatory drugs
- Cyclophosphamide and corticosteroids to treat severe vasculitis.

CRYSTAL DEPOSITION DISEASE

These diseases occur when crystals are laid down in the joints and other organs. Gout is the most common of these conditions but they also include pseudogout or pyrophosphate arthropathy.

Gout

Gout may develop as a result of a disorder of purine metabolism that leads to hyperuricaemia. Urate crystals are deposited in the joints especially of the big toe. There appears to be a genetic and familial association with the incidence of gout.

Epidemiology

Gout is one of the oldest diseases known to man and has been described and catalogued since the time of Hippocrates. It is recognised world wide and in males over 40 years old is the most common inflammatory arthropathy. Life style changes, drugs and an increasing elderly population are thought to be relevant factors leading to the increased incidence of gout (Cohen & Emmerson 1994).

Aetiology

The common causes of hyperuricaemia are a high dietary intake of purines and under excretion of urate. Thiazide diuretic therapy can decrease the excretion of urate thus raising the serum urate and precipitating gout (Gibson 1988).

Pathology

A high level of urate in the blood (hyperuricaemia) is a risk factor but it does not necessarily lead to the condition. Uric acid is retained in the synovial fluid and forms uric acid crystals. Occasionally uric acid calculi occur in the kidneys. Radiological examination reveals bony erosions related to tophi formation around the joints.

Presentation

The peak onset is in males between 40 and 50 years. Females are usually affected later in life. Acute attacks of gout present suddenly, with severe pain in the big toe, heel or ankle that builds up to a peak over several days. Usually only one joint is affected but further joints may be involved during subsequent attacks. Episodes of exacerbation and remission result in chronic gout particularly when hyperuricaemia is not controlled. Attacks of gout can be precipitated by acute illness, trauma, surgery, alcoholic excess and drugs which alter the plasma urate concentration (salicylates, thiazides, frusemide and pyrazinamide).

Clinical features

- Swollen red joint often the big toe
- Severe and unremitting pain in the affected joint
- Fever may be present
- Tophi (nodular swellings) on the fingers, toes and ears which often produce a chalky exudate.

Management

Gout is the one rheumatic disease that can be fully controlled by drug therapy. Patient education and dietary advice enable patients to understand and control their disease.

Therapy may include:

- Non-steroidal anti-inflammatory drugs – indomethacin in high doses to treat acute attacks
- Daily allopurinol or colchicine to reduce hyperuricaemia
- Probenecid when allopurinol is not tolerated.

Pseudogout (pyrophosphate arthropathy)

Pseudogout occurs when crystals of calcium pyrophosphate are deposited in the joints. The disease may be acute or chronic, the knee being the most commonly affected joint. Unlike gout, the big toe is rarely affected but the shoulders, elbows, wrists, hips and ankles may be involved. In acute disease, attacks last for months and usually recur. The chronic disease is progressive and can be similar to OA.

Management usually involves:

- Aspiration and injection of the affected joints with corticosteroids
- Non-steroidal anti-inflammatory drugs
- Rest.

JOINT FAILURE
Osteoarthritis (OA)

OA means inflammation of bone and joint. This disease causes destruction of the hyaline cartilage of the articular surfaces of the bone and varies in severity causing little inconvenience to some patients but chronic pain and disability in others.

Epidemiology

In the past OA was labelled a wear and tear arthritis and was associated with ageing. Today it is described as joint failure (Symmons & Bankhead 1994) and is recognised as the most common rheumatic disease in the UK. Radiographic evidence shows the disease to be present in 80% of the population over the age of 75 years (Cooper 1994). More women than men are affected.

Aetiology

There is no known aetiology or cure for this chronic disease but OA may be related to a genetic factor, trauma or previous joint disease. Obesity, occupation and previous injury often determine which joints are affected and the severity of the disease. It can affect any joint but those most commonly affected are the DIPs, carpometacarpal of the thumb, knees, spine and hips.

Although efforts have been made to classify subsets, the term osteoarthritis covers a range of heterogeneous diseases.

The disease is classified as primary, where there is no apparent cause, and secondary where the cause may be metabolic, anatomic, traumatic or inflammatory (Dieppe 1994).

Secondary OA may be caused by:

- Metabolic diseases – acromegaly, calcium crystal deposition
- Structural disorders – Perthes' disease, congenital hip dislocation
- Trauma – surgical procedures such as menisectomy
- Previous inflammatory arthropathy such as rheumatoid arthritis
- Hypermobility causing a lax joint capsule leading to recurrent dislocation
- Fractures
- Occupational hazards.

Pathology

OA causes thinning, fibrillation (flaking) and destruction of the articular cartilage. The growth of fibrocartilage and bone at the joint margins produces osteophytes that are visible on X-ray. Other radiological changes are the loss of joint space, bony cysts and sclerosis in the subchondral bone. Loss of joint space affects the integrity of the joint causing pain, stiffness, deformity and disability.

Presentation

The peak age of onset is between 50 years and 60 years

and is usually gradual with an increase in pain and stiffness in the affected joints. Often, patients do not seek medical advice until their symptoms are severe and require surgical intervention.

Clinical features

- Pain related to movement although it may be present at rest
- Pain – severe and unremitting especially when the hip is affected
- Stiffness and gelling of joints – relieved by movement
- Restricted range of movement – crepitus and swollen joints
- Hands – Heberden's nodes of the DIPs, squaring of the thumb (Z thumb), Bouchard's nodes of the PIPs (Fig. 2.20)
- Knees – crepitus, Baker's cyst
- Hips and spine are commonly involved
- Feet – hallux valgus (bunion).

The patient often experiences great pain, loss of mobility and an inability to perform everyday functions. In severe cases loss of bone as well as cartilage affects the stability of the joints.

Management

The aim of treatment is to ensure that the patient remains as active and pain free as possible. Education

is a priority to enable the patient to understand the disease and use measures for symptomatic relief (see Ch.15).

Therapy includes:

- Exercise to maintain function and relieve stiffness
- Analgesia and NSAIDs to control pain and stiffness
- Weight reduction where obesity is a problem
- Education and information to enable patients to cope with pain and stiffness and to ensure an awareness of the implications of obesity and lack of exercise
- Major joint replacement – surgery of the hips, knees, shoulders and elbows to increase mobility and reduce pain in severely affected joints.

METABOLIC BONE DISEASE
Osteoporosis

Osteoporosis or loss of bone mass is one of the most common metabolic disorders of the skeleton. Loss of bone leads to fractures of the hip, wrist and spine (Dieppe et al 1985d).

Epidemiology

Osteoporosis is more prevalent in the Anglo-Saxon, Japanese and Indian races and affects more women than men. The incidence of osteoporosis is increasing, possibly due to decreased physical activity in females and an increased life span (Badley 1991). The socio-economic implications of the increased disability and morbidity associated with fractures occurring as a result of osteoporosis cannot be ignored (Woolf & Dixon 1988).

Aetiology

It is known that age, hormonal changes in women, lack of dietary calcium and lack of exercise all increase the risk of osteoporosis. Cardiac, respiratory, renal, neurological, gastrointestinal and rheumatic disease may lead to this condition.

   Osteoporosis must always be considered in patients with rheumatic disease, particularly females who are predominately affected. Inflammatory joint diseases such as RA induce thin bones (osteopenia) and associated factors such as immobility and steroid therapy further increase the risk of osteoporosis. Risk factors in younger women are anorexia and exercise induced amenorrhoea. Alcoholism, hypogonadism and bone

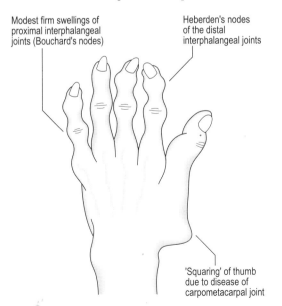

Figure 2.20   The hand in generalised OA (adapted from Dieppe et al 1985, with permission).

tumours are additional underlying causes of osteoporosis in men (Dixon 1991).

Pathology

Loss of the bone mineral, hydroxyapatite, causes both cortical and trabecular bone to become osteopenic and susceptible to fracture. Bone turnover is reduced as the osteoclasts reabsorb bone more quickly than the osteoblasts can produce it. There is a negative calcium balance and breakdown of bone increases the urinary output of calcium (Dieppe et al 1985d).

Peak bone mass is reached in young adulthood, and is always higher in men than women. This level is consolidated from the age of 25 to 30 after which it slowly reduces. In the ten years following the menopause, bone loss accelerates in women and then levels out. Men start to loose bone mass after the age of 60.

Presentation

Diagnosis does not usually occur until problems arise from fractures of the bones. Crush or wedge fractures of the vertebrae produce severe pain that usually resolves after a few months, although deformity of the spine may result. The most common fracture associated with osteoporosis is that of the proximal femur. Hospitalisation is inevitable and the implications of surgical operation are serious, with the risk of venous thrombosis, pulmonary embolism and pneumonia in the elderly. Fracture of the distal radius (Colles' fracture) is also common and results in temporary loss of independence.

Clinical features

- Severe pain due to neurological compression as a result of a spontaneous fracture of the vertebrae.
- Fracture of a long bone such as the femur or radius with resulting loss of independence.
- Loss of height and thoracic kyphosis (Dowager's hump) especially in elderly women who may not have any other symptoms (Fig. 2.21).
- Breathing difficulties and symptoms of hiatus hernia often occur, caused by reduction of the space between the pelvis and rib cage due to spinal kyphosis.

Management

The management of osteoporosis should be directed at prevention. It is important for both health professionals and the public to be aware of the implications

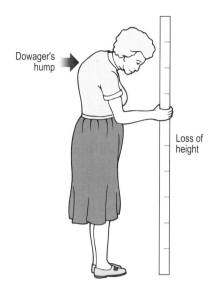

Figure 2.21 Senile osteoporosis — dowager's hump (adapted from Dieppe et al 1985, with permission).

of this disease, risk factors and methods of prevention. An integral part of management is prevention through education.

Risk factors and advice:

- Lack of calcium – information about the dietary requirements of calcium intake.
- Alcohol – excessive intake should be discouraged by education.
- Smoking should be discouraged and information should be given about the harmful effects of this habit.
- Lack of exercise – the benefits of exercise should be explained and exercise encouraged.
- Falls and the risk of broken bones – elderly patients should be reminded that the majority of accidents occur in the home often as a result of poorly fitting footwear, inadequate lighting, loose rugs, steep stairs, slippery floors, and pets.
- Poor eyesight – eyesight should be tested regularly and spectacles worn when prescribed.
- Dizziness or unsteadiness due to conditions such as postural hypotension, transient ischaemic attacks, epilepsy, Ménière's disease and Parkinson's. Patients with these diseases should be advised to take care when standing up or mobilising. Some patients may need walking aids.
- Drugs, which cause dizziness, headache or drowsiness, should be prescribed only if really necessary and patients advised to take care when mobilising.

- Steroid therapy should be discussed with the patient and gradual withdrawal attempted.
- Thyroid therapy should be regularly monitored to ensure that the dosage of thyroxin is correct and does not need reduction.

Drug therapy may include:

- Hormone replacement therapy (HRT), for post-menopausal women and those who have undergone a hysterectomy or oophorectomy.
- Supplemental calcium, didronel and vitamin D may be prescribed and can be very helpful in preventing further loss of bone density.

CONNECTIVE TISSUE DISEASES

Although distinctive conditions, the diseases in this group have many common features, such as vasculitis. They are more common in women than men and there appears to be a genetic predisposition. Some of the diseases overlap, for instance progressive systemic scleroderma and systemic lupus erythematosus.

Systemic lupus erythematosus

Systemic lupus erythematosus also known as SLE, is the most common of the connective tissue diseases (Symmons & Bankhead 1994). It is a chronic, inflammatory, systemic disorder of unknown aetiology which affects the joints and skin and may also involve the kidneys, lungs, heart, gastrointestinal tract and nervous system.

Epidemiology

Although it is found globally, it is most prevalent in the United States. Women are affected more than men at a ratio of 13:1. Afro-Caribbeans and Asians show the greatest incidence of this disease (Emery 1994). For some patients with systemic lupus erythematosus, the prognosis is poor. However, survival rates have increased from less than 50% in 1955 to over 90% in 1990 (Gladman & Urowitz 1994), possibly due to earlier diagnosis and treatment. Black patients fare worse than white patients due to an increased incidence of renal problems. Kidney and central nervous system involvement are associated with a poor prognosis.

Pathology

Skin biopsy reveals epidermal thinning and micro-infarcts due to deposits of immunoglobulin in the tissues. Evidence of an association with HLA B8, DR2 and DR3 antibodies and complement deficiency genes has been found. Blood tests may show an elevated ESR, positive ANA and DNA, reduced neutrophils and platelets. Bone erosion and joint destruction do not normally occur.

Presentation

Patients present with a variety of symptoms ranging from fatigue, malaise and weight loss to rash and arthritis. Proteinurea, pleurisy and Raynaud's phenomenon may also be present at onset.

Clinical features

- Butterfly rash of the face – raised, malar erythema lasting from days to weeks which may be pruritic, painful and photosensitive
- Subacute cutaneous erythema
- Discoid lesions – erythematous plaques which become thick, adherent and scaly
- Alopecia – related to exacerbation of disease activity or due to scarring from discoid lesions. Hair growth normally resumes when the disease remits
- Vasculitis – purpura, nail fold lesions, digital ulceration and subcutaneous nodules
- Polyarthritis of fingers, wrists, knees, ankles, elbows and shoulders which is usually flitting and rarely destructive
- Myalgia secondary to joint inflammation. Systemic lupus erythematosus is often associated with polymyositis
- Tenosynovitis leading to tendon ruptures
- Mucous membrane lesions – mouth and vagina
- Renal involvement – nephritis and proteinurea. The prognosis is worse if the kidneys are affected
- Pulmonary involvement – pleurisy, pleural effusions, pneumonitis and dyspnoea
- Cardiac involvement – pericarditis, pericardial effusions, hypertension and myocarditis
- Gastrointestinal effects – abdominal pain, loss of appetite, nausea, and vomiting caused by peritoneal inflammation
- Neurological effects – migraine-like headaches, chorea, vascular accidents, peripheral neuropathy and cranial nerve lesions causing visual problems
- Psychiatric features – severe depression, paranoia, anxiety, confusion, schizophrenia, dementia and fits.

The distribution of organ involvement is shown in Figure 2.22.

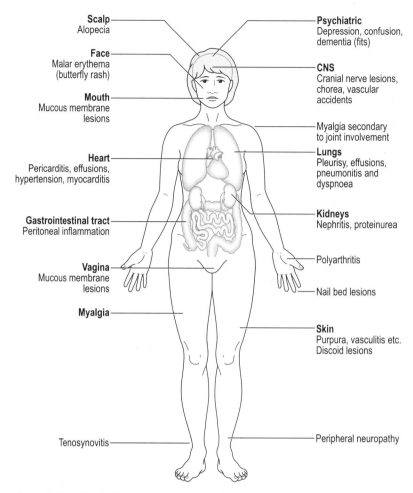

Figure 2.22 The distribution of clinical organ involvement in SLE (adapted from Dieppe et al 1985, with permission).

Photosensitivity can produce exacerbation of skin lesions and systemic features of the disease. Patients run an increased risk of infection. Although systemic lupus erythematosus does not prevent conception, hormonal changes may result in spontaneous abortion. Certain drugs can induce a type of systemic lupus erythematosus in patients with a genetic predisposition to the disease.

They include those listed in Box 2.16.

Once the drug is stopped, the symptoms usually disappear, although evidence of the disease may be present in the blood for some years.

Management

Therapy depends on which organs are affected and patients may require referrals to the dermatologist,

Box 2.16 Drugs inducing systemic lupus erythematosus	
Procainamide	(antiarrhythmic)
Hydralazine, methyldopa	(antihypertensive)
Phenytoin	(antiepileptic)
Isoniazid	(antituberculous)
Oral contraceptives	
Penicillin, sulphonamides	(antibiotics)
Tetracycline, streptomycin	
Griseofulvin	(antifungal)
Phenylbutazone, penicillamine	(antirheumatic)

renal physician, neurologist, haematologist and psychiatrist. The disease needs to be treated as early as possible and the risk of infections and subsequent complications should always be considered. The monitoring of disease activity is important, as acute flares require immediate treatment.

Therapy may include:

- Steroid creams to heal skin lesions
- Non-steroidal anti-inflammatory drugs to relieve arthralgia, arthritis and myalgia
- Antimalarial drugs are used for their anti-inflammatory and immunosuppressive effect
- Methotrexate may be prescribed as an alternative to antimalarials
- Corticosteroids are often used in low doses to reduce disease activity and alleviate fatigue and loss of appetite
- Azathioprine acts as a steroid sparing agent once disease stability has been achieved
- Cyclophosphamide is used when patients have vasculitis, severe thrombocytopenia and renal disease.

Education

Patients need to understand their disease and they should be aware of the risks associated with unexplained weight loss, fatigue, fever and infections. The problems of photosensitivity should be discussed and ways of avoiding exposure to harmful solar radiation, such as covering up and the use of sunscreens should be encouraged. Birth control, the risks of pregnancy relating to the disease and the teratogenic effects of drug therapy (Table 12.3) need to be emphasised.

Scleroderma (progressive systemic sclerosis or PSS)

Progressive systemic sclerosis is a rare disease that affects the skin and internal organs. Over-production of collagen results in fibrosis with consequent tightness and tethering down of the skin, especially of the hands and face. This disease is associated with a high mortality due to obliterative microvascular lesions occurring in the kidney, lung, bowel and heart.

Epidemiology

The aetiology is unknown but there is some evidence that there may be a link with silica, vinyl chloride and silicone surgical implants. Women are affected more frequently than men at a ratio of 3:1. The peak age of onset is between the fourth and fifth decade (Siebold 1994).

Pathology

Initially the small blood vessels of the body are affected, causing inflammation of the sub-cutaneous connective tissue which leads to atrophy and fibrosis of the skin and other organs. Blood tests show a raised ESR, positive rheumatoid factor and ANA. X-ray examination reveals soft tissue calcification, joint space narrowing and periarticular osteoporosis.

Presentation

The initial presentation and course of the disease varies between individuals. Most commonly, patients present with inflamed joints that resolve as the disease progresses. These patients require careful monitoring to ensure that any complications due to involvement of the kidney, bowel, oesophagus, heart and lungs are treated as they arise.

Clinical features

- Pain, swelling and stiffness of joints especially in the hands
- Flexion deformities of the fingers with reddened and ulcerated PIPs, DIPs and finger tips
- Nail fold capillary infarcts
- Oedema of the skin resulting in puffy fingers and hands
- Skin that is dry, tight, wasted, hard and tethered to underlying structures, especially on the hands and face
- Early morning stiffness
- Telangiectasia (see page 57) of the face and neck affects many of these patients
- Arteritis of the renal vessels leads to renal failure with proteinurea and malignant hypertension
- Raynaud's phenomenon is usually present
- Sjögren's syndrome may be present
- Dysphagia caused by fibrosis of the oesophagus is common
- Fibrosing alveolitis
- Microvascular lesions of the lung and heart.

Management

Symptomatic measures are used as problems occur. However, the various complications of this disease call for integrated and empathetic care. Skin changes, especially to the face cause patients distress and loss of self esteem.

Therapy may include:

- Non-steroidal anti-inflammatory drugs and analgesia for inflamed joints
- Creams to relieve tight, dry skin

- D Penicillamine has been shown to halt the progress of the fibrosis but the risk of kidney involvement makes screening essential
- Steroid therapy
- Special make-up for patients with telangiectasia of the face.

CREST syndrome

CREST syndrome is an acronym of:

Calcinosis
Raynaud's
Esophageal dysmotility (using the American spelling)
Sclerodactyly
Telangiectasia

This condition is similar to scleroderma but systemic involvement, apart from oesophageal disturbance, is not apparent until later in the disease. The initial presenting symptom is Raynaud's phenomenon with swollen fingers and hands.

Polymyositis and dermatomyositis

Two major forms of inflammatory myopathy are recognised. They are polymyositis and dermatomyositis.

Polymyositis is a connective tissue disorder that causes weakness of the proximal musculature due to inflammation. When a characteristic skin rash is present with polymyositis, the condition is known as dermatomyositis. The aetiology of these diseases is unknown.

Pathology

Blood tests show an elevated ESR and creatinine phosphokinase (CPK), and rheumatoid factor and ANA may be positive. Monitoring the level of CPK is a useful indicator of disease activity and the efficacy of drug therapy.

Presentation

The peak age of onset is between 30 and 60 years. Patients may present with arthritis of the hands, wrists, elbows, shoulders, knees and ankles. Symmetrical wasting and weakness of limb girdle muscles is common, as is restriction of movement. Some patients develop joint contractures. Respiratory failure is common and 15% of those affected die from this cause (Huskisson & Dudley Hart 1987).

Clinical features

- Joints may be swollen, warm and tender with effusions
- Early morning stiffness
- Malaise and weight loss
- Muscular weakness with muscular pain or tenderness
- Sjögren's syndrome may be present
- Dysphagia – oesophageal involvement
- Raynaud's phenomenon is common
- Skin lesions – malar, lilac rash which may be photosensitive.

Management

High dose prednisolone (60 mg daily) is used initially and the dose gradually reduced once the arthritis has remitted and the muscle weakness has resolved. Therapy with immunosuppressive drugs such as azathioprine or cyclophosphamide is used where remission does not occur. Physiotherapy exercises help to improve muscle weakness and function.

NON-ARTICULAR CONDITIONS

Non-articular conditions are those rheumatic diseases associated with muscle weakness and pain rather than joint involvement.

Polymyalgia rheumatica and giant cell arteritis

Polymyalgia rheumatica, also called PMR, is a common disorder of the middle-aged and elderly which causes symmetrical pain and stiffness in the neck, shoulder and pelvic girdle. It is associated with giant cell arteritis that can affect the temporal artery and result in blindness (Hazelman 1992, Hazelman 1994).

Epidemiology

Both polymyalgia rheumatica and giant cell arteritis are diseases of the elderly and are rarely diagnosed in persons younger than 50 years. Giant cell arteritis mostly affects whites of European background although some cases have been reported in the American black population.

Pathology

Blood tests show an extremely elevated ESR and raised alkaline phosphatase levels. Thyroid and liver function abnormalities may also be apparent from blood tests. Temporal artery biopsy often shows the temporal artery to be inflamed, enlarged, nodular and with a narrow lumen (temporal arteritis). Thromboses may develop at sites of inflammation.

Presentation

The onset is usually acute with patients complaining of extreme pain and stiffness in the shoulder, hips and thighs. The shoulder girdle is more commonly affected than the pelvic girdle. Early diagnosis may be hindered by initial symptoms of fever, fatigue, weight loss, anorexia and depression. Arteritis of the temporal artery can occur and needs immediate treatment with oral steroids to prevent blindness.

Clinical features

- Early morning stiffness in the shoulders, neck and pelvis which is usually symmetrical and worse after rest
- Myalgic pain in the neck, shoulders and pelvic girdle which is aggravated by movement and is often worse at night
- Limited range of movement of shoulders and hips
- Synovitis which is usually mild and resolves quickly
- Malaise, low grade fever and weight loss
- Temporal headache radiating into the occiput is common when giant cell arteritis occurs
- Sleep disturbance caused by scalp tenderness around the temporal and occipital arteries
- Pain in the mouth and throat when chewing, tingling of the tongue and loss of taste
- Visual disturbances or even loss of vision if untreated. Blindness occurs suddenly and painlessly and is permanent.

Management

Corticosteroids are always used to reduce the risk of arteritis and subsequent blindness. Pain and stiffness are relieved quickly within a few days by this treatment. High doses of steroids are used initially and then decreased slowly as symptoms subside. The reduction of steroids is often seen as too slow by some patients who want to stop the treatment as soon as they feel better. Because of this, patient education is important to ensure that patients understand the need for the slow reduction of steroid treatment as symptoms can recur. Most patients will remain on steroid therapy for at least two years, but for some it may be longer. Monitoring of ESR levels should be carried out once therapy has ceased, to detect any relapse. Patients should be warned to seek advice should their symptoms return.

Raynaud's phenomenon

Raynaud's phenomenon was first described by Maurice Raynaud over 120 years ago. It is marked by episodic vasospasm in which the fingers go white, cyanosed and then red.

Aetiology

It is thought that cold, emotion, trauma, hormones and chemicals such as nicotine produce this effect. Raynaud's phenomenon is often associated with scleroderma, systemic lupus erythematosus, RA, dematomyositis and polymyositis. Occupation plays a part in the incidence of this condition, especially manual work and work involving the packing of frozen food, the use of vinyl chloride, ammunition and nitrates.

Pathology

Systemic vasospasm restricts the blood flow to the hands, fingers and in some cases the nose, tip of the tongue and ear lobes. Raynaud's phenomenon is present in 5–10% of the population in varying degrees of severity (Blech 1987). It affects nine times more women than men and may be a precursor of systemic illness.

Presentation

This varies from mild to severe disease and usually presents as pallor and cyanosis of the fingers as the digital blood vessels go into spasm. This is then followed by rubor (redness) as the circulation returns to normal. Pain may be present depending on the amount of vasospasm. In more severe cases, digital ulceration and gangrene can occur.

Management

The management of this condition is predominately educational:

- Information about cold avoidance measures such as thermal socks and gloves, electrically heated gloves, chemical hand warmers and padded or fleece lined shoes
- Patients should be strongly advised to stop smoking
- Nifedipine may be used to increase the peripheral blood supply

- The Raynaud's Association is a support group that provides useful patient information.

Sjögren's syndrome

Sjögren's syndrome affects the exocrine (secretory) glands. Damage and inflammation to the lachrymal and salivary glands causes dry eyes and dry mouth (Venables 1988).

Epidemiology

Sjögren's syndrome is the second most common rheumatic disease and affects more women than men.
  There are three classifications:

- Primary Sjögren's syndrome
- Sjögren's associated overlap syndromes
- Secondary Sjögren's syndrome with RA.

Primary Sjögren's syndrome. This condition mainly affects the exocrine glands and is usually so mild that medical advice is rarely sought. Other conditions such as non-erosive arthritis, Raynaud's phenomenon and purpuric rash of the lower legs may be associated.
  Sjögren's associated overlap syndromes. Besides affecting the exocrine glands, this condition often has features associated with systemic lupus erythematosus and other autoimmune rheumatic diseases such as scleroderma and polymyositis.
  Secondary Sjögren's syndrome with RA. The features of this classification are dry eyes, dry mouth, vasculitic changes such as nailfold infarcts, ulcers and rheumatoid nodules.

Pathology

Investigations have shown that the disease seems to start as a persistent viral infection of the salivary glands, which results in an attack on the salivary epithelium. The Epstein-Barr virus is often present on biopsy of the salivary epithelium. Schirmer's tear test can confirm the diagnosis of dry eyes (keratoconjunctivitis sicca). Dry mouth (xerostomia) can be detected by tests that reveal a reduced salivary flow rate. Blood tests often show a raised ESR, raised rheumatoid factor and hypergammaglobulinaemia.

Presentation

Onset can be between 15 and 65 years and patients complain of dry, gritty, sore eyes and a dry mouth that causes difficulty in swallowing food.

Management

- Dry eyes can be treated with artificial tears (hypermellose eye drops)
- Sucking sweets and chewing gum increases the salivary flow and eases a dry mouth. In more severe cases artificial saliva may be prescribed.

SOFT TISSUE RHEUMATISM

Soft tissue rheumatism describes those conditions that affect the muscles, tendons, tendon sheaths and nerves.

Fibromyalgia syndrome

This is the term used for a collection of symptoms of which musculoskeletal pain is the most predominant (Doherty 1993). Fatigue is common and headache, abdominal pain and bowel disturbance may also be present. Investigations are undertaken to exclude other conditions such as systemic lupus erythematosus, hypothyroidism, polymyalgia rheumatica and carcinoma. In the past, patients with these symptoms were often classed as having psychological rather than physical problems.

Aetiology

The aetiology remains unknown but is likely to involve more than one factor. The condition occurs mainly in women aged between 25 and 45 years. A recent study has indicated that it affects 3.4% of women and 0.5% of men (Wolfe et al 1995).

Presentation

The patient complains of fatigue and tenderness in the upper and lower limbs, base of the skull, lower cervical spine, shoulders and hips. These hyperalgesic or tender sites are distributed symmetrically and firm digital pressure upon them causes the patient to wince and withdraw.

Clinical features

- Pain – tender sites or sometimes more widespread
- Morning stiffness which is generalised
- Fatigue, inability to sleep properly, tiredness on waking
- Irritability, weepiness
- Headache, forgetfulness, poor concentration
- Numbness, pins and needles of hands and feet
- Inability to perform daily living activities.

Management

The prognosis of fibromyalgia is poor and some patients experience their symptoms for many years with little or no relief. Education of the patient and family enables most patients to cope with their condition. Some patients may benefit from counselling. Low dose amitriptyline (25–75 mg) taken at night helps to induce sleep. Although it may be initially painful, patients should be encouraged to undertake a personal exercise programme to improve fitness and enable them to take control of their condition.

Carpal tunnel syndrome

Carpal tunnel syndrome occurs when there is compression of the median nerve at the wrist, resulting in tingling and paraesthesia of the fingers (Hawkins et al 1985).

Pathology

The median nerve runs through the carpal tunnel and compression of the nerve produces tingling and sometimes loss of sensation to the thumb, index, second and half of the third finger. It usually occurs in middle-aged women and may be due to synovitis of the wrist, bony lesions, obesity or fluid retention.

Presentation

A numb, tingling sensation in one or both hands which occurs mainly at night. Features:

- Pain spreading up the forearm.
- Tingling and numbness in the thumb, index, second and half of the third fingers, which is usually present at night but may occur during the day.
- Wasting of the thenar eminence, due to motor involvement with a resultant loss of power and muscle wasting.

Management

A nerve conduction study often helps to verify the diagnosis.

Therapy may include:

- Diuretics if caused by fluid retention
- Wrist splints may relieve symptoms in mild cases
- Local steroid injection and the use of wrist splints for 48 hours
- Surgical decompression when other more

conservative measures have failed to bring relief. Surgery is usually successful and involves division of the flexor retinaculum.

Lateral and medial epicondylitis (tennis and golfer's elbow)

These common rheumatic conditions cause pain and tenderness around the lateral epicondyle (tennis elbow) and medial epicondyle (golfer's elbow). The condition occurs in individuals whose occupation involves repeated gripping and twisting movements of the forearm.

Pathology

Inflammation or damage is present at the enthesis of the carpi radialis component of the extensor tendon (tennis elbow) or the flexor tendon (golfer's elbow).

Presentation

The peak age of onset is between 40 and 60 years. The affected epicondyle is tender and varying degrees of pain are present. Gripping and twisting movements exacerbate the pain that varies from mild discomfort to severe pain.

Clinical features

- Pain – may be bilateral and radiates down the posterior aspect of the forearm (tennis elbow) or down the flexor aspect of the forearm (golfer's elbow)
- Pain on palpation of the lateral or medial epicondyle
- Soft tissue swelling around the area.

Management

These conditions can persist for a year or more. Conservative measures such as elbow splints and ultra sound therapy are used initially. Where the condition persists, a local corticosteroid injection into the affected area followed by a few days' rest usually brings relief. In more chronic cases, manipulation of the elbow under general anaesthetic helps to break down fibrous adhesions and restore mobility. Surgical intervention to divide the tendon (tenotomy) may help when the condition is severe (Golding 1986).

OTHER CONDITIONS
Amyloidosis

Amyloidosis often occurs in patients with long standing RA. Males and females are affected equally with the peak age of onset being between 50 and 60 years. Amyloid deposits are found in the liver, spleen, kidneys, gastrointestinal tract, heart, tongue, nervous system and joints. These deposits are made up of an insoluble protein-like substance. Peripheral neuropathies and heart failure often result. The prognosis for this condition is poor.

Baker's cyst

A Baker's cyst is a swelling that develops at the back of an inflamed knee. This may rupture allowing synovial fluid to track down into the back of the calf. Patients presenting with such a rupture may be misdiagnosed as having a deep vein thrombosis.

Bursitis

Bursitis is inflammation of a bursa that may be due to rheumatic disease or trauma. Pain and swelling is present around the site, the most common being the knee (housemaid's knee), shoulder, elbow (olecranon bursitis), hip (trochanteric bursitis) and ankle.

Treatment with analgesia and rest may help, but in persistent cases aspiration and injection of corticosteroid is necessary.

Calcaneal spur

A calcaneal spur is a bony growth protruding from the calcaneus, which causes great pain and discomfort on walking. Relief can be obtained through protective heel pads inserted into the shoe.

Chondromalacia patellae

Chondromalacia patellae refers to softening of the articular cartilage of the patella, causing anterior pain in the knee. Isometric quadriceps exercises and hamstring stretching will help to build up the surrounding musculature and strengthen the joint.

Erythema nodosum

Erythema nodosum presents as tender nodules in the skin of the lower leg. It is commonly seen in sarcoidosis but may occur with Behçet's syndrome, Crohn's disease, infections, malignant disease and drug reactions. Arthritis is often present with this complaint and usually presents a few weeks before the nodules appear.

Fasciitis

Fasciitis is inflammation of the enthesis of the fascia.

In particular, plantar fasciitis is associated with rheumatic disease especially the spondoarthropathies. A heel pad in the shoe may help to relieve the pain associated with this condition.

Hypermobility syndrome

Hypermobility is caused by ligamentous laxity that may be inherited and is common in many dancers, gymnasts and athletes. Patients with this syndrome are able to over extend the range of movement in their joints. The knees and hands are commonly affected. Hypermobility often leads to OA in later life. Treatment is centered on advice about the benefits of exercise, joint protection and the use of analgesia.

Rheumatoid nodules

Rheumatoid nodules are small growths that are characteristic features of destructive rheumatoid arthritis. They occur subcutaneously over bony prominences and tendons, for example elbows, Achilles tendons, shoulder blades, and fingers. They may also be present inside organs such as the heart and lungs. At the centre of these nodules is an inner core of necrotised collagen, fibrin and cell debris. In some instances subcutaneous nodules discharge and care must be taken to ensure that they do not become infected.

Repetitive strain syndrome

This refers to inflammation of joints or tendons, usually of the hands, caused by repetition of the same action. Typists, check-out till operators and machinists are prone to this condition. Rest and the use of nonsteroidal anti-inflammatory drugs can obtain relief. When inflammation is persistent a steroid injection into the tendon sheath may also help.

Sarcoidosis

Sarcoidosis is a systemic disease in which epithelial cell granuloma can be found in the lungs, lymph glands, spleen, joints and skin. It often presents as a polyarthritis with erythema nodosum and may be acute and transient, or chronic and persistent.

Septic arthritis

Septic arthritis may be due to diabetes, RA, joint trauma, steroid therapy or an infection elsewhere in the body. The affected joint is infected with a pyogenic bacterium and will show the typical signs of inflammation. The joint rapidly becomes swollen and painful and fever is usually present. Treatment should be started immediately and comprises aspiration of the affected joint, rest, and antibiotic cover. Culture of synovial fluid and blood is usually positive. If left untreated, this condition leads to destruction of the joint, septicaemia and death.

Telangiectasia

Telangiectasia is often found in patients with progressive systemic scleroderma or the CREST syndrome. Dilated capillaries and venules, which blanch on pressure, can be seen on the hands, lips, tongue and mucous membranes.

Tenosynovitis

Tenosynovitis is inflammation of the synovial lining of the tendons and is common in inflammatory joint diseases such as RA. Rupture of the extensor tendon or tendon slip often occurs in patients with inflammatory joint disease especially in the hands.

Trigger finger

In trigger finger, the flexor tendon sheaths of the fingers become inflamed and rough. Crepitus and nodules are common, inhibiting the smooth movement of the tendon within the sheath and causing the finger to stick. A steroid injection into the sheath usually relieves this condition.

Action points for practice:

1. Mr. Partridge is a 76-year-old man who is experiencing great difficulty in doing up his shirt buttons. He has tingling and loss of sensation in the thumb and first three fingers of both hands.

- What do you think is wrong with him
- How might the multidisciplinary team help him?

2. Doreen is a 60-year-old lady who was seen in clinic complaining of pain in her shoulders and upper arms. A blood test revealed an ESR of 100 mm/h.

- What is her probable diagnosis?
- What action should be taken to help this lady?
- What problems may ensue?
- How should she be managed in the future?

3. Peter is 28 years old and has ankylosing spondylitis. He has found difficulty in coping with his disease, especially as he has increasing stiffness and restriction in his spine.

- What measures should be taken to help him?
- Write a care plan.

REFERENCES

Arnet F C, Edworthy S M, Bloch D A et al 1988 The American rheumatism association 1987 revised criteria for the classification of rheumatoid arthritis. Arthritis Rheumatism 31: 315–324

Arthur V 1994 Nursing care of patients with rheumatoid arthritis. British Journal of Nursing 3(7): 325–331

Badley E M 1991 Population projections and the effect on rheumatology. Annals of Rheumatic Disease 50: 3–6

Barnes C G 1991 Behçet's syndrome. In: Collected reports on the rheumatic diseases. Arthritis and Rheumatism Council, Chesterfield, p 109–114

Blech J J F 1987 Raynaud's phenomenon. In: Collected reports on the rheumatic diseases. Arthritis and Rheumatism Council, Chesterfield, p 101–104

Buchanan W W, Dequeker J 1994 History of rheumatic diseases. In: Klippel J H, Dieppe P A (ed) Rheumatology. Mosby, St Louis, ch 6, p 1–8

Campion G, Maddison P J 1986 Felty's syndrome. In: Collected reports on the rheumatic diseases. Arthritis and Rheumatism Council, Chesterfield, p 52–55

Cohen M G, Emmerson B T 1994 Gout. In: Klippel J H, Dieppe P A (ed) Rheumatology. Mosby, St Louis, ch 7.12, p 1–15

Cooper C 1994 Osteoarthritis epidemiology. In: Klippel J H, Dieppe P A (ed) Rheumatology. Mosby, St Louis, ch 7.3, p 1–4

Dieppe P A 1994 Osteoarthritis. In: Klippel J H, Dieppe PA (ed) Rheumatology. Mosby, St Louis, ch 7.2 p 1–6

Dieppe P A, Klippel J H 1994 Introduction. In: Klippel J H, Dieppe P A (ed) Rheumatology. Mosby, St Louis, ch 1, p 1–2

Dieppe P A, Doherty M, Macfarlane D G, Maddison P 1985a Rheumatological medicine. Churchill Livingstone, Edinburgh, ch 4, p 56–57

Dieppe P A, Doherty M, Macfarlane D G, Maddison P 1985b Rheumatological medicine. Churchill Livingstone, Edinburgh, ch 5, p 84–90

Dieppe P A, Doherty M, Macfarlane D G, Maddison P 1985c Rheumatological medicine. Churchill Livingstone, Edinburgh, ch 5, p 80–86

Dieppe P A, Doherty M, Macfarlane D G, Maddison P 1985d Rheumatological medicine. Churchill Livingstone, Edinburgh, ch 17, p 333–340

Dixon A St J 1991 Osteoporosis and the family doctor. In: Collected reports on the rheumatic diseases. Arthritis and Rheumatism Council, Chesterfield, p 122–125

Doherty M 1993 Fibromyalgia syndrome. In: Collected reports on the rheumatic diseases. Arthritis and Rheumatism Council, Chesterfield, p 83–86

Emery P 1994 Systemic lupus erythematosus. In: Collected reports on the rheumatic diseases. Arthritis and Rheumatism Council, Chesterfield, p 87–92

Espinoza L R, Cuellar M L 1994 Psoriatic arthritis: management. In: Klippel J H, Dieppe P A (ed) Rheumatology. Mosby, St Louis, ch 3.33, p 1–6

Firestein G S 1994 Rheumatoid arthritis and spondyloarthropathy, rheumatoid synovitis and pannus. In: Klippel J H, Dieppe P A (ed) Rheumatology. Mosby, St Louis, ch 3, p 12.1–12.30

Gibson T 1988 The treatment of gout: a personal view. In: Collected reports on the rheumatic diseases. Arthritis and Rheumatism Council, Chesterfield, p 69–71

Gladman D D, Urowitz M B 1994 Systemic lupus erythematosus – clinical features. In: Klippel J H, Dieppe P A (ed) Rheumatology. Mosby, St Louis, ch 6, p 2.1–2.20

Golding D N 1986 Tennis and golfer's elbow. In: Collected reports on the rheumatic diseases. Arthritis and Rheumatism Council, Chesterfield, p 152–155

Hawkins C, Currey H, Dieppe P 1985 Carpal tunnel syndrome. In: Collected reports on the rheumatic diseases. Arthritis and Rheumatism Council, Chesterfield, p 148–151

Hazelman B L 1992 Polymyalgia rheumatica and giant cell arteritis. In: Collected reports on the rheumatic diseases. Arthritis and Rheumatism Council, Chesterfield, p 97–100

Hazelman B L 1994 Polymyalgia rheumatica and giant cell arteritis. In: Klippel J H, Dieppe P A (ed) Rheumatology. Mosby, St Louis, ch 6, p 18.1–18.8

Helliwell P S, Wright V 1994 Psoriatic arthritis: clinical features. In: Klippel J H, Dieppe P A (ed) Rheumatology. Mosby, St Louis, ch 3, p 31.1–31.8

Hill J 1997 The expanding role of the nurse in rheumatology. British Journal of Rheumatology 36(4): 410–412

Hill J 1992 A nurse practitioner rheumatology clinic. Nursing Standard 7(11): 35–37

Huskisson E C, Dudley Hart F 1987 Joint disease and all the arthropathies. Wright, Bristol

Keat A 1986 Reiter's syndrome and reactive arthritis. In: Collected reports on the rheumatic diseases. Arthritis and Rheumatism Council, Chesterfield, p 61–64

Khan M A 1995 Ankylosing spondylitis. In: Klippel J A, Dieppe P A (ed) Rheumatology. Mosby, St Louis, ch 3, p 25.1–25.10

Lawrence R 1994 Rheumatoid arthritis, classification and epidemiology. In: Klippel J H, Dieppe P A (ed) Rheumatology. Mosby, St Louis, ch 3, p 3.1–3.4

Leak A M 1991 Juvenile chronic arthritis. In: Collected reports on the rheumatic diseases. Arthritis and Rheumatism Council, Chesterfield, p 72–77

Matteson E L, Cohen M D, Conn D L 1994 Rheumatoid arthritis. Clinical features – systemic involvement. In: Klippel J H, Dieppe P A (ed) Rheumatology. Mosby, St Louis, ch 3, p 5.1–5.8

Rai A. Struthers G. 1994 Ankylosing spondylitis. In: Collected reports on the rheumatic diseases. Arthritis and Rheumatism Council, Chesterfield, p 65–68

Seibold J R 1994 Systemic sclerosis: clinical features. In: Klippel J H, Dieppe P A (ed) Rheumatology. Mosby, St Louis, ch 6, p 8.1–8.14

Symmons D, Bankhead C 1994 Health care needs assessment for musculoskeletal diseases. Arthritis and Rheumatism Council, Chesterfield

Symmons D P M, Barrett E M, Bankhead C, Chakravarty K, Scott D G I, Silman A J 1994 The incidence of rheumatoid arthritis in the United Kingdom; results from the Norfolk arthritis register. British Journal of Rheumatology 33: 735–739

Toivanen A 1994 Reactive arthritis. In: Klippel J H, Dieppe P A (ed) Rheumatology. Mosby, St Louis, ch 4, p 9.1–9.8

Venables P 1988 Sjögren's syndrome. In: Collected reports on the rheumatic diseases. Arthritis and Rheumatism Council, Chesterfield, p 93–96

White P 1994 Juvenile chronic arthritis. Clinical features. In: Klippel J H, Dieppe P A (ed) Rheumatology. Mosby, St Louis, ch 3, p 17.1–17.10

Wilson J W K, Waugh A 1996 Ross and Wilson Anatomy and Physiology in Health and Illness, 8th edn, p 29, 373, 376, 380, 381, 383, 386, 388, 389, 391, 399, 407, 415. Churchill Livingstone, Edinburgh

Wolfe F, Ross K, Anderson J, Russell I J, Herbert L 1995 The prevalence and characteristics of fibromyalgia in the general population. Arthritis Rheumatism 38: 19–28

Woolf A D, Dixon St. J 1988 Osteoporosis – a clinical guide. Martin Dunitz, London

Wright V, Helliwell P S 1992 Psoriatic arthritis. In: Collected reports on the rheumatic diseases. Arthritis and Rheumatism Council, Chesterfield, p 56–58

Yazici H 1994 Behçet's syndrome. In: Klippel J H, Dieppe P A (ed) Rheumatology. Mosby, St Louis, ch 6, p 20.1–20.6

FURTHER READING:

Arthritis and Rheumatism Council 1991 An introduction to the musculoskeletal system: a handbook for medical students. Arthritis and Rheumatism Council, Chesterfield

Arthritis and Rheumatism Council 1995 Collected reports on the rheumatic diseases. Arthritis and Rheumatism Council, Chesterfield

Boyle A C 1986 A colour atlas of rheumatology. Wolfe Medical Publications, London

Dieppe P A, Bacon P A, Bamji A N, Watt I 1986 Atlas of clinical rheumatology. Gower Medical Publishing, London

Dieppe P A, Doherty M, Macfarlane D G, Maddison P 1985 Rheumatological medicine. Churchill Livingstone, Edinburgh

Golding D N 1989 A synopsis of rheumatic diseases. 5th edn. Wright PSG, Bristol

Hamilton Hall 1983 The new medicine rheumatology. MTP Press, Boston

Huskisson E C, Dudley Hart F 1987 Joint disease and all the arthropathies. Wright, Bristol

Klippel J H, Dieppe P A 1994 Rheumatology. Mosby, St Louis

Smith Pigg J, Driscoll R W, Caniff R 1985 Rheumatology nursing: a problem-oriented approach. John Wiley, New York

Wilson K J W, Waugh A 1996 Ross and Wilson anatomy and physiology in health and illness, 8th edn. Churchill Livingstone, New York

Winwood R S, Smith J L 1985 Sears's anatomy and physiology, 6th edn. Edward Arnold, London

3

Immunology and investigative techniques

Jane Douglas

The aim of this chapter is to provide a basic understanding of the immune system and its role in rheumatic diseases. The common investigations used in the rheumatic diseases will also be discussed. After reading this chapter you should be able to:

- **Describe the immune system and its function**
- **Summarise the role of the immune system in rheumatic diseases**
- **Discuss the investigations commonly performed on rheumatic patients**
- **Discern the relevance of the results of investigations to the disease process**
- **Describe the action of drugs used in the treatment of rheumatic diseases in relation to the immune system.**

To clearly understand the problems faced by patients with rheumatic disease, it is necessary to develop an appropriate knowledge of anatomy and physiology. This knowledge enables the nurse to understand the disease processes involved and interpret the patient's symptoms in a way that will influence the planning and administration of care.

Many rheumatological disorders, such as rheumatoid arthritis (RA), are autoimmune in nature (Fye & Sack 1991). They occur due to the immunological action of one's own cells or antibodies on components of the body (Weller 1989).

This chapter discusses the relevant normal physiology of the immune system, and contrasts this with the disordered physiology that occurs in some rheumatic diseases. The focus of the chapter is upon RA and it also discusses investigations, methods of testing and the significance of results. A case study is used to aid understanding and enable nurses to relate theory to practice.

Explanatory overviews of the main areas are discussed, but for a more in depth study, the reader should refer to specialist textbooks or to the references cited in the text. It should be noted that the field of immunology is constantly being questioned, debated and researched.

THE IMMUNE RESPONSE

The immune response of the body is a protective mechanism essential to survival. The mechanisms of this response are based primarily on the ability of the body to recognise invasion by any potentially harmful substance. Defence and protection of the body's cells and tissues are achieved by the initiation of complex chemical and mechanical processes (Langelaan 1988, Weller 1989).

The environment in which we live exposes us to infectious microbial agents, that if left uncontrolled by our bodies, could multiply causing pathological damage. These agents include:

- Bacteria
- Viruses
- Fungi
- Parasites.

The immune system has two functional systems that work in conjunction with each other. They are the:

- Innate system
- Adaptive system.

The innate system forms the first line of defence, affording protection through the skin, mucosa and body fluids. It is also known as natural immunity because it is present from birth.

The adaptive system is activated when the innate system is violated and normally eliminates the infection by the production of a specific response to each infectious agent. Lifelong immunity, such as to diphtheria or measles, is achieved by recognition of the same infection by the immune system should it attack once again. Specificity and memory can therefore be seen to be key features of the adaptive response. A variety of cells and soluble factors distributed throughout the body make up and play a part in both the innate and adaptive immune systems (Brostoff et al 1991, Goodman 1991a). (see Fig. 3.1).

ANTIGENS AND ANTIBODIES

An agent or substance that the body recognises as

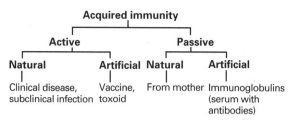

Figure 3.1 Summary of the types of acquired immunity (from Wilson and Waugh 1996, with permission).

'foreign' is known as an antigen. Most antigens are proteins but certain carbohydrates may act as weak antigens.

The recognition of these antigens sets in motion complex chemical and mechanical activities within the body, to protect the cells and tissues. The most common means of protection is either the production of further protein, called an antibody, or the production of special lymphocytes that carry a substance on their cell surface that resembles an antibody. The result of the antigen and antibody meeting, is a specific chemical interaction, in which antibody binds to the active site of the antigen, so destroying it. The result is the formation of a complex, often referred to as an immune complex. This occurs when the antibody binds to the active site of the antigen. Further destruction occurs due to an increase in the susceptibility of the immune complex to phagocytosis by leucocytes (Langelaan 1988).

THE CELLS OF THE ADAPTIVE IMMUNE SYSTEM

The body contains a set of organs collectively known as the lymphoreticular organs, in which the cells making up the immune system are particularly found. These organs include lymph nodes, the spleen, bone marrow, the thymus, and within the gastrointestinal and respiratory tracts the mucosa associated lymphoid tissues. Immune system cells are also located in extravascular tissues occupying the interstices of a network of reticular cells and fibres, that interlock and are supported by a framework of reticular cells (Kamani & Douglas 1991).

A cell from the lymphoid series is known as an immunocyte (Weller 1989) if it can:

- Produce an antibody by reacting with an antigen
- Participate in delayed hypersensitivity reactions
- Participate in cell-mediated immunity.

The predominant immunocytes are lymphocytes, but monocyte-macrophages, endothelial cells, rare eosinophils and mast cells also have functions in the immune system. The bone marrow contains self-renewing stem cells that are able to develop in any one of several ways (pluripotent) and it is from these that the cells of the immune system originate.

Approximately one percent of total body weight is made up of lymphocytes. Lymphocytes are found in:

- Lymph nodes
- Spleen
- Peyer's patches of the ileum.

Lymphocytes recirculate continuously through the lymphatic and vascular channels in the blood and tissues and are in dynamic equilibrium.

Macrophages are derived from monocytes and are highly phagocytic components of the reticuloendothelial system. Inflammation can stimulate these usually immobile cells into being actively mobile and they can facilitate the production of antibodies by interacting with lymphocytes. Macrophages are located in the:

- Lymphoid organs
- Lungs
- Liver
- Nervous system
- Serous cavities
- Connective tissues
- Bones
- Joints.

The lymphoid tissues are sometimes categorised into one of two groups tissues (Kamani & Douglas 1991, Weller 1989).

Primary or central lymphoid organs:

- Bone marrow
- Thymus.

Secondary or peripheral organs:

- Peyer's patches
- Lymph nodes
- Spleen.

Functions of the adaptive immune system

Pathogenic microorganisms carry antigens and recognition of these antigens is the function of the adaptive immune system. Once they have been recognised the source of the antigen is then eliminated by the appropriate immune response.

Due to the great variety of forms of pathogens, with different life cycles, the immune system must cope with many challenges (Brostoff et al 1991).

CELL-MEDIATED IMMUNITY AND HUMORAL IMMUNITY

Two broad categories can be used to describe the immune response:

1. Mediated immunity, which responds against intracellular pathogens, for example a virus infected cell.
2. Humoral immunity which responds against extracellular microorganisms.

The immune system is most effective when both types of response are involved. The pathogens that infect cells need to move between cells via the blood or tissue fluids. Because of this, a part of their life cycle is spent in the extracellular environment. This is illustrated by the case of the influenza virus. T lymphocytes of the cell-mediated immune system destroy infected cells, whilst antibody produced by the humoral immune system limits reinfection by controlling the spread of the virus via the blood.

Cell-mediated immune system

Cell-mediated immunity involves a variety of activities concerned with the destruction or containment of cells recognised to be harmful or foreign.

Lymphocytes processed by the thymus gland are known as T lymphocytes. They leave the bone marrow around the time of birth and pass to the thymus gland. The precise nature of the process that occurs is unknown, but it results in them carrying the genetic information that enables them to react with many possible antigens. T lymphocytes recognise the intracellular antigens that are present on the surface of the cells of the body and every lymphocyte is able to react with a specific antigen.

Antigens of the body's own cells are excluded, enabling the T lymphocytes to recognise 'self' and 'non-self' cells. Consequently, lymphocytes will not react against 'self' cells. However, in the case of autoimmune diseases, a problem occurs with recognition and 'self' cells can be wrongly recognised and destroyed.

After being programmed to interact with a specific antigen, the T lymphocytes begin permanent circulation between the blood and lymphatic systems. Movement into secondary lymphoid tissue, for example into lymph glands, spleen or bone marrow, occurs upon recognition of an antigen by one or more of the T lymphocytes. It or they then divide to form two types of cells:

1. Memory cells, that are processed in the same way as themselves.
2. Killer cells, that interact with the antigen.

A highly specific chemical interaction occurs when the antigen is recognised by the receptors on the surface of the T lymphocyte (Bell et al 1980, Kamani & Douglas 1991, Langelaan 1988).

Humoral immune system

Humoral immunity is concerned with antibody and complement activities. Recognition of extracellular antigens is by antibodies produced by B lymphocytes which are conveyed to their destination by the blood.

B lymphocytes are derived from the bone marrow but are not processed in the thymus gland but in lymphoid tissue elsewhere in the body. The site of this processing is unknown, but some evidence suggests that it may occur in the bone marrow itself. The lymphoid tissue of birds has been located in the bursa of Fabricus, hence the 'B'.

B lymphocytes do not neutralise or destroy the antigens themselves. Surface receptors enable recognition of an appropriate antigen. They then move into secondary lymphoid tissue and in the same way as they themselves were processed, they proliferate to form daughter lymphocytes, which can also be referred to as memory cells. In addition, they form plasma cells that remain in the lymphoid tissue, and it is these cells that produce and secrete the appropriate antibody.

The humoral response can be divided into primary and secondary. In the primary response, the immunoglobulin 'M' class predominates and an antibody is produced 48 to 72 hours following initial contact with the antigen. In the secondary response, the immunoglobulin 'G' class predominates, occurring within 24 to 48 hours and lasting much longer than the primary response. This response is a consequence of repeated contact with the antigen and forms the basis for consecutive immunisation (Fig. 3.2).

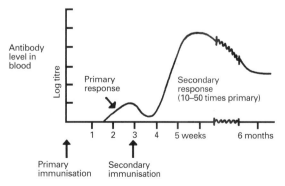

Figure 3.2 The antibody response to immunisation (from Wilson and Waugh 1996, with permission).

B lymphocytes and memory cells circulate in the humoral system. This is summated in Figure 3.3 (Bell et al 1980, Brostoff et al 1991, Kamani et al 1991, Langelaan 1988, Weller 1989).

ANTIBODIES

Antibodies circulating in blood are protein molecules that have a specific amino acid sequence. It is this property that enables the antibody to adhere to and interact only with that antigen that instigated its synthesis. This antigen specific property is the foundation of the antigen–antibody reaction fundamental to the humoral immune response.

Antibodies are often referred to as immunoglobulins because they are usually found in the gammaglobulin fraction of plasma proteins. They may have two or more antigen binding sites enabling them to clump together (Chapel & Haeney 1993, Weller 1989).

Immunoglobulin/antibody biological activities

Immunoglobulins are bifunctional and can:

- Bind to antigens
- Initiate other biologic phenomena independent of antibody specificity.

Immunoglobulins are divided into five classes separated by structure and function.

1. Immunoglobulin G (IgG)
2. Immunoglobulin A (IgA)
3. Immunoglobulin M (IgM)
4. Immunoglobulin D (IgD)
5. Immunoglobulin E (IgE).

Immunoglobulin G (IgG)

IgG can be found in all fluid compartments of the body and in the blood and in normal adults, it constitutes approximately 75% of the total serum immunoglobulins. These molecules are passed from mother to fetus because their small size allows them to cross the placenta. It is the only immunoglobulin capable of doing this and is responsible for providing the newborn child with protection during its first few months of life. Antibodies are able to exert their protective function through an innate response known as the inflammatory response. The IgG antibody initiates the non-specific defence mechanism known as the complement system and is the predominant antibody in the secondary humoral response.

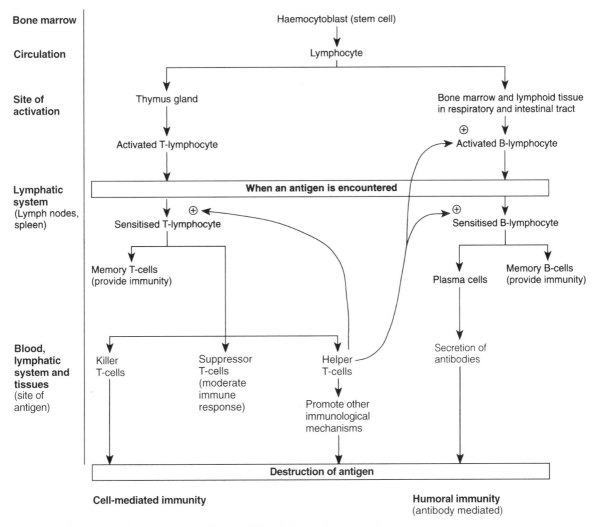

Figure 3.3 Summary of immunity (from Wilson and Waugh 1996, with permission).

Because it is bivalent, IgG is able to bind to two identical antigens and using its third arm is able to bind to special receptor sites on particular cells, for example phagocytes. If a cell is the foreign substance, antibodies cover its surface by binding to surface antigens. Foreign cell destruction occurs when phagocytes and other cells carrying appropriate surface receptors bind to the cell binding sites of the antibodies. This is thought to be the sequence of events when transplants are rejected, or when the body's own cells are damaged due to an autoimmune disease (Goodman 1991b, Langelaan 1988, Weller 1989).

Immunoglobulin A (IgA)

Immunoglobulin A constitutes approximately 15% of the total serum immunoglobulins and is predominant in the mucosal immune system. Found in mucous secretions it is produced by plasma cells in the mucous membranes and passes into the lumen of the tract, with mucous. This secretory IgA is found in copious amounts in:

• Tears
• Saliva
• Nasal mucosa

- Bronchial secretions
- Vaginal secretions
- Mucous secretions of the small intestine
- Prostatic fluid
- Blood.

It provides the primary defence mechanism against local infections. Its protective action is believed to be by coating the surface of the invading pathogens so preventing them from adhering to the mucous lining (Goodman 1991b, Langelaan 1988, Weller 1989).

Immunoglobulin M (IgM)

Immunoglobulin M is the largest of the immunoglobulins. It is short lived and its production is initiated when the body confronts a new antigen. Found in blood, it constitutes 10% of normal immunoglobulins and is prominent in early immune responses to most antigens. It predominates certain antibody responses, for example 'natural' blood group antibodies and causes agglutination of blood due to its ten antigen binding sites. One molecule of IgM, bound to an antigen, is sufficient to initiate the complement cascade, as it is the most efficient complement-fixing antigen (Goodman 1991b, Langelaan 1988, Weller 1989).

Immunoglobulin D (IgD)

Found only in blood, these large antibodies are normally present in serum and constitute 0.2% of total serum immunoglobulins. The main function of this immunoglobulin has not yet been defined. Nevertheless it has been suggested that IgD, with IgM, may be involved in the differentiation of human B lymphocytes since it is the predominant immunoglobulin on their surface, at certain stages of their development (Goodman 1991b, Langelaan 1988, Weller 1989).

Immunoglobulin E (IgE)

Immunoglobulin E constitutes only 0.004% of the total serum immunoglobulins. It has a very high affinity for mast cells that are found mainly around capillaries and is also found attached to basophils. Both of these contain granules of histamine. The cell binding sites of this antibody allows it to bind to mast cells and basophils, resulting in the release of large quantities of histamine, causing allergic reactions such as hay fever and asthma. Allergists use the alternative name 'allergen' for any antigen that stimulates the production of IgE. Wheal and flare reactions are characteristic manifestations when allergic individuals have their skin exposed to allergens. This is because IgE stimulates the release of pharmacological mediators from mast cells, when certain specific allergens are combined. IgE is thought to be significant in the defence of the body against parasitic infections (Goodman 1991b, Langelaan 1988, Weller 1989).

THE COMPLEMENT SYSTEM

A key role is played in the host defence process by a group of plasma and cell membrane proteins, known collectively as complement (Frank 1991). These serum proteins usually exist as inactive precursors, but when activated, behave as enzymes. An antigen complex, such as IgG or IgA activates an enzyme known as 'C1'. This is the first in a series and the remaining enzymes are then activated sequentially, to form a cascade. IgM is the most potent of these activators of 'C' (Chapel & Haeney 1993, Frank 1991).

The complement system acts as a mediator for both adaptive and innate immunity. Activated by antibody in immune complexes, known as classic pathway activation or, in the presence of certain microbial surfaces, as in the alternative pathway, the complement system is one of the main mediators of inflammatory reactions (Brostoff et al 1991).

The complement system has three main functions:

1. Lysis (destruction) of cells, bacteria and enveloped viruses. This provides a dramatic example of the activation of the complement cascade.

2. Opsonisation, where bacteria and other cells are prepared for phagocytosis (engulfing of microorganisms and other cells). The microorganisms are coated with one or both immunoglobulin and complement which enables them to be more easily recognised by macrophages and phagocysed.

3. Regulation of characteristics of the inflammatory and immune responses. At the site of inflammation, these proteins perform a function in vasodilation, cohesion of phagocytes to the endothelium of blood vessels and expulsion of the phagocyte from the vessel. They also direct phagocytic cells into inflamed areas and function in the clearance from the body of infectious agents (Chapel & Haeney 1993, Frank 1991).

HYPERSENSITIVITY

When antibodies recognise antigen, their intended response is its destruction. However, if this adaptive response is exaggerated or occurs inappropriately, tissue damage can also occur with severe or even fatal effects. This inappropriate response is often referred to as hypersensitivity. There are three types of hypersensitivity:

1. Immediate hypersensitivity
2. Delayed hypersensitivity
3. Contact hypersensitivity.

Immediate hypersensitivity reactions

An agent such as histamine, released during an antibody–antigen interaction, can bring about an immediate reaction. Examples include anaphylaxis and atopy.

Delayed hypersensitivity reactions

Delayed hypersensitivity reactions can occur after about 24 hours. This response involves the reaction of T lymphocytes with antigens and is referred to as a cell mediated response. Examples include autoimmune diseases and graft rejection.

Contact hypersensitivity reactions

Contact hypersensitivity occurs when skin comes into contact with a chemical substance that has the properties of an antigen (Brostoff et al 1991, Chapel & Haeney 1993, Hollingworth 1988, Langelaan 1988).

Five types of hypersensitivity reaction are recognised. However, not all are involved in the pathogenesis of rheumatic diseases.

Type I

Type I reactions are immediate. Mast cells and basophils, sensitised with IgE, interact with the antigen (allergen). Pharmacological mediators of inflammation are released, resulting in the clinical effects of allergy. Hay fever and extrinsic asthma are examples of this type of hypersensitivity. This reaction is also referred to as anaphylactic hypersensitivity. This is relevant to reactions to medications, which may not occur on first contact with a drug, acting as the allergen, but possibly at a second or subsequent dose. (Brostoff et al 1991, Chapel & Haeney 1993, Hollingworth 1988, Langelaan 1988).

Type II

IgM and IgG are involved in type II hypersensitivity reactions. This reaction is initiated when antigenic determinants, forming part of the cell membrane, react with antibody. Phagocytosis occurs and the complement system is activated. Clinical examples include immune haemolytic anaemia and organ specific auto-

immune diseases. Autosensitised T cells may result in organ specific autoimmune diseases. T cells are thought to have a primary role in RA and multiple sclerosis and autoreactive T cells have been cloned from patients with these diseases. Type II hypersensitivity is also referred to as antibody dependent cytotoxic hypersensitivity (Brostoff et al 1991, Chapel & Haeney 1993, Hollingworth 1988, Langelaan 1988).

Type III

Type III reactions occur as a result of immune complexes being present in the tissues or in the circulation. The immune complexes (antigens and antibodies), bring about various degrees of tissue damage when deposited in various tissues. Localisation of immune complexes is dependent on several factors:

- Charge
- Size
- Local concentration of complement
- Nature of the antigen.

If they amass in large quantities in the tissues, severe tissue damage can occur, by activation of complement and accessory cells. This type is also referred to as immune complex mediated hypersensitivity. Immune complexes are found in a variety of rheumatic disorders, the connective tissue diseases being noteworthy. Soluble immune complexes in the circulation are deposited in blood vessels, joints, glomeruli, the skin and other tissues when there is an excess of antigen. It is the function of the reticuloendothelial system to clear the circulating immune complexes. In the connective tissue disorders, this system may become saturated, favouring deposition in the tissues. Serum sickness serves as another example of this type of reaction. Approximately 10 days following exposure to the antigen, glomerulonephritis, arthralgia and urticaria occur. IgG antibody is produced in response to antigen stimulation. Circulating, soluble immune complexes are formed when the IgG reacts with the antigen. Formation of these complexes results in the concentration of antigen being lowered expeditiously. The process is usually self-limiting continuing only whilst the antigen is present. Other clinical examples are extrinsic allergic alveolitis and systemic lupus erythematosus (Brostoff et al 1991, Chapel & Haeney 1993, Hollingworth 1988, Langelaan 1988).

Type IV

T lymphocytes rather than antibodies are responsible for initiating type IV reactions. The T lymphocytes react with the antigen and as a result lymphokines are released. The lymphokines attract other cells especially macrophages. These macrophages then set free lysosomal enzymes. The reaction is delayed for 24 to 48 hours following exposure to the antigen. This delayed hypersensitivity is demonstrated in the experimental Mantoux test (Heaf test) when a reaction occurs after 24 hours. Various bacteria such as streptococci and salmonella can also cause this type of reaction. When the response involves the skin, such as in reactions to metals or plants, it is called contact dermatitis. Drug and viral rashes also serve as examples. Type IV response is also known as a cell-mediated reaction (Brostoff et al 1991, Chapel & Haeney 1993, Hollingworth 1988, Langelaan 1988).

Type V

In a type V reaction, also referred to as an antibody and cell-mediated reaction, an antibody attacks a target cell. Lymphocytes may then also become attached to the cell binding site of the immunoglobulins. Lysis of the target cell may also occur if phagocytic cells are attracted. This type of reaction can occur when, for example, the herpes simplex virus infects cells, or in antibody coated tumours such as melanoma. A further example is where thyrotoxicosis occurs due to IgG antibodies reacting with thyroid stimulating hormone receptors of the thyroid gland. This results in the production of excessive amounts of thyroid stimulating hormone, a stimulatory hypersensitivity (Hollingworth 1988, Langelaan 1988).

THE MAJOR HISTOCOMPATIBILITY COMPLEX (MHC)

For the immune system to provide effective protection against hostile elements present in the environment, such as viruses and bacteria, it must be able to respond appropriately. This means that it must distinguish between antigens it would be harmful to respond to and those that it would be beneficial to respond to; that is to have the ability to discriminate between 'self' and 'non-self'.

The major histocompatibility complex is responsible for this discrimination. In humans the histocompatibility antigens are known as human leucocyte antigens (HLA). The locus for the HLA is located on the sixth chromosome and important aspects of immune function are controlled by a group of several thousand genes, on the short arm of this chromosome. The gene products of the sixth chromosome are divided into three classes: Classes one and two are histocompati-

bility antigens, so named because of their strong antigenicity, or ability to react with an antibody in transplant rejection. They are also known as human leucocyte antigens. Class three comprises components that initiate pathways of complement.

Everyone inherits a unique combination of a number of genes for these cell surface proteins. Receptors for these antigens, carried by T cells, survey tissues. If a cell is normal and healthy, recognition is by normal histocompatibility antigens. If a cell is diseased, foreign antigen is present enabling it to be recognised as such.

Recognition of a cell carrying a foreign antigen, by a helper or cytotoxic T cell, is determined by the histocompatibility antigen. Cytotoxic/suppressor T cells recognise class one antigens present on most nucleated cells. Only helper T cells recognise the class two antigens that are almost exclusively antigen presenting macrophages and the B cells. The presence of foreign antigen directs the appropriate immune response by histocompatibility antigens (Brostoff et al 1991, Chapel & Haeney 1993, Hollingworth 1988, Schwartz 1991).

AUTOIMMUNE DISEASES

For many years it was believed that the body would not react against itself, causing damage. It was considered that the body would always recognise its own proteins and never respond against itself by producing antigens. Tolerance mechanisms that render the body unresponsive to self-antigens are in situ to prevent the disastrous effects of autoimmunity. However, it is now well established that under some conditions, it is possible for the immune system to cause the body to react against itself, by not recognising its own proteins as 'self'. This lack of recognition results in the production of autoantibodies and in common with normal immune responses, both humoral and cellular responses are involved. In the normal response, invasion by foreign organisms results in destruction of cells by the activity of complement and antibodies and through the cytotoxic effects of lymphocytes. In the case of an autoimmune disease however there is excessive or abnormal activity by the components of the immune system.

The spectrum of autoimmune disease spans from organ specific to non-organ specific. Hashimoto's thyroiditis is an example of an organ specific disease, with antibodies and the invasive destructive lesion being targeted on one organ. Systemic lupus erythematosus is an example of a non-organ specific disease, in which antibodies are directed to antigens and characteristic lesions of the disease are widely distributed throughout the body (Brostoff et al 1991, Hollingworth 1988, Luckmann & Sorenson 1980).

THEORIES FOR AUTOIMMUNE RESPONSES

There is much speculation about why autoimmunity occurs and the question of whether a disease is truly autoimmune can be controversial. In some cases, when a patient presents with manifestations of a given disease, it is possible to speculate that a virus, for example, has provoked a response. The autoimmune response and disease manifestations may not possess a causal relationship. On some occasions a secondary response can occur when 'self' molecules are released through the disease process, exacerbating an antibody response. The term autoimmune disease is used when the process of autoimmunity itself appears to be the primary cause of the disease.

Hollingworth (1988) gives some possible explanations of proposed or demonstrated mechanisms:

- A possible example of a virus causing an autoimmune response or the likely cause of methyl-dopa induced haemolytic anaemia. Cell surface components are modified rendering them autoantigenic, or 'altered self'.
- Muscle fibres may be rendered autoantigenic in polymyositis as histocompatibility antigens, usually lacking on normal muscle fibres, are found to be present in polymyositis. This is known as aberrant expression of histocompatibility antigens.
- A possible mechanism is molecular mimicry. It is thought that an infecting microorganism and a 'self antigen' may possess antigenic similarity, which results in an immune response directed against 'self'. Reiter's disease, which can be caused by a number of infections, serves as a possible example and in this case the 'self antigen' is HLA-B27.
- Using the Epstein-Barr virus as an example, it is considered possible for autoreactive lymphocytes to be activated through direct activation of B cells. Certain IgM producing B cells are known to be directly activated by bacterial lipopolysaccharides.
- It is suggested that autoreactive cells would proliferate if T suppressor activity was eliminated. This is referred to as T suppressor failure. In the case of systemic lupus erythematosus there is impaired suppressor T cell activity and some viruses prefer to infect certain lymphocyte subclasses.

RHEUMATIC DISEASES

It has been known for a long time that RA and systemic lupus erythematosus have immunological mechanisms associated with them. The immune system is responsible for many of the characteristics of rheumatic diseases such as inflammation and damage to joints and surrounding structures. Most rheumatic diseases appear multifactoral in origin, but their exact aetiology is unknown. Sjögren's syndrome, dermatomyositis, scleroderma and mixed connective tissue diseases along with certain types of vasculitis also have immunological features.

It is believed that genetic factors make certain individuals susceptible so that in response to a stimulus, such as infection or other exogenous challenge, pathological processes occur. In these people, tissue inflammation or abnormal function can result from persistent or exaggerated immune responses.

Circulating autoantibodies, such as rheumatoid factor and antinuclear antibodies, are common in these diseases, and it is their presence that demonstrates that abnormal immunological activity is occurring. They are not always responsible for causing the damage to joints and tissues but they assist in diagnosis and prognosis (Chapel & Haeney 1993, Pisetsky 1994).

Classification of immunological mechanisms

Eisenberg & Cohen (1988) and Pisetsky (1994) classified four types of immunological mechanisms that have been characterised by the effectors of immune injury. In the case of rheumatic diseases type 2–4 reactions are usually responsible. However, it is possible that more than one mechanism may be in action at the same time.

Type 1, IgE-mediated/allergic

A high affinity Fc receptor enables antibodies to bind to basophils or tissue mast cells. These IgE mediated allergic reactions stimulate vasomotor and bronchospastic changes that lead to asthma, urticaria or anaphylaxis. IgE autoantibodies that include rheumatoid factors and antinuclear antibodies have been found. However, the role of type 1 in autoimmune rheumatic diseases, remains unproven.

Type 2, antibody-mediated effects on cells, cytotoxic

Autoantibodies, usually IgG or IgM can activate the complement system. The effects of inflammation can accompany this. These cytotoxic reactions, mediated by autoantibodies, can cause injury to cells.

Type 3, immune complexes

Activation of the complement system and generation of proinflammatory mediators occurs when the immune complexes from the circulatory system are deposited in tissues. Antibodies can also bind to antigens that have been bound or trapped in tissues, enabling immune complexes to form in situ. Systemic lupus erythematosus has immunological manifestations that resemble immune complex mediated injury. However, it has yet to be proved that the circulating immune complexes in this condition have direct immunological effects.

Type 4, cellular reactivity/mediated

Immune injury can be caused by T cells (products of B cells) acting directly upon tissue containing foreign antigen or bearing autoantigens. Tissue injury may be caused by cytotoxic effects of T cells killing cells directly or by cell growth and function being disturbed by the development of cytokines.

An overview of immunological findings in five common rheumatic diseases can be seen in Table 3.1.

TESTS AND INVESTIGATIONS

The following section aims to promote a basic understanding of the tests and investigations used in rheumatology. It is important to appreciate that there is more than one way to perform certain tests and that results may be stated in a variety of units. In addition, terminology and ranges of values that are considered normal may differ between hospitals and from consultant to consultant.

Rheumatoid factor

In this test two circulating immunoglobulins, IgM / IgG complex, are referred to for clinical purposes. They are present in 80% of patients with RA (Bird et al 1985). In this test, antibodies cause agglutination of sheep red cells, bacteria or latex, coated with IgG fraction. Examples are:

- RA latex fixation test – a titre of 1:40 or more is significant
- Rose-Waaler test – positive at a titre of 1:32 or more
- Particle agglutination test – normal range being 0–40.

The rheumatoid factor can be affected by age in the older adult patient and also by a variety of other clinical problems, such as liver cirrhosis and cancer (McGhee 1993, Maclean et al 1991, Stites & Rodgers 1991).

Antinuclear antibodies

This test is an assessment of tissue-antigen antibodies that is regularly used in the diagnosis of the autoimmune collagen disease, systemic lupus erythematosus. The immunoglobulins IgM, IgG and IgA are the antinuclear antibodies that react with the nuclear part of leucocytes forming antibodies to deoxyribonucleic acid (DNA) and ribonucleic acid (RNA) as well as others (Kee 1987). A technique known as immunofluo-

Table 3.1 The immunological findings in five rheumatic diseases (Brostoff et al 1991, Chapel and Haeney 1993, Fye and Sack 1991, Kamani and Douglas 1991)

Condition	Rheumatoid factor	Antinuclear antibodies	Immuno-globulins	Human leucocyte antigen (HLA) associations	C-reactive protein	C3. C4.	Erythrocyte sedimentation rate (ESR)
Rheumatoid arthritis	80% patients	30% patients	IgM	DR4 and DR1 (approx. 80% of patients)	Raised (disease active)	Normal or raised	Raised
Systemic lupus erythematosus	50% patients	95% patients (can be negative does not exclude)	IgG, IgM	B8, DR3	Usually normal (disease active)	Decreased or normal	Raised or maybe lowered
Systemic sclerosis	30% patients	80% patients		B8, DR3			Maybe raised
Ankylosing spondylitis	Seronegative	Not seen		B27 (approx. 95% of patients)			Maybe raised when disease active
Sjögren's syndrome	90% patients	60% patients	raised	B8, DR3	Can be normal		Maybe raised

rescence is used to detect their presence. In this test a specific antibody or antigen is labelled with a fluorescent compound (fluorochrome) that can then identify the location of an antibody or antigen. A titre > 1:25 is considered positive in systemic lupus erythematosus (Kee 1987, Weller 1989). It is a test considered useful in the diagnosis of systemic lupus erythematosus where it is found to be positive in approximately 95% of patients. It is also found in 20–40% of patients with RA and its presence is a strong indication that a patient may have Felty's or Sjögren's syndrome. Antinuclear antibodies can also occur in patients with certain connective tissue disorders:

- Progressive systemic sclerosis
- Mixed connective tissue disease
- Myositis
- Juvenile chronic arthritis.

In addition, relatives of patients with systemic lupus erythematosus can be found to have antinuclear antibodies. In the healthy population, the incidence of antinuclear antibodies increases in older adults and can be affected by certain drugs (Kee 1987, Maclean et al 1991, McGhee 1993).

Erythrocyte sedimentation rate (ESR)

The erythrocyte sedimentation rate is a measurement, of the rate at which erythrocytes settle in unclotted blood. The test is non-specific and can be affected by physiological factors and is therefore considered by some to be unreliable. It is raised in RA. This measurement is used as a disease marker and to monitor disease activity (Evans 1981, Kee 1987, Maclean et al 1991, Weller 1989). The normal ranges are 4–20 mm/h in males and 10–25 mm/h in females (Bird et al 1985).

C-reactive protein (CRP)

C-reactive protein is an acute phase protein used to monitor disease activity and the effectiveness of drug therapy in inflammatory rheumatic diseases. Criteria for using the test are similar to those used for the erythrocyte sedimentation rate test. It is a non-specific test that detects C-reactive protein in the blood during an acute phase inflammatory process and tissue destruction. During inflammation, changes in the C-reactive protein level occur ahead of changes in ESR. In systemic lupus erythematosus and Sjögren's, the CRP can be normal even when the ESR is raised and the disease is active (Kee 1987, Maclean 1991).

Normal range: 0–8 (mg/l) (McGhee 1993).

Plasma viscosity (PV)

Plasma viscosity is often used in preference to the erythrocyte sedimentation rate. It is raised when the erythrocyte sedimentation rate is raised, due to an increased concentration of proteins. Plasma viscosity is found to be raised in inflammatory conditions and in paraproteinuraemias such as myeloma (Evans 1981). The normal range is 1.50–1.72 cp (Weller 1989).

Haemoglobin content (Hb)

This test measures the concentration of oxygen carrying protein in blood cells and so provides a measure of the oxygen carrying capacity of blood (Kee 1987, Evans 1981). The normal ranges are; in males 13.5–18 g/dl and in females 11.5–16.5 g/dl (McGhee 1993).

White blood count (leucocytes)

This test measures the concentration of white cells in the blood. These can be divided into two groups:

1. Polymorphonuclear leucocytes, comprising neutrophils, eosinophils and basophils.
2. Mononuclear leucocytes, comprising monocytes and lymphocytes.

A decreased level can be influenced by drug therapy and is found to be present in systemic lupus erythematosus and Felty's syndrome. An elevated level is found in RA, gout, fever and acute infections (Kee 1987, McGhee 1993). Normal range is $4.9–10.0 \times 10^9/l$.

Platelet count

The main function of platelets is in the process of blood clotting. When the level is low it is known as thrombocytopenia. This can occur in autoimmune diseases, with platelet antibody formation, for example in systemic lupus erythematosus. In some inflammatory conditions such as RA, the level can be found to be high, when it is known as thrombocytosis. (Weller 1989). The normal range is $150–400 \times 10^9/l$ (McGhee 1993).

Complement

The complement system is concerned with the mediation of inflammation and is activated by immunoglobulins IgM and IgG. Once the system has been activated two of its components, C3 and C4, especially act as enzymes. Raised complement levels are found in many inflammatory rheumatic diseases.

A raised C3 and normal C4 indicate an acute phase response. A raised or normal C4 occurs in RA. Low C3 and/or C4 can suggest systemic lupus erythematosus, RA and other connective tissue disorders or a glomerulonephritis caused by immune complex disease (Bird et al 1985, Kee 1987, Maclean et al 1991, Weller 1989).

Normal values: C3, 0.63–1.70 g/l; and C4, 0.11–0.45 g/l (McGhee 1993).

Serum uric acid

Hyperuricaemia is the term generally used to describe an elevated serum uric acid level. In the body, uric acid is produced as a by-product of purine metabolism or oxidation. Gout is the most common condition caused by hyperuricaemia. As well as elevated levels in the patient's blood, urates or salts may crystallise to form deposits, known as tophi, in joints and tissues or to form insoluble stones in the urinary tract (Kee 1987, Weller 1989). Normal values; adult male 3.5–7.8 mg/dl, adult female 2.8–6.8 g/dl (Kee 1987).

HLA B27 (human leucocyte antigen)

This antigen is found to be positive in 95% of patients with ankylosing spondylitis, as well as in Reiter's disease and in juvenile chronic polyarthritis. It is also positive in 5% of the normal population (McGhee 1993, Maclean et al 1991).

Alkaline phosphatase

Alkaline phosphatase is an enzyme found localised on cell membranes that hydrolyses phosphate esters liberating inorganic phosphate. It is produced mostly in bone and in the liver and is therefore a useful test in diagnosing liver and bone diseases. In bone disorders, abnormal osteoblastic activity, or bone cell production, causes elevated levels. It is elevated in Paget's disease, osteitis deformans, osteomalacia and active RA (Bird et al 1985, Kee 1987, Weller 1989). Normal range 100–300 IU/l.

Bence-Jones protein

This protein is of low molecular weight and can be found in the urine of patients with multiple myeloma, other bone tumours, hyperparathyroidism, amyloidosis, leukaemia and metastatic carcinoma. This test requires a specimen of urine for laboratory analysis (Bird et al 1985, Evans 1981, Kee 1987, McGhee 1993).

Synovial fluid examination

This transparent and viscous fluid is found in joint cavities, bursae and tendon sheaths. The synovial membrane that lines joint cavities secretes it and its composition is that of connective tissue. Examination of synovial fluid allows diagnosis through detection of crystals or infection (Bird et al 1985, Weller 1989).

Aspiration

Aspiration is the removal of a sample of synovial fluid from a joint, by means of a needle and syringe using a strict aseptic technique. The fluid can be sent for laboratory tests such as microscopy and bacteriology and if required, biochemical analysis. Its appearance gives an indication of diagnosis; for example, in degenerative conditions it is more sticky or viscous. However, it is found to be more dilute in RA and other polyarthritides. A polarising microscope can be used to look for crystals such as uric acid or calcium pyrophosphate (Bird et al 1985, Maclean et al 1991).

Arthroscopy

Arthroscopy is the examination of the interior of a joint using an optical device called an arthroscope. The most commonly examined joint using this method is the knee. A local or general anaesthetic can be used. A general anaesthetic can allow a more thorough examination and assessment of the menisci, cruciate ligaments, and loose bodies. It also allows synovial biopsies to be taken. It is useful in the diagnosis of, for example, extrasynovial and synovial diseases and to monitor the progress of disease activity. Joint size can be indicative of the diagnosis. In RA and seronegative polyarthritis the joint capacity is often found to be large, whereas in osteoarthritis (OA) the joint capacity is often found to be small (Bird et al 1985, Kee 1987, Maclean et al 1991).

Synovial biopsy

A biopsy is the removal of tissue from a living body for examination under a microscope. During an athroscopy, a needle biopsy of synovium can be performed (Evans 1981, Kee 1987, Maclean et al 1991).

Radioisotope scanning

This technique involves using radioactive substances that are taken up by particular organs, when introduced into the body or a joint, usually intravenously.

A scanner is then used to detect the emission of radiation. Radioisotope scans can assist in the early diagnosis of ankylosing spondylitis, the assessment of inflammation, detection of infection, secondary malignant deposits and Paget's disease (Bird et al 1985, Goldman 1978, Maclean et al 1991).

Radiographs (X-rays)

Film, specially sensitised to X-rays or gamma rays, is used to make records of internal structures of the body. In rheumatology patients, radiological examination is an integral part of the assessment of clinically affected joints and for consideration of surgical intervention. In early RA, feet, hands and wrists are the most usual joints to be examined in this way. They often show early changes, such as soft tissue swelling around an affected joint and enlargement of the joint cavity. In contrast, in OA, cartilage is lost and the two bones are found to have moved closer together. In RA, later changes can be seen, such as the development of bony erosions (osteopenia) and a decrease in the joint space, with the erosion and loss of cartilage (Bird et al 1985, Carter 1984, Maclean et al 1991).

Case study 6.1 Rheumatoid arthritis and the immune system

This case study is included to illustrate the relevance of the immune system to rheumatic disease and to show the way in which tests and investigations are used. It concerns a fictitious patient, Mrs Owen who is 56 years old and lives with her husband aged 54 and their 15-year-old son.

Mrs Owens's general practitioner referred her to a consultant rheumatologist in August describing the onset of her disease to have been 4 months earlier. Following tests, he had made the diagnosis of RA on the presence of a positive rheumatoid factor. He described her as complaining of considerable pain in her hands and knees and that her symptoms were not responding to non-steroidal anti-inflammatory drugs. He had prescribed piroxicam 30 mg to be taken at night and nabumetone 500 mg twice a day. Mrs Owen was also starting to develop some swelling and deformity of her metacarpophalangeal joints in her hands. Her blood tests showed a slight anaemia and a raised erythrocyte sedimentation rate.

Her consultant at the out-patient clinic saw Mrs Owen in November. He described her as presenting with a classic, symmetrical, inflammatory, peripheral, nodular polyarthritis. He also reported that she had lost weight and was feeling depressed. Her weight at this time was 61.3 kg and her height 1.53 m. Examination of her musculoskeletal system showed local and generalised inflammation, developing contractures of her elbows and that her knees were already badly affected. As a result of his examination an admission to hospital was arranged, to review her medical management.

On admission to the rheumatology ward in December, Mrs Owen described how her problems had started in April. Her feet had become swollen and over the 2 months prior to her admission her left knee had been swollen and painful, especially when she was mobilising. She had also been suffering some back pain. The severity of her symptoms fluctuated but they never went away completely. Her morning stiffness lasted for up to one hour and she described no pain at night. Her ability to walk in a way normal to her had been reduced and the pain became worse on standing. Her hand function was also affected and she found herself unable to open jars and tins and experienced difficulty when cooking. Because her hands were painful, her appetite had been affected and she had lost 9.5 kg in weight.

On admission to hospital, Mrs Owen was able to attend to her own personal hygiene and dressing needs. She reported no other medical or surgical problems past or present and before the onset of her arthritis, she had been fit and healthy.

The philosophy of the ward was to provide holistic multidisciplinary care. During her stay she was referred to the:

- Dietician about her weight loss
- Physiotherapist with regard to her mobility problems
- Occupational therapist for her problems with manual dexterity.

All members of the ward multidisciplinary team assess the patients for their educational needs and respond as appropriate with verbal education supported by the provision of relevant literature and group sessions.

Mrs Owen was able to be self caring while in hospital. The nursing care provided focused on meeting educational and psychological needs. Rest was encouraged during the first few days in order to prevent damage to her joints and to allow the inflammation to settle.

Drug therapy

Mrs Owen's medical management during her hospital admission was focused on the review of her current medication that had been prescribed to relieve the symptoms of her disease. The symptom control approach had apparently been unsuccessful and after a full medical review comprising, verbal history, blood tests and X-ray reports, it was decided to choose a drug that would modify the disease process.

Prior to admission Mrs Owen had been prescribed an analgesic agent, co-proxamol and a non-steroidal anti-inflammatory agent, piroxicam. This non-steroidal anti-inflammatory drug was ineffective and a second, nabumetone, was tried prior to admission to hospital. This also proved unsuccessful and so it was decided to prescribe the next avenue of a second line or long term agent, sulphasalazine.

Co-proxamol (dextropropoxyphene hydrochloride B.P 32.5 mg and paracetamol 325 mg)

Co-proxamol is an analgesic that is taken regularly as a prophylactic measure, or when pain starts to build up. The dose is two tablets three or four times per day. The paracetamol component has an analgesic and anti-pyretic effect. When given alone the dextropropoxyphene component is a mild analgesic somewhat less potent than codeine. However when combined with paracetamol its power is potentiated. Dextropropoxyphene acts on the central nervous system as a depressant (AHFS 1992, Reynolds 1993).

Piroxicam and nabumetone

These drugs are non-steroidal anti-inflammatory drugs which reduce inflammation and pain. They are believed to act by inhibiting the synthesis of prostaglandins; fatty acids that act as mediators of inflammation. The recommended daily dose of piroxicam is to start at 10 mg per day and adjust to 20 mg or to 30 mg as necessary. The recommended daily dose of nabumetone is 1g (AHFS 1992, Reynolds 1993).

Sulphasalazine

Sulphasalazine is classed as a long-term agent or second line drug. This group of drugs is thought to act by modification of disease activity rather than the relief of symptoms. The exact action of sulphasalazine is presently being assessed in several research studies. This class of drug is well recognised to be slow acting and takes two months or more to demonstrate any effects. Sulphasalazine requires very close monitoring for unwanted side effects including blood dyscrasias. Full blood count should be checked monthly and liver function tests carried out 3-monthly (protocols may vary between consultants) (AHFS 1992, Reynolds 1993).

Triamcinolone

During her admission, Mrs Owen was also prescribed a steroid intra-articular injection for her left knee. Triamcinolone belongs to a group of drugs known as pure anti-inflammatory agents. The absorption of this drug is slow and its anti-inflammatory effects last for several weeks (AHFS 1992, Reynolds 1993).

Rheumatoid arthritis and Mrs Owen

RA is a systemic disease that can become particularly painful and disabling. Inflammation of the synovium and tendon sheaths occurs and can eventually lead to the joint becoming damaged or even destroyed. The disease process may progress until all joints in the body are involved (Chapel & Haeney 1993, Fye & Sack 1991, Kumar & Clark 1990). Mrs Owen complained of this type of inflammation when she referred to the pain in her feet, hands and knees.

She described experiencing weight loss and feeling depressed. The extreme tiredness, malaise, weight loss, depression and other psychological and social effects commonly found in chronic, unpredictable disabling diseases are also associated with RA (Le Gallez 1993, Shipley & Newman 1993).

All blood test results must be evaluated within the context of the full clinical picture. Mrs Owen had a positive rheumatoid factor measuring > 640 titre (normal 0–40). This indicates presence of the immunoglobulin classes of antibodies IgM, IgG and IgA. If one of these antibodies is detected, the arthritis is referred to as seropositive RA. In seronegative RA the IgM immunoglobulin class is undetectable. However, this does not mean that the patient does not have RA, since approximately 74% of seronegative patients become seropositive (Stites & Rodgers 1991, Waterlow 1992).

Raised erythrocyte sedimentation rates were also detected. These were 53 mm/h on 6th November and later, 12 mm/h on 19th December, compared with a normal range of 10–25 mm/h in females. A raised erythrocyte sedimentation rate is an indication of inflammation (Bird et al 1985).

Mrs Owen was also found to be anaemic, with her haemoglobin 10.3 g/dl compared with a normal range of 11.5–16.5 g/dl in females (McGhee 1993.) Anaemia is the most common extra-articular manifestation seen in this disease and it is usually normocytic, normochromic. The excessive uptake of iron by the reticuloendothelial system is largely responsible and results in iron being unavailable for use in developing red cells (Hart & Clarke 1993).

She had a C reactive protein level of 99 mg/l compared with the normal level of 0–8 mg/l, (McGhee 1993). This plasma protein is one of the acute phase proteins of the inflammatory response. It binds to the cell and bacterial walls and activates complement (Hollingworth 1988).

Mrs Owen presented with swollen knees. This problem will now be used to relate the immunological pathogenesis of RA.

The synovial lining of the knee possesses two cell types, mucosal and phagocytic, which function as a barrier to serum proteins and as a means of disposal of unwanted material. A normal knee joint is shown in Fig. 2.8. Inflammation of small blood vessels occurs in RA and is known as vasculitis. This is the earliest synovial change to occur and is accompanied by oedema caused by an increase in capillary permeability. Because the cause of the immune response in this condition is unknown it must be assumed that a primary stimulus caused the production of IgG by synovial lymphocytes and that an immune response was initiated by the recognition of this as foreign. We know this to have occurred, as she was positive for rheumatoid factor. The complement system by the classic pathway would then have been activated due to the presence of IgG aggregates or IgG rheumatoid factor. Stimulation of the alternative pathway would have been due to the accumulation of the complement breakdown products in the knee joints. A number of inflammatory phenomena will have occurred due to the activation of the complement system:

- Release of histamine
- Production of factors chemotactic to polymorphonuclear neutrophils and to mononuclear cells
- Cell lysis, causing damage to the synovial membranes
- Leucocytes crowding into the synovial space.

Inflammatory cells produce leukotrienes and prostaglandins and are thought to have a leading role in the arbitration of the inflammatory process. The inflammatory and proliferative response of the synovium is expanded by the release of activated lysosomes and enzymes.

Certain characteristic elements can be observed in the mononuclear infiltrate of the synovium of an affected joint and for the purpose of this study we shall assume them to be present. They include:

- Perivascular collections of helper T cells
- Interstitial collections of suppressor T cells
- B lymphocytes
- Lymphoblasts
- Plasma cells
- Macrophages.

Continued rheumatoid factor and immunoglobulin synthesis and accumulation of macrophages occurs due to the liberation of lymphokines as a result of the immunological interaction.

The release of proteases and collegenases could have already or could potentially cause damage to Mrs Owen's joints due to the attraction of polymorphonuclear neutrophils by the immune complexes. An inflammatory exudate overlying synovial cells (pannus) can form due to hypertrophy of the inflamed synovium (Weller 1989). This pannus extends over the articular cartilage surface. Erosion of cartilage and bone can occur due to the release of enzymes by local infiltrating macrophages (Chapel and Haeney 1993, Fye & Sack 1993). The stages of RA leading from the normal joint to the destructive phase are shown in Fig. 3.4.

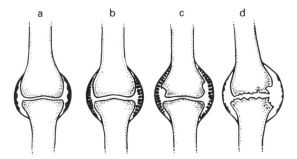

Figure 3.4 The three stages of rheumatoid arthritis. (A) The normal joint. (B) Stage 1, cellular phase. (C) Stage 2, inflammatory phase. (D) Stage 3, destructive phase. (From Davis 1994, with permission.)

Action points for practice:

- Write a case study on a patient with systemic lupus erythematosus focusing on the immunological aspects, incorporating the role of the patient's present drug therapy (see Ch. 12). If this stimulates your interest why not carry out similar studies on a variety of rheumatic diseases.
- Reflect upon your current practice and assess how knowledge of the immunological processes involved in rheumatic diseases could enhance or develop the nursing care that you give.
- Review your staff and patient education programmes (see Ch. 15), and develop them as appropriate to disseminate your new knowledge and to provide a better understanding of rheumatic diseases.

REFERENCES

AHFS 1992 American Society of Hospital Pharmacists, USA

Bird H A, Le Gallez P, Hill J 1985 Combined care of the rheumatic patient. Springer-Verlag, Berlin

Bell G H, Emslie-Smith D, Paterson C R 1980 Textbook of physiology, 10th edn. Churchill Livingstone, Edinburgh

Brostoff J, Scadding G K, Male K D, Roitt I M 1991 Clinical immunology. Mosby, London

Carter P H 1984 An introduction to diagnostic radiography. Churchill Livingstone, Edinburgh

Chapel H, Haeney M 1993 Essentials of clinical immunology, 3rd edn. Blackwell Scientific Publications, London

Davis P S 1994 Nursing the orthopaedic patient, p 218. Churchill Livingstone, Edinburgh

Evans D M D 1981 Special tests and their meanings, 12th edn. Faber, London

Eisenberg R A, Cohen P L 1988 The role of immunological mechanisms in the pathogenesis of rheumatic diseases. In: Primer on the rheumatic diseases, 9th edn. The Arthritis Foundation, Atlanta GA, Chap. 8, p36–44

Frank M M 1991 Complement and kinin. In: Stites D P, Terr A I (eds) Basic and clinical immunology, 7th edn. Appleton and Lange, USA, ch 14, p161–174

Fye K H, Sack K E 1991 Rheumatic diseases. In: Stites D P, Terr A I (eds) Basic and clinical immunology, 7th edn. Appleton and Lange, USA, ch 36, p 438–463

Goodman J W 1991a The immune response. In: Stites D P, Terr A I (eds) Basic and clinical immunology, 7th edn. Appleton and Lange, USA, ch 3, p 34–44

Goodman J W 1991b Immunoglobulin structure and function. In: Stites D P, Terr A I (eds) Basic and clinical immunology, 7th edn. Appleton and Lange, USA, ch 9

Goldman M, 1978 A guide to the X-ray department. John Wright & Sons, Bristol

Hart D H, Clarke A K 1993 Clinical problems in rheumatology. Martin Dunitz Ltd, Australia

Hollingworth P 1988 Rheumatology. Heinmann Medical Books, London

Kamani N R, Douglas S D 1991 Structure and development of the immune system. In: Basic and clinical immunology, 7th edn. Appleton & Lange, USA, ch 2, p 9–33

Kee J L 1987 Laboratory and diagnostic tests with nursing implications, 2nd edn. Appleton and Lange, USA

Kumar P G, Clark M L 1990 Clinical medicine, 2nd edn. Baillière Tindall, London

Langelaan D G 1988 Acquired defences. In: Hinchliff S, Montague S (eds) Physiology for nursing practice. Baillière Tindall, London, ch 6.2, p 579–598

Le Gallez P 1993 Rheumatoid arthritis effects on the family. Nursing Standard 7(39): 30–34

Luckmann J, Sorenson K C 1980 Medical-surgical nursing, 2nd edn. W B Saunders Company, Philadelphia

Maclean D, Bateson M, Pennington C 1991 Lecture notes on clinical investigation. Blackwell Scientific Publications, London

McGhee M 1993 A guide to laboratory investigations, 2nd edn. Radcliffe Medical Press, Oxford

Pisetsky D S 1994 Rheumatic disease etiology: immune mediated inflammation. In: Klippel J H, Dieppe P A (eds) Rheumatology. Mosby, St Louis 1;13. 1–6

Reynolds J E F 1993 Martindale the extra pharmacopia, 30th edn. Pharmaceutical Press, London

Schwartz B D 1991 The human major histocompatibility human leukocyte antigen (HLA) complex. In: Stites D P, Terr A I (eds) Basic and clinical immunology, 7th edn. Appleton & Lange, USA, ch 4, p 45–60

Shipley M, Newman S P 1993 Psychological aspects of rheumatic diseases. Baillieres Clinical Rheumatology 7(2): 215–219

Stites D P, Rodgers R P C 1991 Clinical laboratory methods for detection of antigens and antibodies. In: Stites D P, Terr A I (eds) Basic and clinical immunology, 7th edn. Appleton & Lange, USA, ch 18, p 217–262

Waterlow J 1992 Positive attitude will aid treatment. A guide to rheumatoid arthritis. Professional Nurse 7(4): 242–247

Weller B F (ed)1989 Baillière's encyclopaedic dictionary of nursing and health care, 1st edn. Baillière Tindall, London

Wilson K J W, Waugh A 1996 Ross and Wilson Anatomy and Physiology, 8th edn, p 65, 66. Churchill Livingstone, Edinburgh

Addressing the patient's problems

People who have rheumatic diseases encounter many physical, psychological and social problems. This section will enable the nurse to assess these problems systematically and describes effective methods of intervention. The RCN Rheumatology Nursing Forum Problem Model is used as a framework in order to provide a logical and structured format for the large amount of information presented.

4

Assessing rheumatic patients

Catherine Sturdy

The aim of this chapter is to describe the most commonly used methods of assessment in the rheumatic diseases. An illustration of their use in planning, delivering and evaluating care for the patient with rheumatoid disease will also be outlined.

After reading this chapter you should be able to:
- **Describe a variety of standard clinical assessment tools in current use**
- **Discuss their value in following the course of disease and efficacy of treatment**
- **Demonstrate understanding of how such tools can be used to monitor and audit delivery of care**
- **Carry out a nursing assessment on which to base a plan of care.**

In 1986, Chamberlain stated 'Without accurate assessment, comprehensive and appropriate help may be denied to a patient and increasing dependency will go unrecognised, even if the accompanying despair is witnessed'.

The most obvious need for assessment is to monitor the progress of the disease and the efficacy of treatment, but this is only one part of the requirement. More important from the patient's viewpoint, is how they feel, rather than how the doctor thinks they should feel on the basis of clinical and biochemical measurements. Bowling (1991) suggested that for chronic or life threatening conditions, symptom response and survival rates are no longer adequate measures. Therapy has to be evaluated by the extent to which it is likely to lead to an outcome of life worth living in social and psychological, as well as physical terms.

The first part of the chapter describes a variety of assessment tools. These include clinical assessments, measures of disability and assessments of the impact that chronic diseases have on quality of life, both physically and psychologically. Within the scope of this chapter it is possible to look at only a selection of tools and questionnaires. New ways of assessment are being developed continually, particularly in the area of quality of life measurement and outcome observations (see Further Reading).

The second part of the chapter illustrates the use of nursing assessment as a basis for planning the delivery of care.

CLINICAL ASSESSMENTS

Hill (1991a) has stated that a good clinical assessment should:

- Be capable of detecting small changes accurately
- Demonstrate the trends of change
- Require only tools that are quick and easy to use
- Not involve expensive equipment
- Be scientifically sound and well validated.

As well as measuring the activity and progress of the disease, and the efficacy or non-efficacy of treatment, it is necessary to assess the effect that the disease is having on the patient. To this end assessment tools are described which will monitor not only a patient's disability but also their attitude and well-being.

Assessing pain

Pain is a complex and individual response, making it extremely difficult to assess. Seers (1989) considers that its complexity should be seen as a challenge, not an obstacle. Camp & O'Sullivan (1987) believe that nurses have not found pain sufficiently important to merit complete assessment and documentation. The nurse's perception of pain may differ from that of the patient and several studies have demonstrated that nurses underestimate the degree of pain experienced by the patient (Seers 1989, Bondestam et al 1987). However, in order to treat pain effectively, it is essential to assess it accurately.

A detailed discussion of pain is included in Chapter 8, but the following are some examples of pain assessment measures that can be used both for judging the need for intervention and monitoring the efficacy of those interventions.

The Visual Analogue Scale (VAS)

A Visual Analogue Scale is shown in Figure 4.1a. It comprises a line, usually 10 cm long, which can be either horizontal or vertical. It is marked at one extremity 'no pain' and at the other 'pain as severe as it could be', or 'intolerable pain'. The patient is asked to place a mark on the line to illustrate the level of pain experienced over a given period of time, for example during the past 7 days. The distance of the mark from the end of the scale is then measured in centimetres to provide a measure of pain experienced.

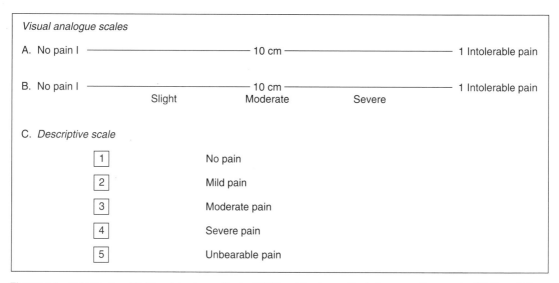

Figure 4.1 Pain Scales. (A) Visual Analogue Scale. (B) Visual Analogue Scale incorporating words. (C) Descriptive Pain Scale.

Patients often find the concept of the Visual Analogue Scale difficult to grasp initially, and they tend to place their marks towards either the end of the scale, particularly to the left (Bird & Wright 1982, Hill 1991a). Their understanding can be assisted by adding such indications as 'slight', 'moderate' and 'severe' along the 10 cm line, as shown in Figure 4.1B.

However Bird et al (1985) report that patients appear to relate more easily to a descriptive scale, such as that shown in Figure 4.1C, graduated 1 to 5, from 'no pain' through to 'unbearable pain' than they do to an ungraduated 10 cm Visual Analogue Scale.

The Body Map

A Body Map is shown in Figure 4.2. Either the 10 cm Visual Analogue Scale or the five point scale can be combined with a Body Map to indicate the area and severity of pain. Many pain assessment charts and questionnaires have been developed combining the above tools with descriptive words and records of interventions, both pharmaceutical and non-pharmaceutical. Examples of these include the London Hospital Pain Observations chart (cited by Raiman 1986) and the McGill Pain Questionnaire that was developed in Canada by Melzack (1975) and revised by Jamieson (1988). Although not specifically designed for patients with rheumatoid disease they are useful and well-validated tools, and have been used unmodified in rheumatic diseases. They could form a basis from which to develop more specific questionnaires and assessments.

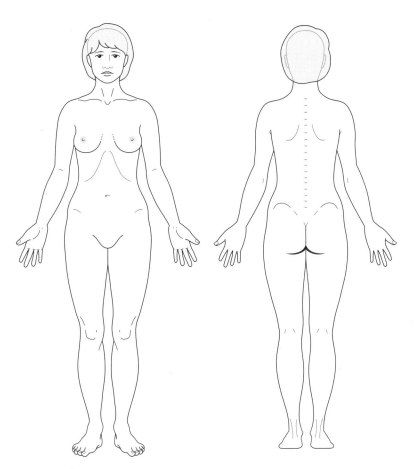

Put an 'X' on the above body outline where you feel pain
Put an 'O' after the 'X' if you feel the pain is on the outside of your body
Put 'I' after the 'X' if it is an internal pain

Figure 4.2 Body Map.

Daily Diary Cards

A simple Daily Diary Card (Figure 8.4), filled in by the patient either at home or whilst a patient in hospital, is an invaluable assessment tool. Its advantages are that it:

- Provides the nurse with data needed for the management of the disease
- Serves as a basis for discussion and planning future interventions
- Enables the patient to be an active participant in treatment and decision making
- Forms an invaluable educational tool, allowing the patient to identify those factors which influence their symptoms.

A Diary Card should include:

- A simple pain scale
- A record of analgesia required, in addition to regular medication
- Space to record what made the pain worse and what reduced it
- Space to record duration of morning stiffness.

Early morning stiffness

The most convenient way of assessing morning stiffness is by means of a Daily Diary Card. Early morning stiffness has been used as an assessment of disease activity for many years and it is the duration of the stiffness rather than its intensity that correlates with disease activity (Hill 1991a). Steinberg (1978) defines stiffness as 'the discomfort or restriction perceived by the patient when attempting the first part of an easy movement of a joint, after a period of inactivity. For some patients, stiffness is a sensation of no greater discomfort than the sensation that the fingers contain too much fluid.'

Morning stiffness can create many difficulties for the patient; some report having to get up much earlier than the rest of the family in order to prepare for the day; washing, dressing and breakfasting can all take longer. Because of this, the implications of early morning stiffness must be considered during a hospital admission, particularly when planning such activities as physiotherapy and occupational therapy assessments. A slow release anti-inflammatory medication taken late in the previous evening, a warm shower first thing in the morning, as well as gentle massage, can all be helpful.

Initially patients may find the duration of early morning stiffness difficult to judge and some find it difficult to differentiate between pain and stiffness.

Consequently, some patients may require encouragement when first using a diary card, until they gain the confidence that they can record consistent data.

A more detailed discussion of stiffness is given in Chapter 8.

Grip strength

The appearance of a hand is not always a true indicator of functional ability. The patient with a hand devastated and disorganised by disease activity has often learned strategies of maintaining some grip, whereas an apparently normal hand can have its grip weakened by painful joints. This can lead not only to difficulties with activities of living, but can also have safety implications.

Grip strength is measured using a dynamo-sphygmomanometer. A small bag, similar to a sphygmomanometer cuff is attached to a mercury manometer graduated from 20–300 mm Hg. The bag is inflated to a pre-decided pressure, usually 20 or 30 mm Hg, to ensure that it is comfortable for the patient to grip. The patient is then asked to squeeze the bag with one hand whilst holding the elbow away from the body. The peak pressure is recorded. Peak pressure is used in preference to sustained pressure, as the latter would possibly cause the patient more discomfort. The exercise is repeated with the other hand.

It is advised that three readings are taken from each hand and the mean pressure is recorded. Ideally, to avoid discrepancies, the recordings should be taken at approximately the same time of day, as diurnal variations can occur. To avoid observer variations, the same assessor should perform the test each time, using the same equipment.

There is no 'normal' range of grip strength, although a healthy adult has no problem obtaining readings of over 300 mm Hg. A person with hands affected by rheumatoid disease may record readings as low as 30–40 mm Hg during periods of high disease activity.

Once a baseline for a particular patient is established, serial improvement can be demonstrated when treatment is effective.

The Ritchie Articular Index

The Articular Index (Ritchie et al 1968) was developed as a simple scoring system to assess joint tenderness in patients with rheumatoid arthritis (RA). It has been shown, along with grip strength, to correlate with biochemical parameters such as C-reactive protein as an indicator of disease activity (Rhind et al 1980). As well as being a valuable research tool it also highlights

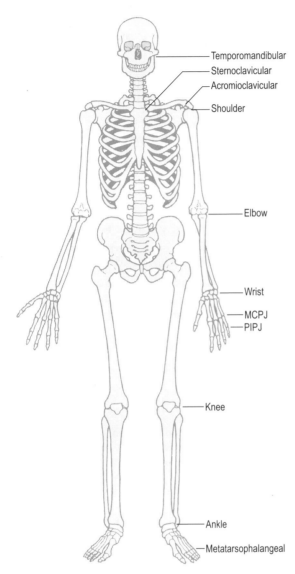

Figure 4.3 The joints included in the Ritchie Articular Index.

experienced when lying in bed at night. If so the patient is asked to say if this is mild, moderate or severe, and it is scored accordingly.

The patient's response to firm pressure on the joint margin is scored as follows:

No pain or tenderness reported	0
The patient says that pain is felt	1
The patient feels pain and winces	2
The patient feels pain, winces and withdraws the joint	3

The following joints are treated as single units for scoring purposes:

- Temporomandibular joints
- The cervical spine
- Sternoclavicular joints
- Acromioclavicular joint
- Metacarpophalangeal joints of each hand
- Proximal interphalangeal joints of each hand
- Metartarsophalangeal joints of each foot.

The highest scoring joint from each unit is taken as the score for the whole of that unit. The maximum possible is 78. However a score of 30 or more is considered high, and indicates that reassessment of all therapies is required.

Swollen and Tender Joint Count

The Ritchie Articular Index looks solely at joint tenderness. A further measure of disease activity can be obtained by assessing the number of joints that have active synovitis present, in addition to those which are tender. Information can be recorded on a joint count outline such as that illustrated in Figure 4.4. Serial counts give a valuable indication of the efficacy or otherwise of therapeutic interventions. This method is often used as part of the assessment strategy in clinical and drug trials.

Steinbrocker Functional Scale

The Steinbrocker Functional Scale was originally developed and described in the 1940s. It divides patients into four classes based on ability for self care (Steinbrocker et al 1949).

- Class One: Complete functional capacity with ability to carry out all usual duties without handicaps
- Class Two: Functional capacity adequate to conduct normal activities, despite handicap of discomfort or limited mobility of one or more joints
- Class Three: Functional capacity adequate to

specific problem areas. Unfortunately, extra pain may be inflicted when this assessment is carried out, so it is essential that a full explanation is given to the patient.

The joints studied are illustrated in Fig. 4.3. Tenderness is elicited by firm pressure over the joint margin. In the case of the cervical spine, the hip joints, the talocalcaneal joints and the mid tarsal joints, this is impracticable and so passive movement is used. If the assessment is taking place in an outpatient clinic, it is not always possible to lie the patient down to assess hip movement. Bird et al (1985) suggest that it is adequate to ascertain from the patient whether pain is

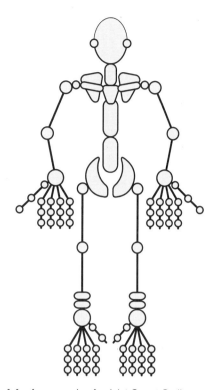

Figure 4.4   An example of a Joint Count Outline.

perform only little or none of the duties of usual occupation or of self care
- Class Four: Largely or wholly incapacitated with patient bedridden or confined to a wheelchair, permitting little or no self care.

This is a broad classification and not very sensitive to change. The majority of patients with rheumatic disease fall into categories two and three. However it is sometimes used in clinical research trials as a criterion for inclusion and exclusion of patients. It is a simple grading and is quick to apply, but needs to be used in conjunction with other assessments.

The Stanford Health Assessment Questionnaire (HAQ)

The original Stanford Health Assessment Questionnaire was devised and evaluated by Fries et al (1980) at the Stanford Arthritis Center in California. It includes five categories of measures:

- Death
- Disability
- Discomfort (pain)
- Drug toxicity
- Dollar cost.

It has been modified for use in other countries, including Britain (Kirwan &Reeback 1986). A typical section of the questionnaire is shown in Appendix 1.

The disability section is the most commonly used. The short form contains 20 questions and includes a 15 cm visual analogue pain scale. It provides a format for assessment of current disability, progress of disability and improvement in ability.

The 20 questions are divided into eight categories:

- Dressing/grooming
- Arising
- Eating
- Walking
- Hygiene
- Reach
- Grip
- Activities.

The patient is asked to tick the answer which best describes their usual ability over the past week, and to indicate if any aids are used or help required from another person.

The replies are scored as follows:

Without difficulty	0
With some difficulty	1
With much difficulty	2
Unable to do	3

The score for an individual item is adjusted when assistive devices or help from another person is required. For example, if the answer to the question 'Can you dress yourself . . .?' is 'With some difficulty' the score is 1. However, if the use of dressing devices is indicated, this score is increased to 2. The highest score within any category determines the score for that category. The total functional ability index is calculated by adding the scores of each category and dividing by the total number of categories answered. This gives a final score in the 0–3 range with higher scores indicating higher levels of disability. The 15 cm Visual Analogue Scale pain scale is measured from the left hand side, and the result divided by 5, to give a score in the 0–3 range.

Tennant et al (1996) point out that the 20 items provide a useful scale but vital information can be lost, and the changes in disability may be masked, by the way in which the Stanford Health Assessment Questionnaire is scored.

The information gained from the responses to individual sections on this questionnaire enables the care team to plan which are the most appropriate measures to introduce. The need for occupational therapist and physiotherapist input may be indicated, as may intervention from other agencies. It is also a useful tool when supporting patients applying for social, domestic and financial assistance and benefits. When used at initial diagnosis, it provides a baseline and the efficacy or otherwise of a period of in-patient treatment can be demonstrated by comparing scores on admission and discharge or subsequent follow up appointment.

As well as being a practical outcome measure and an evaluation tool the health assessment questionnaire is widely accepted as a research tool. Tennant et al (1996) refers to over 100 papers in which the Stanford Health Assessment Questionnaire is cited.

The Arthritis Impact Measurement Scales (AIMS)

The Stanford Health Assessment Questionnaire does not include a psychological component, but the Arthritis Impact Measurement Scales combine function, pain and psychological assessments within one questionnaire.

The Arthritis Impact Measurement Scales were developed in Boston, USA and first published in 1980 by Meenan et al. They are now used in many countries worldwide. Hill et al (1990) modified them for use in the UK. Forty-five questions form the basic scales, measuring:

* Mobility
* Physical activity
* Activities of daily living
* Pain
* Anxiety
* Depression.

An additional three items are useful for obtaining general estimates of health status and there are further questions to assist in assessing general health perceptions. The final item is a Visual Analogue Scale to estimate the overall impact of arthritis on the patient. This makes a total of 53 items on the questionnaire, but if required, further items can be added concerning use of medication, co-morbidity and demographic data.

The questionnaire is self administered and takes 10–15 minutes to complete. A sample question is shown in Figure 4.5. Scoring also takes 10–15 minutes. This first involves decoding the responses. The order of the responses varies from item to item, so that the first does not always indicate poor health status. The scores for each item within the scale are then totalled. The range of possible scores in a given scale depends on the number of items included in that scale, so a normalisation procedure is performed, so that all scores are expressed in the 0–10 range, with 0 representing good health status, and 10 representing poor status.

Each of the basic scales can be used alone or in

Please circle one number for each question.

34. During the past month, how much of the time have you enjoyed the things you do?

All of the time	1
Most of the time	2
A good bit of the time	3
Some of the time	4
A little of the time	5
None of the time	6

Figure 4.5 Completing the AIMS Questionnaire – a sample question.

combination, depending on which are most appropriate to the users needs.

The Hospital Anxiety and Depression Scale (HAD)

Psychological well being is an important dimension when looking at quality of life (see Chapter 5). Studies indicate that people with rheumatoid disease have a higher incidence of depression than the general population (DeVellis 1993). The Hospital Anxiety and Depression Scale is an instrument developed in the UK to examine states of depression in a general medical outpatient setting (Zigmond & Snaithe 1983). It contains seven items on anxiety and seven on depression, with higher scores indicating higher levels of anxiety or depression.

Each question has four response options, in order to discourage the patient from opting for the mid point. As anxiety may be increased by a clinic visit or hospital admission, the patient is asked to indicate the response that relates most accurately to feelings over the past week. The score is added up using the scoring grid. Anxiety and depression are scored separately. A typical question and its method of scoring are shown in Figure 4.6.

The Hospital Anxiety and Depression Scale can be used as a tool to assess clinical effectiveness, as a research tool, and also for audit purposes. Although self report questionnaires are not adequate for diagnosing clinical depression (Rodin et al 1991), some authors believe that this tool can be useful in guiding treatment, and for giving an indication of when to refer to a clinical psychologist or to seek psychiatric assistance. A score of 8–10 is suggested as borderline, with a score of over 11 indicating the necessity for further intervention.

The Rheumatoid Attitudes Index (RAI)

The Rheumatoid Attitudes Index was adapted from

Example of anxiety question

I feel tense and 'wound up'.

Most of the time	3
A lot of the time	2
Time to time, occasionally	1
Not at all	0

Example of depression question

I still enjoy the things I used to enjoy:

Definitely as much	0
Not quite so much	1
Only a little	2
Hardly at all	3

Items extracted from HOSPITAL ANXIETY AND DEPRESSION SCALE © R P Snaith and A S Zigmond 1983, 1992, 1994. Reproduced by permission of the publishers NFER-NELSON, Darville House, 2 Oxford Road East, Windsor SL4 1DF. All rights reserved. Record form items originally published in 'Acta Psychiatrica Scandinavica 67, 361–70 © Munksgaard International Publishers Ltd, Copenhagen, 1983.

Figure 4.6 Hospital Anxiety and Depression Scale – sample questions and scoring.

the Arthritis Helplessness Index (Callahan et al 1988). It looks at learned helplessness and loss of control. It has been demonstrated that greater helplessness correlates with:

• Greater age
• Lesser education
• Lower self esteem
• Lower internal locus of control
• Higher anxiety and depression
• Higher impairment in performing activities of daily living.

This was demonstrated using the health assessment questionnaire. Over one year, it was found that changes in helplessness correlated with changes with difficulties with performing activities of living (Callahan et al 1988).

The questionnaire comprises 15 questions. The patient is requested to tick one of five boxes, ranging from 'strongly disagree' to 'strongly agree'. The answers are scored according to the grid as shown in Figure 4.7.

The score range is 15–60 with a score of 15 indicating the greatest control and one of 60 indicating the least control.

This tool can be used for research and audit purposes, but is particularly useful as a guide to where further educational input and empowerment strategies are required. For example, if the answer to the question 'I have considerable ability to cope with my pain' is 'strongly disagree' this would provide a basis

for further exploration of mechanisms for controlling and coping with pain.

Clinical assessments used for specific rheumatological conditions

Systemic lupus erythematosus

There are several clinical assessment tools available for measuring disease status in systemic lupus erythematosus, but none are sufficiently sensitive and specific to be relied upon entirely (Hay et al 1993). Because of the variety of clinical manifestations in this disease, the number of specialities involved in its management, and the fact that it is characterised by 'flares' and remissions, it is difficult to evolve one instrument that is not too complicated and unwieldy to be practical. Those tools available are used in conjunction with the laboratory indicators.

The British Isles Lupus Assessment Group (BILAG) index was evolved by a group of British rheumatologists and scores disease activity in different organ groups, separately. It has been tested for validity along with other tools (Liang et al 1989) and was modified by Hay et al (1991).

The tool comprises 86 items, related to eight organ based systems. The scoring is based on a five point ordinal scale and each system is scored separately. A total score is not produced. If carried out manually, it is a lengthy and time consuming assessment to complete, but there is now a computer programme available for this purpose. The content of the index and a sample of questions are shown in Figure 4.8.

Systemic sclerosis

There are as yet no internationally agreed standards for assessing disease activity and severity in systemic sclerosis. However an assessment that is sometimes used is a 'skin score'. Work carried out in Denmark (Zachariae et al 1994) demonstrated that increase in a simple skin score, correlated with an increase in Type III procollagen, and thus Type III collagen. The degrees of skin thickening and pliability are judged over each of the areas as shown in Figure 4.9 and scored 0–3 as follows:

Normal skin	0
Skin which is thickened	1
Thickened, unable to pinch the skin	2
Thickened, unable to move the skin (it is tethered)	3

Ankylosing spondylitis

Several assessment strategies are employed when

	Strongly disagree	Disagree	Neither agree nor disagree	Agree	Strongly agree
My condition is controlling my life	1	2	2.5	3	4
Managing my condition is largely my own responsibility	4	3	2.5	2	1
I can reduce my pain by staying calm and relaxed	4	3	2.5	2	1
Too often my pain just seems to hit me out of the blue	1	2	2.5	3	4
If I do all the right things I can successfully manage my condition	4	3	2.5	2	1
I can do a lot of things myself to cope with my condition	4	3	2.5	2	1
When it comes to managing my condition I feel I can only do what my Doctor tells me to do	1	2	2.5	3	4
When I manage my personal life well my condition does not flare up as much	4	3	2.5	2	1
I have considerable ability to control my pain	4	3	2.5	2	1
I would feel helpless if I couldn't rely on other people to help with my condition	1	2	2.5	3	4
Usually I can tell when my condition will flare up	4	3	2.5	2	1
No matter what I do or how hard I try, I just can't seem to get relief from my pain	1	2	2.5	3	4
I am coping effectively with my condition	4	3	2.5	2	1
It seems as though fate and other factors beyond my control affect my condition	1	2	2.5	3	4
I want to learn as much as I can about condition	4	3	2.5	2	1

Figure 4.7 Rheumatoid Attitudes Index (from Callahan et al 1988, with permission).

caring for patients with ankylosing spondylitis. A Visual Analogue Scale may be used to assess pain and stiffness.

One of the characteristics of ankylosing spondylitis is chronic enthesitis and the pain this causes. An Enthesis Index was developed in Newcastle by Mander et al (1987), and is a convenient and non-invasive measure of disease severity.

The scoring is based on the patient's response to firm palpation over the enthesis points as illustrated in

Groups of questions included in the BILAG index

General
Mucocutaneous
Neurological
Musculoskeletal
Cardiovascular and respiratory
Vasculitis
Renal
Haematology

A total of 86 questions, with each group totalled
individually

Figure 4.8 The BILAG Index.

A Sample set of questions from the BILAG index

VASCULITIS
Answers: 1 = improving, 2 = same, 3 = worse, 4 = new or yes/no

60.	Major cutaneous vasculitis including ulcers	( ) (1.2.3.4.)
61.	Major abdominal crisis due to vasculitis	( ) (1.2.3.4.)
62.	Recurrent thromboembolism (excluding strokes)	( ) (1.2.3.4.)
63.	Raynaud's	( ) (1.2.3.4.)
64.	Livedo reticularis	( ) (1.2.3.4.)
65.	Superficial phlebitis	( ) (1.2.3.4.)
66.	Minor cutaneous vasculitis	( ) (1.2.3.4.)
67.	Thromboembolism (excluding stroke – first episode)	( ) (Y/N)

Score method for systemic sclerosis

Observer .... Patient details

Name ....

Date ....

Skin score

0 : normal
1 : thickened
2 : thickened, unable to pinch
3 : thickened, unable to move

Please score as appropriate

	Right		Left
Face	....	.... Upper arms	....
Anterior chest	....	.... Forearms	....
Abdomen	....	.... Dorsum of hand	....
		.... Fingers	....
		.... Thighs	....
		.... Lower legs	....
		.... Dorsum of feet	....

Figure 4.9 A Skin Score for patients with systemic sclerosis.

Figure 4.10. Some of the sites are scored as a group, the highest scoring site within that group being the score recorded for the group as a whole. These groups are:

• Nuchal crests
• Costochondral joints
• Sacroiliac joints
• Cervical spinal processes
• Thoracic spinal processes
• Lumbar spinal processes.

The remaining sites are scored individually left and right.

The scoring is as follows:

No pain	0
Mild pain	1
Moderate tenderness	2
Wince or withdraw	3

The total possible score is 90.

To enable the patient to differentiate between the sensation of firm palpation and the discomfort or pain caused by enthesitis, it is suggested that a control point is selected where enthesitis does not occur. The mid point of the clavicle is an example. The pressure on this point is demonstrated to the patient at the start of the procedure.

There will be inter-observer variability, so the same practitioner should carry out the observations on the same patient on subsequent visits.

The Enthesis Index has been found to correlate with severity of pain and stiffness, and reductions in scores have been demonstrated when the patient is taking non-steroidal anti-inflammatory medication.

The effects of the disease on posture can be difficult to quantify. Measurements used include the distance between the wall and the patient's tragus or occiput. Forward flexion of the lumbar spine can be measured by the use of the modification of Schober's technique (McRae 1969). The lumbar-sacral junction is identified between the dimples of Venus, and with the patient upright a point is taken 5 cm below this and 10 cm above. The patient is then asked to flex as far forward as possible, and the difference above initial 15 cm separation is noted. This technique measures skin distraction, but this relates to true lumbar flexion. In the healthy spine the distraction will be around 5 cm

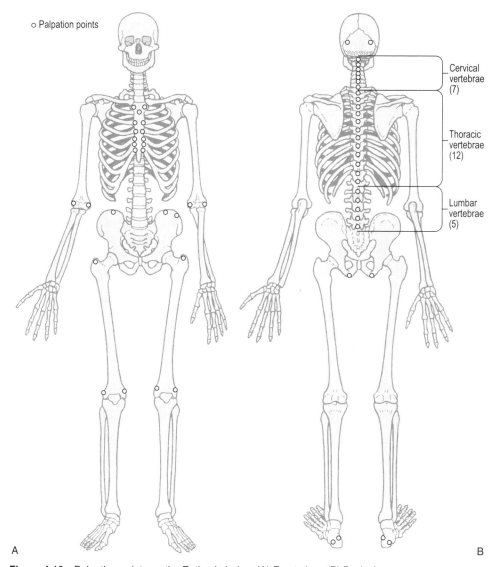

o Palpation points

Cervical
vertebrae
(7)

Thoracic
vertebrae
(12)

Lumbar
vertebrae
(5)

A

B

Figure 4.10   Palpation points on the Enthesis Index. (A) Front view. (B) Back view.

but in the patient with ankylosing spondylitis this is reduced.

Fibromyalgia

The assessment of fatigue and sleep disturbance is discussed in Chapter 9. However, in addition to these problems, patients with fibromyalgia present with several distinct hyperalgesic sites, which may be determined by digital palpation. These sites, which are illustrated in Figure 4.11 are normally uncomfortable to firm pressure, but the patient with fibromyalgia will experience marked tenderness and will wince or withdraw. In addition, negative control points are used where there should be no tenderness, for example the forehead or distal forearm. If tenderness is present wherever the patient is touched the diagnosis may be one of fabrication of symptoms or psychiatric disturbance (Doherty 1993). For a diagnosis of fibromyalgia to be confirmed, the patient will experience pain at ten or more of the tender points illustrated, in a symmetrical pattern.

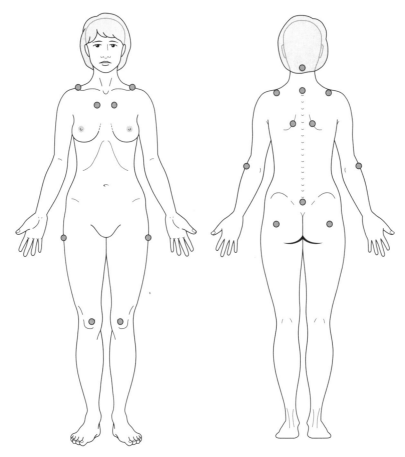

Figure 4.11 Body Map illustrating the tender points used in the assessment of fybromyalgia.

NURSING ASSESSMENT

For the purpose of this example the 1990 Roper, Logan and Tierney model of nursing based on Activities of Living (AL), has been used as a framework to illustrate some of the problems that patients with rheumatoid disease may experience. In this model, activities of living are listed as:

- Maintaining a safe environment
- Communicating
- Breathing
- Eating and drinking
- Eliminating
- Personal cleansing and dressing
- Controlling body temperature
- Mobilising
- Working and playing
- Expressing sexuality
- Sleeping
- Dying.

This is not an exhaustive list of problems. Every patient is an individual with an individual set of difficulties.

Maintaining a safe environment

Loss of joint function may lead to a patient with inflammatory joint disease becoming unsafe in the performance of everyday activities such as lifting kettles and pans, turning on and off cooker and water taps, operating machinery or driving a car. An admission to hospital is an opportunity to assess these activities, and the occupational therapist's involvement is invaluable. The use of the Stanford Health Assessment Questionnaire on admission, provides a structured way of highlighting where the patient is experiencing problems and where intervention is appropriate.

Being admitted to hospital, to an alien environment, can in itself increase safety risk factors. It increases anxiety levels that in turn can increase the risk of accidents. The person with long-standing disease may already have appropriate adjustments to the home. Chairs and beds will be of the correct height for safety and comfort, toilet facilities modified and required objects will be in familiar and suitable positions. Moorat (1983) examined accident reports in an English general hospital over a 2-year period. Forty-nine percent of accidents occurred whilst patients were getting out of bed or using the commode or toilet. Early morning was shown to be the peak period. Patients with RA experiencing early morning stiffness are especially at risk, and for this reason all patients should complete a Daily Diary Card to assess morning stiffness.

Walking aids, which may be safe in home surroundings, may be less so on shiny ward floors. Although the patient may be perfectly safe moving from room to room in the familiar surroundings of home, ward areas can appear vast and daunting. Bed tables and lockers may not be as stable as furniture at home when used as extra support.

The importance of control of infection in hospitals is well recognised. Patients who are receiving immunosuppressant drug therapy have increased risk of hospital acquired infection.

Communicating

When a patient is admitted to hospital, the social dimensions of his communicating change. As Roper (1990) points out, the problem is that the patient has joined a group of unfamiliar people, some of whom, the patients, are present all the times whilst others, the nurses, are in his vicinity some of the time, and a whole variety of others who come and go. It is of little wonder that even the most confident individual experiences some difficulty in trying to make sense of such an environment, which is alien to most people.

The family, social and work group is no longer around the patient, and difficulties with ALs, needs, abilities and disabilities have to be explained afresh. Self consciousness, fear, poor body image and depression are among barriers to effective communication.

In addition to information-giving about the specific episodes of care, part of the empowerment strategy for patients with chronic disease is education about the condition and its treatment. For this to be carried out effectively, it is necessary to assess the patient's knowledge and here tools such as the Patient Knowledge

Questionnaire (Hill et al 1991) will prove useful. Patient education is dealt with in more depth in Chapter 15.

The nurse must also be aware, through her assessment of the patient, of any barriers to communication that could include:

• Difficulty with reading
• Difficulty with writing
• Problems with holding pens and leaflets
• Impaired vision
• Poor hearing
• Impaired speech.

Breathing

Problems with breathing should be noted. In systemic rheumatoid disease, pleural effusion, occurrence of nodules and a diffuse interstitial fibrosis can cause these. Systemic lupus erythematosus, systemic sclerosis, polyarteritis nodosum and ankylosing spondylitis all have potential for involvement of the respiratory system.

Methotrexate therapy can occasionally lead to pulmonary fibrosis. Steroid therapy can mask infection.

Does the patient smoke cigarettes or a pipe and if so, why? Some patients reward themselves with a cigarette after struggling to perform what is, to a fit person, a simple activity. Others use smoking as a mechanism to relax or cope with pain. However it must be part of our education package to inform them of the dangers of tobacco smoking.

Eating and drinking

Eating and drinking frequently prove problematic and difficulties in this area should be assessed. An articular index will help to pinpoint any problems.

Do upper limb problems make it difficult to transfer food to the mouth? If so, an assessment of grip strength could be valuable. Manipulation of cutlery may be difficult and lead to inability to cut up food. Loss of dexterity may make it nearly impossible to open individual packs of butter, cheese or biscuits, all of which are often served in hospitals. A full or heavy cup may be difficult and dangerous to lift to the mouth, especially if it has a small handle. Some patients have their own adapted cutlery and special cups, which they feel more comfortable using. If so, they should be encouraged to bring these from home. Otherwise the occupational therapist will be able to assist by assessing for suitable equipment (see Ch. 11).

Some patients find it difficult to eat in public because they are embarrassed, feeling that they are 'messy eaters'. They may prefer to eat by the bed rather than sitting at a table with other patients, especially if they need to take frequent sips of water or mouth sprays when the dry mouth of Sjögren's syndrome is a problem.

When it is difficult and painful to get to the toilet, patients may be reluctant to maintain an adequate fluid intake.

Medications can cause indigestion or nausea. Steroid therapy, along with the disease process can make the patient more vulnerable to osteoporosis and advice regarding dietary intake of calcium and supplements may be required (see Ch. 10).

Some patients with aggressive disease may be underweight, but conversely, reduction in mobility and 'comfort' eating may lead to weight gain in others, with all its attendant problems.

Nutrition is covered in Chapter 10

Elimination

Roper et al (1990) points out that one of the more interesting characteristics of this AL is that, by custom, it is performed in private. Even in societies that emphasise the communal nature of living, eliminating is normally a private activity and the products of elimination are concealed from the public eye.

The potential for problems in this area should be assessed. It may be difficult for the patient to get on and off the toilet, to cleanse herself and adjust clothing. Whilst at home, she may have aids to assist her independence, but the situation could be very different in the ward. It may be difficult to accept help from a close relative or familiar carer, but even more difficult and embarrassing to explain one's problems to a stranger, even if that stranger is a care professional!

Great care is required when assisting patients on and off bedpans. It is an undignified procedure, but also can be a very painful activity for the patient with rheumatoid disease. By careful assessment of the situation, by listening to and working with the patient, the discomfort should be minimised.

Hospital admission, with its change of environment, routine and diet can disrupt normal elimination patterns. In addition, some medications can cause diarrhoea or constipation, so it is essential to establish the patient's normal elimination pattern.

Personal cleansing and dressing

The inability to attend to one's own hygiene needs, to be unable to cut one's own finger and toe nails or do one's own hair can have a devastating effect, espe-

cially on body image. So too can be the fact that one may have to adapt the styles of clothing worn. Fashionable footwear may be a thing of the past! Foot problems and pain in the feet can be assessed when carrying out an Articular Index. Footwear can be checked at the same time, as it can become ill fitting and be a potential cause of further damage as the disease progresses.

Patients should be encouraged to wear the correct footwear around the ward and at home. If the patient already has equipment at home to assist with washing and dressing, it is important that it is brought into hospital. This will help to minimise the difficulties the patient may experience in a strange environment. It will assist in maintenance of independence, and allow for further assessment. The Stanford Health Assessment Questionnaire or Arthritis Impact Measurement Scales will provide valuable information here (Hill 1991b).

Skin integrity

Great care needs to be taken when assisting rheumatoid patients with paper-thin skin with hygiene or to dress. Nurses' rings, buckles and long finger nails can cause much damage.

This subject is discussed in greater depth in Chapter 10.

Controlling body temperature

Some patients with inflammatory joint disease find they are more comfortable in a warm ambient temperature whilst others prefer to be cool. Some find that warm weather, cold weather or dampness aggravate their pain or stiffness. Knowledge of individual patient's preferences allows the use of appropriate clothing or bed covers. Several light layers of clothing are better than a heavy garment. A duvet is often more comfortable to painful joints than blankets.

Mobilising

It is important to ascertain the extent to which mobility is limited by pain and stiffness, what walking aids are used, and whether they are appropriate and safe. The use of the Arthritis Impact Measurement Scales or the Stanford Health Assessment Scale will be of use.

When moving up and down the bed, the use of a 'monkey pole' should be avoided wherever possible. Even if there is no obvious disease present in the upper limbs, the potential is there; for example, 90% of patients with rheumatoid disease develop wrist involvement. Damaged upper limbs affect many ALs and use of a 'monkey pole' could compound early problems.

Grip strength is often diminished early in the disease, so safety is a factor that needs to be considered.

If the patient is unable to stand unaided, from sitting position, a high seat, ejector chair or electrically rising chair may be beneficial.

It is important to discover if the patient takes any regular exercise. The physiotherapist, as part of her treatment regime, will be giving the patient a series of exercises to continue at home. Does the patient have the motivation, and understand the importance, of continuing with these?

Working and playing

Has the patient had to give up a preferred occupation because of the ways in which the disease affects him or her or is the patient struggling against fatigue and pain to continue to work? A workplace assessment may be required. A change of direction may be necessary in order to maximise abilities rather than struggling against disabilities.

Does the patient have the appropriate knowledge and understanding of the importance of pacing of activities and can she recognise the warning signs of a flare? The Daily Diary Card is a useful assessment tool here, providing a basis for discussion and information giving.

Chronic disease affects not only going out to work and household tasks, but also leisure pursuits. It can be devastating to be prevented from playing sport, painting, handicrafts, or even walking the dog. Socialising can become difficult and poor self esteem and body image can lead to social isolation.

How much is the disease affecting the patient's outlook on life? Does she feel 'in control'? Valuable information can be gained from the use of Arthritis Impact Measurement Scales and the Rheumatoid Attitudes Index. The Hospital Anxiety and Depression Scale will indicate whether intervention should be sought from a clinical psychologist.

Expressing sexuality

Has self esteem suffered? Has the patient lost interest in appearance?

Relationships can be placed under great strain. Any sexual activity can be painful and difficult and the use of the Articular Index will highlight any problems with the hips, knees or hands that can cause positional difficulties.

Sexuality is rarely an AL that can be assessed on first meeting a patient. However, it is important that the patient is aware that understanding, help and information is available, for both them and their partner, should they want it (see Ch. 6).

Sleeping

It is important to establish what the patient feels is her normal sleep pattern. If sleep is disturbed, what causes this? If it is disturbed by pain, which pain relief measures have been explored? Perhaps an adjustment in the timing of medication is required. This information can be obtained, in a structured way, by the use of a pain assessment questionnaire, possibly combined with a Daily Diary Card and Visual Analogue Scale. Assessment of tender and swollen joints can provide valuable guidance when assisting patients to position themselves for rest. The correct placing of pillows and the weight of bedclothes can make the difference between a beneficial period of relaxation and a time of great discomfort. However, a good night's sleep, although essential for well-being, can lead to an increase in early morning stiffness.

In order to pace activities and combat fatigue, is the patient in the habit of resting during the day? Many rheumatology wards, aware of the problems caused by fatigue, include a rest period as part of the daily routine.

An in-depth account of sleep and fatigue is given in Chapter 9.

Dying

Although RA is rarely a life threatening disease, it may be life changing. Other diseases within the speciality may have a poorer prognosis, for example systemic lupus erythematosus or scleroderma.

How does the patient view the future? What can we do, as part of a multiprofessional team, to empower the patient and family to cope with that future?

SUMMARY

Each of the diseases and conditions that affect patients cared for by a rheumatology team has its own set of assessment tools to monitor and record various aspects of disease severity and progress of treatment. In addition, there are many other assessments available for use in planning, monitoring, researching and auditing the care of patients with RA. Of necessity, this chapter is not comprehensive, but it describes a range of assessments which will give an indication of disease progress, pain, ability and disability, of psychological well-being and coping skills and of quality of life. These assessments will provide a basis for planning interventions and, by serial recording, a demonstration of benefit or otherwise of these interventions. They also have proven validity for use in research.

Action points for practice:

- A patient is admitted to hospital with a 'flare' of RA. Using the model of your choice, carry out a nursing assessment on which to base a plan of nursing care.
- A patient is newly diagnosed as having RA. Which assessments and measurements would you wish to record as a baseline?
- You are setting up a database of the patients with RA cared for by the multiprofessional team.

Which assessment tools would you select to provide ongoing information about disease activity, efficacy of treatment, alterations in ability and quality of life? Consider not only those mentioned in this chapter, but also, using the reference and further reading lists, explore other possibilities. Discuss your reasons for making your selection.

REFERENCES

Bird H, Le Gallez P, Hill J 1985 Clinical assessments in rheumatology. In: Combined care of the rheumatic patient. Springer Verlag, Berlin, p 204

Bird H, Wright V 1982 Assessments in the rheumatic diseases. In: Applied drug therapy in the rheumatic diseases. John Wright, Bristol, p 43

Bondestam E, Hovgren K, Gaston Johannsen F et al 1987 Pain assessment by patients and nurses in the early phase of myocardial infarction. Journal of Advanced Nursing 12: 677–682

Bowling A 1991 Measuring health, a review of quality of life measurement scales. Open University Press, Buckingham, p 1

Callahan L, Brooks R, Pincus T 1988 Further analysis of learned helplessness in rheumatoid arthritis using a rheumatology attitudes index. Journal of Rheumatology 15: 418–426

Camp L D, O'Sullivan P S 1987 Comparisons of medical surgical and oncology patients' descriptions of pain and nurses' documentation of pain assessments. Journal of Advanced Nursing 12: 593–598

Chamberlain A 1986 Assessing disease activity and disability. In: Reports on rheumatic diseases. Practical Problems 4, Arthritis and Rheumatism Council, Chesterfield

DeVellis B M 1993 Depression in rheumatological diseases. In: Newman S, Shipley M (eds) Psychological aspects in rheumatic disease. Baillière's clinical rheumatology, Baillière Tindall, London, 7(2): 241–258

Doherty M 1993 Fibromyalgia syndrome In: Reports on rheumatic diseases. Arthritis and Rheumatism Council, Chesterfield, Series 2: 23

Fries J F, Spitz P, Kraines R G, Holman H 1980 Measurement of patient outcomes in arthritis. Arthritis and Rheumatism 23: 137–145

Hay E, Gordon C, Emery P 1993 Assessment of lupus, where are we now? Annals of the Rheumatic Diseases 52: 169–172

Hay E M, Bacon P, Gordon C et al 1991 Development and testing of BILAG index (version 3). British Journal of Rheumatology 30: 23

Hill J 1991a Assessing rheumatic disease. Nursing Times 87(4): 33–35

Hill J 1991b Health status in rheumatic disease. Nursing Standard 6(1): 25–27

Hill J, Bird H A, Hopkins R, Lawton C, Wright V 1991 The development and use of a patient knowledge questionnaire. British Journal of Rheumatology 30: 45–49

Hill J, Bird H A, Lawton C W, Wright V 1990 The arthritis impact measurement scales: an anglicised version to assess the outcome of British patients with rheumatoid arthritis. British Journal of Rheumatology 29: 193–196

Jamieson A H 1988 The McGill pain questionnaire thirteen years on. Journal of Drug Development 1: 8–14

Kirwan J, Reeback J S 1986 Stanford health assessment questionnaire modified to assess disability in British patients with rheumatoid arthritis. British Journal of Rheumatology 25: 206–209

Liang M H, Socher S A, Larson M G, Schur P H 1989 Reliability and validity of six systems for the clinical assessment of disease activity in systemic lupus erythematosus. Arthritis and Rheumatism 32: 1107–1118

Mander M, Simpson J M, McLellan A, Walker D, Goodacre J A, Dick W C 1987 Studies with an enthesis index as a method of clinical assessment in ankylosing spondylitis. Annals of the Rheumatic Diseases 46: 197–202

McRae I F, Wright V 1969 Measurement of back movement. Annals of the Rheumatic Diseases 28: 584–593

Meenan R, Gertman P, Mason J 1980 Measuring health status in arthritis. Arthritis and Rheumatism 23(2): 146–152

Melzack R 1975 The McGill pain questionnaire: major properties and scoring systems. Pain 1: 277–299

Moorat D 1983 Accidents to patients. Nursing Times 79(20): 59–61

Raiman J 1986 Towards understanding pain and planning for relief. In: Nursing 11. Baillière Tindall, London, p 411–422

Rhind V, Bird H A, Wright V 1980 A comparison of clinical assessments of disease activity in rheumatoid arthritis. Annals of the Rheumatic Diseases 39: 135–137

Ritchie D, Boyle J, McInnes J et al 1968 Clinical studies with an articular index for the assessment of joint tenderness in patients with rheumatoid arthritis. Quarterly Journal of Medicine 147: 393-406

Rodin G, Craven J, Littlefield C 1991 Depression in the medically ill, an integrated approach. Brunner Mazel, New York, p 4

Roper N, Logan W, Tierney A 1990 The elements of nursing. Churchill Livingstone Edinburgh

Seers K 1989 Assessing pain. Nursing Standard 3(15): 33–35

Steinberg A D 1978 On morning stiffness. Journal of Rheumatology 5: 3–7

Steinbrocker O, Traeger C, Batterman R C 1949 Therapeutic criteria in rheumatoid arthritis. Journal of the American Medical Association 140(8): 650–652

Tennant A, Hillman M, Fear J, Pickering A, Chamberlain M A 1996 Are we making the most of the Stanford health questionnaire? British Journal of Rheumatology 35: 574–578

Zachariae H, Bjerring P, Halkier-Sorensen L, Heickendorff L, Sondergaard K 1994 Skin scoring in systemic sclerosis: a modification-relations to subtypes and the aminoterminal propeptide of type 111 procollagen (P111NP). Acta Dermatological Venereolgica 74: 444–446

Zigmond A S, Snaith R P 1983 The hospital anxiety and depression scale. Acta Psychiatrica Scandinavica 67: 361–370

FURTHER READING

Long F, Scott D 1996 Measuring outcomes in rheumatoid arthritis. Royal College of Physicians, London

5

Psychological aspects

Sarah Ryan

The aim of this chapter is to promote an understanding and emphasise the importance of addressing the psychological aspects of rheumatological disorders. This will help to prevent the negative consequences of helplessness and depression developing. After reading this chapter you should be able to:

- Describe the different models of control theory
- Discuss the features of chronic illness
- Discuss why control is important to well-being
- Understand the depression associated with rheumatological disorders
- Describe the role of the nurse in the assessment and management of psychological symptoms.

CHRONIC ILLNESS

Chronic conditions such as rheumatoid arthritis (RA), ankylosing spondylitis and osteoarthritis (OA) have a global impact on an individual's life, affecting not only physical functioning but also their:

- Self esteem
- Role
- Relationships
- Control perceptions
- Level of mood.

Consequently, care management should not simply concentrate on disease suppression, but should enable patients to come to terms with the emotional and psychological impact of illness. In the case of RA, the course of the disease is difficult to predict and it has no known cure. A patient learns quickly that treatments are only palliative and that stressful flare ups can be encountered frequently (Parker & Wright 1995). If the psychological consequences of chronic disability are neglected, negative control mechanisms can become established, increasing depression and social isolation (Parker & Wright 1995).

The features of chronic illness

Chronic illness has been defined as an altered health state that will not be cured by a single surgical procedure or a short course of medical therapy (Miller 1992). It has been described as the fourth world made up of millions of people alienated from everyday life and deprived of interaction because of the effects of the disease and its treatment (Copper 1976).

Three main features of chronic illness have been identified (Reif 1975):

- Disease symptoms interfere with normal activities and routines
- The medical regime is limited in its effectiveness
- Treatment, although intended to mitigate the symptoms and long term effects of the disease, contributes substantially to the disruption of the usual pattern of living.

These features could apply to a person with a rheumatic disease such as RA.

The effect of chronic illness on the individual

Rheumatic disease, such as RA, causes pain, stiffness, fatigue and in some cases deformity. The mainstay of treatment, the use of disease modifying anti-rheumatic drugs such as intramuscular gold or methotrexate, is variable in its effectiveness and does not always suppress the condition. Often the individual feels unwell due to the systemic nature of the condition, which in turn effects control perception. For example, the patient feels unable to influence, events, which contributes to depression and poor coping.

The patient may also have to deal with the discontinuation of medication that is helping to suppress the condition, due to a toxic reaction. This can exert a heavy psychological toll. As symptoms increase, feelings of helplessness and hopelessness can occur which can cause the patient to lose faith in care management. In this situation, the role of the nurse is crucial. Support, explanation and reassurance will be needed to ensure that the patient remains an active participant in care and does not perceive further treatment modalities as useless.

The uncertainty that patients face with rheumatological disorders is often derived from the inability to arrive at meaning in the illness related event (Mishel 1981). Sources of uncertainty are rife and include:

- Inconsistency in symptom patterns
- Differences between expected and experienced illness related events
- Unfamiliarity with the situation.

A patient's perception of uncertainty will be influenced by their education, degree of social support from significant others and the relationship between the patient and the health care professional.

Patients require information about their condition so that they can begin to exercise cognitive and behavioural control. A patient will feel less threatened by a flare if they have been taught what symptoms to expect if the disease moves into a more active phase and which self help methods to implement, for example:

- Application of an ice pack to an inflamed area
- Resting the affected joint
- Maximising analgesic intake.

Although this does not prevent the flare, it reduces the uncertainty by emphasising that although it is unpleasant, it is normal to experience certain symptoms in this situation. This information will enable the patient to take on an active role in care management, thus increasing the perception of control and removing feelings of helplessness that can occur in the face of such events.

Patients will require different psychological support at different stages of their illness, and they must know whom to contact for advice, should they enter an unfamiliar illness episode. Support will help to minimise the uncertainty of illness. Group work with family members can also be advantageous, as chronic illness can be bewildering for all concerned and sharing knowledge can help all parties to work together.

Disability

Disability has been characterised as four successive stages (Pope & Tarlov 1991):

1. Pathology – the cellular abnormalities which accompany illness or injury.
2. Impairment – the dysfunction of organ systems which can accompany disease.
3. Functional limitations – the restriction of activities in everyday life due to illness or disease.
4. Disability – the limitations in performance of social roles due to environmental or societal constraints.

It is at this last stage that the patient perceives their illness through the effect it has on their role and their ability to carry out activities meaningful to them. From this perspective, disability is determined by more than the purely biomedical aspects of disease. Disability can be minimised if psychological functional status can be preserved and if environmental and societal constraints can be minimised.

Krueger (1984) likens disability to loss and states that patients will go through several stages which include:

• Shock
• Retreat, denial or disbelief
• Grief, mourning or depression
• Hostility and anger
• Adjustment.

Often, the initial lack of success of treatment leads to mourning that is analogous to normal grief such as at the death of a loved one. A feeling of hopelessness may also be experienced. For some patients it is the worsening of symptoms, despite taking the prescribed treatment that can adversely affect hope and lead to a negative perception of control. Here, the nurse has a vital role to play in educating patients about how they can live with the condition. Through empowering individuals and their families the nurse will be endorsing a shared responsibility and enabling the patient to move towards the state of adjustment (Box 5.1).

Box 5.1   Characteristics of adjustment in arthritis

• Living with the illness
• Seeking information
• Employing self management techniques such as pacing activities
• Remaining socially active
• Valuing oneself and one's contribution to society
• Sharing feelings with family and friends
• Working in partnership with health care professionals
• Seeking help and advice when required

The road to mastery

Shaul (1995) conducted in depth interviews with women with arthritis and concluded that they experienced three different stages before achieving an element of mastery over the condition.

1. Becoming aware. The initial stage was one of 'becoming aware'. The perception of the condition as a problem occurred when the symptoms did not go away, became worse or interfered with daily living. For many the first few years were the worst. As they struggled with the severe physical effects of their RA their emotional well-being suffered.

2. Learning to live with it. The second stage 'learning to live with it' was characterised by a sense of disconnectedness and a feeling of alienation from the family. Some emerged from this stage knowing that certain strategies worked for particular problems, for instance pacing when fatigued, to conserve energy and reduce pain. These women incorporated the illness into themselves and although they could not predict its course, or when another flare would occur, they were better able to cope when an unfavourable situation did arise.

3. Mastery. The final stage was one of 'mastery'. The women revealed a new identity, a different perspective on health. Knowledge was acquired about the disease and how to live with it. 'The women began as novices and emerged as experts in living with RA' (Shaul 1995).

The achievement of mastery involves a learning process which includes how to:

• Set goals and expectations
• Ask for help from others
• Marshal and manage energy
• Maintain connections with the family and community
• Work with health care professionals.

To achieve a sense of mastery the individual must gain a sense of control over the situation and develop a repertoire of control strategies to enable them to cope with the changes in the process and context of the illness.

During the nursing assessment, it should be possible to determine which of the three stages the patient has reached by the use of open ended questions as shown in Box 5.2.

Box 5.2   Nursing assessment – The stages of mastery

Stage one	What symptoms does your arthritis cause? What does your arthritis prevent you doing? How do you cope on a daily basis?
Stage two	How do you try to minimise the pain? What would you do if a flare occurs? How often should you exercise?
Stage three	How do you feel about yourself in relation to your arthritis?

Empowering the patient to achieve mastery – implications for the nurse

If the patient is at stage one, (becoming aware) the nurse should give support through explanation of the condition, to minimise natural fear and anxiety. To be most effective, this should be given on an individualised basis, relevant to the patient's frame of reference.

It must be remembered that a chronic illness is ever changing. Mastery of one phase of the illness may be achieved, but if the individual finds themselves in an unfamiliar phase, they will revert to the position of novice as shown in Figure 5.1.

To cope with any rheumatic illness the patient will need to learn how their illness affects their well being. Treating patients as genuine participants, ought to be central to a profession that has human interpersonal relationships at its heart. Instead, participation has sometimes come to be thought of as merely an improbable by-product of involving patients in their own care plans (Ashworth et al 1992). The term participation can only be used correctly when the nurse is aware of the physical, psychological, social and emotional meaning of the illness. At the same time the patient who is genuinely participating in the encounter has some awareness of the nurse as a person with a host of other demands and concerns. Participation involves mutual awareness of the stock of knowledge that constitutes each other's experiences. It would be a mistake for nurses to assume they intuitively know what the lived experience of any patient is like.

Any advice given to a patient will pass through a filter of lay beliefs, which are usually internally consistent and rational in their own terms. They are not static but change in the light of new experiences and the availability of believable information. Providing accurate information to the patient about their condition enhances predictability and a sense of cognitive control.

It is important to encourage patients to participate in as many treatment decisions as possible. When a patient chooses a course of action they are more likely to own it and persist with it, even if the benefits are not immediately apparent. Informing patients about treatment alternatives and allowing them a choice should heighten this sense of control and may play a key role in whether the treatment proves to be beneficial (Wallston 1993). Nurses can help patients develop, secure and use resources that will promote a sense of control through a partnership based on mutual respect

and trust. Knowledge is gained from the sharing of experience and through understanding the psychological and social influences surrounding their lives (Wallerstein & Bernstein 1988).

ASPECTS OF CONTROL

Control

Langer (1983) defines control as 'the active belief that one has a choice among responses that are differentially effective in achieving the desired outcome' and makes the following generalisations:

1. People are motivated to gain control of their environment and like to believe they are actually in control. Control may not be an inherent motivator in all situations but only where it will actually make a difference. Even if the acquisition of control does not make a visible difference the perception of control is the valuable factor or the issue in question. Perceived control may not affect deformity, but it may influence pain perception through cognitive or behavioural interaction, which leads on to Langer's second generalisation.

2. Even the illusion of control is acceptable. People feel unease when they lack control and resent perceived attempts to influence their freedom of choice.

3. People want to be responsible for their success but ascribe failure to chance.

Control is a factor in limitation in insight; lack of control implies that the patient lacks a central ingredient that will enable them to achieve mastery over their rheumatic illness. Lack of knowledge is often the limiting factor and so teaching the patient should help to remedy this deficit. However, any learning process should include the admission between the patient and the professional that information skills and behaviour do not guarantee results. The nurse must not add to the coping burden by seeming to imply that the patient can have control over all situations (Pigg et al 1985). The patient may faithfully follow the management programme yet because of severe active disease, progressively lose function, have uncontrollable symptoms and generally deteriorate.

Theoretical models of control

Locus of control

The concept of locus of control stems from social learning theory which proposes that people relate their behaviour to outcomes and engage in a specific type of behaviour if they believe it will achieve the desired outcome (Rotter 1966). For example a patient will

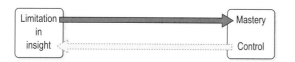

Figure 5.1 The changing pattern of chronic illness.

engage in relaxation if they believe it will influence their pain and they also desire to take an active part in pain management.

The construct of locus of control differs between individuals some of whom believe control is:

- *Internal* – dependent on the individual's own characteristics or behaviour
- *External* – dependent on the actions of other people or simply on chance.

Researchers have shown that an external locus of control is associated with less favourable clinical outcomes (Burckhardt 1985). It is often characterised by passive coping mechanisms such as withdrawal, lack of goal setting, lack of self involvement, denial and lack of information seeking.

Rotter's social learning theory predicts that when an individual finds themselves in a novel situation, for example faced with a chronic illness, it is their generalised expectations that determine behaviour. If so, a person having an internal locus of control would be best able to cope when faced with illness. Having a negative self concept can limit what an individual can achieve and a perception that they have no control over their life (i.e. external locus of control), will make them more prone to feelings of helplessness and depression (Broome 1989).

The onset of a chronic illness may challenge a person's belief that they can influence matters. As a result a change from an internal to an external perception may occur, until a level of mastery is achieved and an internal perception regained. As a person gains more experience of living with rheumatic disease, expectations in a specific situation will become more important predictors of behaviour than the individual's expectations in general. The belief that other people play a significant role in well-being does not necessarily imply a loss of control, especially if powerful others can be influenced to act in the patient's best interests.

Independence is not an issue unless it is threatened; patients require information, support and guidance to enable them to view themselves as normal (Pigg et al 1985).

Learned helplessness

Learned helplessness refers to a state of complete induced passivity. Burish et al (1984) concluded that maintaining a belief during chronic illness could be maladaptive in the face of repeated failures to gain control over the disease. Learned helplessness assumes that as a result of being subjected to uncon-trollable adverse events, the individual acquires the beliefs that actions do not affect outcomes; for example exercise does not influence pain perception. Someone in this situation comes to expect that further responding will be futile and stops trying to control symptoms through behavioural interventions (Bandura 1977, Wallston 1995).

Learned helplessness is related to psychological adjustment in patients with chronic RA (Nicassio et al 1985, Callahan et al 1988) and involves three types of deficit:

- Cognitive deficit – a reluctance to develop new coping behaviours through a lack of information
- Motivational deficit – a reduced effort to engage in the activities of daily living
- Emotional deficit – a low self esteem.

There appears to be a correlation between high levels of helplessness as recorded on the Rheumatology Attitudes Index (Nicassio et al 1985) and low self esteem, lower levels of formal education (Callahan et al 1988), high anxiety and depression scores and impaired ability as assessed by the Stanford Health Assessment Questionnaire (Fries et al 1980). Research on psychosocial adjustment in patients with systemic lupus erythematosus showed a correlation between engagement in activities of daily living and the development of new coping behaviour (Engles et al 1990). There was also a correlation between lower levels of perceived helplessness and longer duration of disease, suggesting that coping behaviour develops over time.

Self efficacy

Self efficacy is based on beliefs about control. It refers to personal judgement of performance capabilities, as distinct from actual accomplishments, in a given domain of activity (Lorig 1989). According to the theory of self efficacy (Fig. 5.2), behavioural change and maintenance are a function of:

- Expectations about the outcomes that will result from engaging in a particular behaviour
- Expectations about one's ability to engage in or execute the behaviour.

It should be emphasised that both outcome and efficacy expectations reflect a person's belief about their capabilities rather than their actual capabilities.

The theory postulates that a person's perceptions of their capabilities affect:

- How they behave, for example what activities will be accomplished

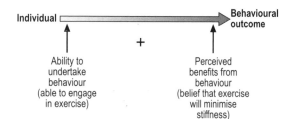

Figure 5.2 The theory of self efficacy.

- The acquisition of new behaviour
- The level of motivation and effort expended on a task
- Emotional reactions such as anxiety, distress and thought patterns.

An individual with a low opinion of their ability to carry out a particular task may ponder about their personal deficiencies rather than think about accomplishing the task in hand (O'Leary 1985, Strecher et al 1986).

Self efficacy is not a personality characteristic which operates independently of contextual factors. An individual's efficacy expectations will vary greatly, depending on the nature of the task which confronts them. Consequently, it is inappropriate to characterise a person as having a high or low self efficacy, without reference to the specific behaviour and circumstances with which the judgement is associated (Strecher 1986).

Skills that may be required to improve self efficacy include:

- Social skills – for example to persuade the family that rest is a necessary component of treatment
- Psychomotor skills – using joints in such a way as to prevent unnecessary pain
- Self regulatory skills – to recognise frustration as a normal response in chronic illness and to adopt techniques such as pacing activities.

Research has shown that patients and their families holding a negative perception of the future may instil a fatalistic attitude towards self management (Hewlett 1994). Although self efficacy is based on self judgement, the views of close associates will be an influencing factor. The motivation to engage in exercise for example will be reduced by lack of family support or their non belief in its value. The time that an individual will persist with exercise may be affected by the fact that it does not always show an immediate result (O'Leary 1985).

Self efficacy theory has been applied to diverse domains of psychosocial functioning including anxiety disorders (Bandura et al 1980, Bandura 1982) and achievement behaviour (Schunk & Carbonaj 1984). These studies have provided evidence that a person's perception of their efficacy significantly affects their level of motivation and psychosocial functioning.

Perceived self efficacy for behaviours that affect health status will predict further health, given that subjects believe that the outcome of their behaviour will be improved health, and improved health is their objective. There may be secondary gains to not achieving health, such as increased social support. The patient's sense of self efficacy in managing the symptoms and problems caused by RA is universally correlated with depression levels (Lorig et al 1989). It has also been found that high self efficacy scores are related to lower joint counts and fewer exhibitors of objectively assessed pain behaviours (Buescher et al 1991).

Factors influencing self efficacy. Providing positive efficacy feedback has been shown to improve tolerance to pain (Neufield & Thomas 1977). This suggests that perceived self efficacy, independent of actual performance in coping tasks, affects the person's ability to cope with discomfort.

Lorig and her colleagues (1989) studied a group of patients who had attended the Arthritis Self Management Course (see Ch. 15). Half of the sample felt their pain and disability had reduced after attending the course and attributed this to an increased sense of influence (which could be termed mastery). But the remainder of the sample experienced no alteration and in some cases their pain levels and state of disability had increased. The findings indicated that the sense of one's personal ability to affect the management of the condition was strong in some subjects but relatively weak in others.

Health beliefs. A person's beliefs about health are influenced by culture, social background, experience of health/illness and social network. These are complex factors and their origins difficult to discover but they play a vital role in health behaviour (McAllister & Farquhar 1992).

Four logic constraints contained in lay theories about causation of illness have been identified (Chrisman 1977). These are:

1. Degeneration (ageing)
2. Balance (diet)
3. Invasion (germs)
4. Mechanical (blockage of blood vessels).

Their importance and dominance will vary from one culture to the another, but must be taken into account when attempting to influence health behaviour and self efficacy.

The concept of illness causation amongst working class mothers was studied by Pitt and Stott (1983) who found that the majority believed 'germs' to be the main causes of illness. These women, who regarded the causes of illnesses as external to the individual, were less likely to feel responsible for being ill. Those who felt some degree of responsibility for their illness were likely to be home owners and have more years of education. Their feelings of control in their lives may account for their greater sense of responsibility for health.

Typology of control

The complex influence of chronic illness on everyday life makes Lewis's typology of control (1986) valuable, in that it distinguishes between degrees of control and discriminates between beliefs and the possession of behavioural competencies. The typology provides the rheumatology nurse with a range of care options to empower the patient to have control.

Processual control

This describes the situation in which a person is consulted but does not necessarily influence the decision. Lack of influence is of less importance to the individual than actually being consulted. Such tokenism can be beneficial even if the belief of control proves to be illusory, because the person believes they have been involved.

The belief that we have control and can influence events that relate to us as individuals, is central to self concept and well-being. A correlation has been found between self concept and control, in that people with higher levels of self esteem are better able to cope with the anxiety caused by illness and are less likely to adopt avoidance behaviour strategies such as denial (Tones 1991).

The environment facilitates the exercise of control. Consequently it is necessary to move away from the classic characteristics of the hospital as a total institution, with its tendency to depersonalise and disempower individuals (Goffman 1961). Control can be situationally determined and feelings of deference in communication with health care professionals can create powerlessness in patients and the perception that their actions will not affect an outcome (Miller 1992).

Cognitive control

Cognitive control occurs where a person cannot influence events but understands their reason and nature. This has clear psychological benefit. For example a patient who understands what is involved in a painful investigative procedure may not be able to influence the level of discomfort but will be in a position to manage the event intellectually and thus reduce its threat. It has been shown that individuals with severe pain reported fewer days of pain limited activity when they were able to derive benefit from the pain (Tennan et al 1992). This phenomenon, where meaning is derived from an adverse stressor is described by Rothbaum et al (1982) as secondary control. This cognitive adaptation addresses the heart of chronic illness and its significance for a patient's life.

Behavioural control

Behavioural control is where a person is able to adopt behaviour that potentially or actually alters the objective qualities of an adverse event. Pain management techniques are examples of this.

Contingency control

This is similar to the concept of locus of control (Rotter 1966). It concerns the extent to which individuals believe that events effecting them are controlled by:

• Their own effort (internal locus of control)
• The influence of choice and powerful others (external locus of control).

Existential control

In existential control, a person perceives they have no control over events but retains some degree of resilience through religious convictions. Newman (1993) views this as a negative coping strategy, as no attempt is made to influence the condition or learn to live with it.

Lewis (1986) makes clear that the essential ingredient in control is that the individual *believes* that they can influence events, even if their perception is incorrect.

Self medication programmes have demonstrated that by involving patients in their own care and enabling them to have responsibility for drug administration within a supportive environment, a higher level of well-being is reported (Bird 1990). Higher levels of psychological well-being have also been reported by patients with arthritis where they attempted to take control of their condition by engaging in physical activities and expressing their feelings (Newman 1993).

Frequently society associates control with independence, power and strength – all positive attributes. Conversely, lack of control is often associated with dependency and viewed negatively. However, dependency is a relative term and can be part of re-normalisation (Wiener 1975) where a person learns to accept new ways of carrying out activities. Patients require help and support to do this; it does not come automatically and patients must have information that will enable them to make informed decisions (Hill 1995).

The rheumatology nurse should be well equipped to support and teach, and so empower patients to manage their own care by sharing responsibility. This is an essential process for improving self esteem and accepting the condition, so that effective coping strategies can be developed which will improve well-being.

Wallston's theoretical model of control for patients with RA (Wallston 1995)

Adaptation to a chronic condition such as RA signifies that the patient and those close to them have mastered the myriad changes brought about by the condition and its treatments. The key to adaptation is perceived control and no matter how one assesses perceived control, the more control one perceives the more successful the adaptation.

Wallston (1995), influenced by the work of Lazarus & Folkman (1984) and Hobfoll (1989), has constructed a theoretical model on the stages influential in determining whether adaptation occurs or not. In this model, the presence of RA and its consequences such as pain and/or dysfunction, constitute a stressor for the patient and the patient's significant others. The threat value of the stressor relates to the amount of adaptation required to deal with the stressor. The individual appraises this and if the stressor is perceived as a threat then a secondary appraisal will occur. This will include a judgement of the adequacy of resources available. Resources can be:

- Internal – the patient's belief about the controllability of the stressor

or

- External – the actual support available from the family.

If the secondary appraisal shows there to be sufficient resources to counter the threat, the person feels in control of the situation and this affects adaptation

positively. Conversely, if the appraisal shows that resources are insufficient, for example if they are no longer able to attend to their hygiene needs and have no family to assist, one of two things may occur:

1. Where the individual is predisposed to accept control, they may engage in a variety of coping behaviours in the hope that something can help the situation.

2. Conversely helplessness may set in and either no coping occurs or the coping is maladaptive.

The model states that both perceived control and coping influence the appraisal of whether the stressor is threatening or non harmful. Both coping and the adaptation are also directly affected by the actual availability of resources, as well as by appraisal of their availability (Hobfoll 1989). Adaptation is an ongoing process in which the outcome of one stage feeds back and influences appraisals made at the next stage.

The health belief model

The health belief model evolved from an exploration of people's failure to take up screening and preventative programmes of health in the United States. It was later applied to the way in which people responded when they were ill, and whether they complied with treatment and advice. In the model, behaviour is dependent on two main variables:

- The value an individual places on a particular goal
- The individual's estimation of the likelihood that a given action will achieve that goal.

The model is constructed from three dimensions:

1. Perceived susceptibility or vulnerability. This is often the strongest predicting factor of the model. However, people often neglect the true risk factors in relation to their situation, behaviour termed unrealistic optimism (Weinstein 1982). An example in chronic rheumatic illness is that whilst lack of mobility will increase the possibility of osteoporosis developing, patients remain reluctant to take responsibility for minimising the chances of this happening, by increasing exercise.

2. Perceived severity. The weakest predictor of behaviour is often cited as perceived severity because people are relatively unthreatened by long term outcomes which are difficult to imagine and unlikely to happen. However this is not the case in RA where perceived severity has been shown to have a strong negative effect on behaviour (Hewlett 1994).

3. Perceived benefits. Motivation plays a key role in the efforts required to influence behaviour and can be considered as the patient's perceptions of the rewards minus the costs. Exercise may be beneficial but it is also painful and an exercise programme may reduce the time available to spend with the family. These factors of benefit and cost, will influence whether a person adopts the recommended exercise regime for their arthritis.

The model does not acknowledge the role of efficacy beliefs to the extent of incorporating them formally, nor does it acknowledge influences on past behaviour (Rutter 1993). The important aspect of the health belief model is that it is based on the patient's perception that it is the correct foundation for approaching control in chronic illness. It is only when the nurse has an understanding of the meaning that RA has to an individual, from their viewpoint, and the effects it has had on societal roles, that care will have meaning and be relevant to the individual concerned.

The theory of reasoned action

The theory of reasoned action differs from the health belief model in that it addresses beliefs and attitudes in general and is not specific to health (Rutter 1993). The model is founded on the concepts of cognition and behaviour that are assumed to be products of reasoned information processing. Patients may fail to comply with medical advice because they do not understand or do not agree with the physician's stated rationale. This may be regarded as unreasoned behaviour, yet it is reasoned within the individual's lay belief system.

To predict behaviour from this model one must measure individual belief on two levels:

1. Personal belief – what is seen as a consequence of a particular behaviour, for example relaxation to ease pain.
2. Normative beliefs – the perception of important others on a particular behaviour, who may view relaxation as time consuming and impinging on family activities.

The importance of normative beliefs is shown by the fact that social acceptance of behaviour relates positively to behavioural change and can influence healthier lifestyles (Jacobson 1986).

However, research shows that personal beliefs more accurately predict behaviour than do normative beliefs. It was found that 20% of a sample of patients with RA ignored professional advice to rest, believing that this would be 'giving in' and 'letting the arthritis win' (Donovan 1991). This research highlighted that patients do not always interpret the information given

to them by doctors in the way it was intended. Patients wanted doctors to understand the severity of their problems as they perceived them, whereas doctors took a routine approach and tried to reassure all patients by stating that their condition was mild and in the early stages. For individual patients this did not make sense. From their perspective they were in considerable pain and feared the future. The idea that this was a mild form of the disease or at an early stage merely heightened anxieties, the opposite of what had been intended. The medical inattention to illness (the lack of appreciation by doctors of the difficulties of living with the results of sickness), is in part responsible for patient non compliance, dissatisfaction with health care and inadequate clinical care (Lazare et al 1975). This has led for a call for the development of a new framework for understanding and treating sickness. Patients weigh up the costs and benefits of various options open to them before choosing the most suitable treatment programme. Medical advice has to compete with a range of other suggestions and if it is not credible it may be dismissed. People's lay beliefs determine what advice is reasonable but actions also have to be possible within the constraints of everyday life. Some patients may reject advice to rest because it makes them stiff or interferes with family commitments. It is important to elicit lay beliefs to understand reasons for poor compliance.

The theory of reasoned action has important implications for nursing care, as it maintains that a person's personal belief will be the main influence on behavioural interventions. It is therefore necessary to discover the patient's beliefs, and explore their explanatory models, so that care, which is both meaningful and relevant to the individual, can be advocated.

A serious limitation of the model is that it applies only to behaviour perceived by the individual to be under their control. For example, a patient may have a positive attitude about attending the rheumatology clinic, but without a means of transport, they will not be able to carry out the behavioural intervention that will match their belief. What is missing is Bandura's element of self efficacy; the conviction that one can execute the behaviour required to produce the outcome. There is also an assumption that all actions are reasoned and therefore rational. However, patients' explanatory models and to some extent those of medicine may be inconsistent and even self contradictory, although they are usually relevant to the individual concerned (Klienman et al 1978).

It is of the utmost importance that the nursing assessment considers control orientation in the planning, implementation and evaluation of care. If patients do not believe that they can influence the symptoms of their arthritis, they will not adapt to their new situation. Advocating self management principles to a patient with an external locus of control will not influence or alter their behaviour. The nurse must elicit individual lay beliefs and plan care accordingly in a shared partnership; if the proposed care does not appear relevant to the patient, it will be rejected. Empowerment can only occur if time is spent understanding our patients as individuals and their roles within their social context.

If the patient enters a new phase of their illness, it could alter their control orientation and return the *experienced* patient to the stage of *novice*. For this reason patients should be provided with a contact name so that they can be given relevant advice.

DEPRESSION

Depression is perhaps the most vexing and possibly the most widespread of the many types of psychological symptoms that can occur secondary to RA (Parker & Wright 1995). Although the precise prevalence of major depression in RA is not known, it has been estimated to affect 21–34% of patients (Creed et al 1990). Significant depression is a fairly common and important complication of RA.

Moldofsky and Chester (1970) describe two types of depression:

1. Depression that is more marked when joint tenderness is at its peak.
2. Depression that is more marked when joint tenderness is reduced.

The latter type has a less favourable outcome.

Major depression has been defined by Parker and Wright (1995) as that which is a 'profound, depressive syndrome of sufficient intensity to impair psychological, social and vocational functioning'. Features of depression are outlined in Box 5.3.

Box 5.3 Features of depression

- Alteration in appetite
- Sleep disturbance
- Altered psychomotor activity
- Decreased energy
- Feelings of worthlessness
- Difficulty with concentration
- Recurrent thoughts of death

Depression can be measured by the Hospital Anxiety and Depression Scale (Zigmond & Snaith 1983) or the appropriate scales from the AIMS ques-

tionnaire (Meenan et al 1980) and both are described in detail in Chapter 4.

The relationship between depression and disability

In RA, psychological factors have been shown to be more accurate predictors of subsequent disability than conventional disease activity measures (McFarlane & Brooks 1988). People with RA who had depressive symptoms performed 12% or fewer of their valued activities compared with patients with RA who were not depressed (Katz & Yelin 1994). A later study found that a loss of 10% or more of individual-valued activity was a significant predictor of late onset of depressive symptoms (Katz & Yelin 1995). It is difficult to be certain of the cause and effect relationship, but it was concluded that the severity of the RA is the causative factor, and that the limitations it imposes on lifestyle heralds the onset of depressive symptoms. However, there were individuals in the study who experienced loss of valued activities who did not develop depressive symptoms, suggesting that other factors influence the relationship between activity loss and depressive symptoms. Control mechanisms may be one such factor. Learning different control mechanisms may enable the individual to undertake activities in other ways. For example, knowledge of joint protection techniques will enable behavioural control to develop and allow household activities to be carried out with minimal discomfort.

Study of the relationships between depression and pain is difficult, as there is no clear way to ascertain if depression exacerbates pain or visa versa. In empirical studies, control of variables such as pain and depression is extremely difficult and other research methodologies such as qualitative content analysis may be useful to explore this relationship. In a qualitative study (Shaul 1995), depression was mentioned as an outcome of physical limitations and as a companion to pain and fatigue. One participant stated:

'It is a vicious cycle with rheumatoid arthritis. You feel depressed so your arthritis acts up more and the more it acts up the more depressed you get until you break it somehow'.

Previous pain and the interaction of pain and sleep disturbances have been shown to be associated with subsequent depression (Nicassio & Wallston 1992).

In RA, the apparent relationship between depression, pain and disability argues for a biopsychosocial approach to care management. Care should extend beyond the traditional approach, to embrace a genuine rehabilitation strategy where the maximisation of psychological and social functioning becomes a major treatment objective.

Chronic illness has a global impact on an individual and their significant others. Treatment of arthritis must not concentrate solely on the physical problems at the expense of the psychological manifestations. For an individual to have perceived control of their condition, all aspects of their arthritis must be considered from the patient's frame of reference. The role of the nurse must incorporate assessing the patient's perception of control from their lay beliefs, then planning or matching interventions to move the patient towards mastery and acceptance. A patient whose arthritis is suppressed by drug therapy yet has little insight into how to live with the condition, will not adapt positively. A shared approach within an holistic framework is the way forward and nurses must not miss the opportunity to enter into a meaningful therapeutic relationship with patients.

Action points for practice:

- Next time you carry out a patient assessment, include questions to illicit the control orientation of the patient. This will influence how much involvement is required of the nurse in care interventions.
- List the characteristics you would expect a patient to exhibit if they had adjusted to living with their arthritis.
- Design an information sheet for patients on self management techniques for pain control. This will influence behavioural control.
- Think about how depression is catered for in your clinical area. Provide a leaflet for colleagues informing them of how to recognise depression in their patients.

REFERENCES

Ashworth P D, Longmate M, Morrison P 1992 Patient participation: its meaning and significance in the context of caring. Journal of Advanced Nursing 17: 1430–1439

Bandura A 1977 Self-efficacy– towards unifying theory of behavioural change. Psychological Review 84(2): 191–215

Bandura A 1982 Self efficacy mechanisms in human agency. American Psychology 37: 122–147

Bandura A, Adams N E, Hardy A B, Howells G H 1980 Tests of the generality of self efficacy theory. Cognitive Therapy Research 4: 39–66

Bird C 1990 A prescription of self help. Nursing Times 86: 52–55

Broome A 1989 Health psychological processes and applications, 2nd edn. Chapman Hall, London

Buescher K L, Johnston J A, Parker J C 1991 Relationship of self efficacy to pain behaviour. Journal of Rheumatology 18: 968–972

Burish T, Carey M, Jamison R, Lyles J, Stein M, Wallston K 1984 Health locus of control and chronic disease; an external orientation may be advantageous. Journal of Social and Clinical Psychology 2: 326–332

Burckhardt C S 1985 The impact of arthritis on quality of life. Nursing Research 34: 11–16

Callahan L, Brooks R H, Pincus T 1988 Further analysis of learned helplessness in rheumatoid arthritis. Using a rheumatology attitude index. Journal of Rheumatology 15(3): 418–426

Chrisman N J 1977 The health seeking process; an approach to the natural history of illness. Culture, Medicine and Psychiatry 1: 351–377

Copper J S 1976 Living with chronic neurological disease. WW Norton, New York

Creed F, Jayson M V, Murphy S 1990 Measurement of psychiatric disorder in rheumatoid arthritis. Journal of Psychosomatic Research 34(1): 79–87

Donovan J 1991 Patient education and the consultation: the importance of lay beliefs. Annals of the Diseases 50: 418–421

Engles E W, Callahan L, Hochberg M, Pincus T 1990 Learned helplessness in systemic lupus erythematosus: using the rheumatology attitude index. Arthritis and Rheumatism 33: 281–286

Fries J F, Holman H R, Kraines R G, Spitz P 1980 Measurement of patient outcome in arthritis. Arthritis and Rheumatism 23: 137–145

Goffman E 1961. Asylums. Doubleday, New York

Hewlett S 1994 Patients' views on changing disability. Nursing Standard 8(31): 25–27

Hill J 1995 Patient education in rheumatic disease. Nursing Standard 9(25): 25–28

Hobfoll S 1989. Conservation of resources. A new attempt at conceptualising stress. American Psychology 44: 513–524

Jacobson D 1986 Types and timing of social support. Journal of Health and Social Behaviour 27: 250–264

Katz P, Yelin L H 1994 Life activities of persons with rheumatoid arthritis with and without depressive symptoms. Arthritis Care Research 7: 69–77

Katz P, Yelin L H 1995 The development of depressive symptoms among women with rheumatoid arthritis, the role of function. Arthritis and Rheumatism 38: 49–56

Klienman A, Eisenberg L, Good B 1978 Culture care and illness. Annals of Internal Medicine 88: 251–258

Krueger D W 1984 Rehabilitation Psychology. Aspin, Maryland

Langer E J 1983 The psychology of control. SAGE, California

Lazare A, Eisenthal S, Wasserman L 1975 The customer approach to patienthood. Archives of General Psychiatry 32: 553–558

Lazarus R S, Folkman S 1984 Stress appraisal and coping. Springer, New York

Lewis F M 1986 The concept of control a typology and health related variable. In: Tones K 1991. Health promotion empowerment and the psychology of control. Journal of the Institute of Health Education 29 (11): 17–25

Lorig K, Chastain R, Holman H, Shoors, Ung E 1989 The beneficial outcomes of the arthritis self management course are not adequately explained by behavioural change. Arthritis and Rheumatism 32: 91–95

McAllister G, Farquhar M 1992 Health beliefs a cultural division. Journal of Advanced Nursing 17: 1447–1454

McFarlane A C, Brookes P M 1988 Determinants of disability in arthritis. British Journal of Rheumatology 27: 7–14

Meenan R, Gertman P, Mason J 1980 Measuring health status in arthritis. Arthritis and Rheumatism 23(2): 146–152

Miller J F, 1992 Coping with chronic illness overcoming powerlessness, 2nd ed. FA Davies, London

Mishel M 1981 The meaning of uncertainty in illness. Nursing Research 30: 258–268

Moldofsky H P, Chester W J 1970 Pain and mood pattern in patients with rheumatoid arthritis. A prospective study. Psychosomatic Medicine 32: 309–318

Neufield R W J , Thomas P 1977 Effects of perceived efficacy of a prophylactic controlling mechanism on self control under pain stimulation. Canadian Journal of Behavioural Science 9: 224–232

Newman S P 1993 Coping with rheumatoid arthritis. Annals of the Rheumatic Diseases 52: 553–554

Nicassio P M, Callahan L F, Herbert M, Pincus T, Wallston KA 1985 The measurement of helplessness in rheumatoid arthritis. The development of the arthritis helplessness index. Journal of Rheumatology 12: 462–467

Nicassio P M, Wallston K A 1992 Longitudinal relationships among pain, sleep problems and depression in rheumatoid arthritis. Journal of Abnormal Psychology 101(3): 514–520

O'Leary A 1985 Self efficacy and health. Behavioural Research and Therapy 23(4): 437–451

Parker J C, Wright G E 1995 The implications of depression for pain and disability in rheumatoid arthritis. Arthritis Care and Research 8 (4): 279–283

Pigg J S, Caniff R, Driscoll P W 1985 Rheumatology nursing. A problem orientated approach. John Wiley, New York

Pitt R, Stott N C H 1983 A study of health beliefs, attitudes and behaviour among working class mothers. Department of general practice. Welsh National School of Medicine, Cardiff

Pope A M, Tarlov A R 1991 Disability in America. Towards a national agenda for prevention. National Academy Press, Washington DC

Reif L 1975 Beyond medical intervention strategies for managing life in the face of chronic illness. Davies M, Kramer M, Straiss A (eds) Nurses in practice. A perspective on work environments. Mosby, St Louis, p 261–273

Rotter J B 1966 Generalised expectancies for internal versus external control of reinforcements. Psychological Monographs 80 (1): 1–28

Rothbaum F, Snyder S, Weisz J 1982 Changing the world and changing the self. A two process model of perceived control. Journal of Personality and Social Psychology 42: 5–37

Rutter D 1993 Social psychological approaches to health. Harvest Wheatsley, London

Schunk D, Carbonaj J 1984 Self efficacy models. In: Matarazzo J (ed) Behavioural health: a hand book of health enhancement and disease prevention. John Wiley, New York

Shaul M P 1995 From early twinges to mastery: The process of adjustment in living with rheumatoid arthritis. Arthritis Care and Research 8(4): 290–297

Strecher V J, Becker M, Devills B, Rosenstock I 1986 The role of self efficacy in achieving health behaviour change. Health Education Quarterly 13(1): 73–91

Tennen H, Affleck G, Higgins P M, Mondola R, Urrows S 1992 Perceiving control, constructing benefits and daily processes in rheumatoid arthritis. Canadian Journal of Behavioural Science 24(2): 86–203

Tones K 1991 Health promotion empowerment and the psychology of control. Journal of the Institute of Health Education 29(1): 17–25

Wallston K 1993 Psychological control and its impact on the management of rheumatological disorders. Baillière's Clinical Rheumatology 7(2): 281–296

Wallston K 1995 Adaptation, coping and perceived control in persons with rheumatoid arthritis Rheumatology in Europe 2: 291–304 (suppl). Eular Publications, Switzerland

Wallerstein N, Bernstein E 1988 Empowerment education. Friere's ideas adapted to health education. Health Education Quarterly 15(4): 379–394

Wiener C L 1975 The burden of rheumatoid arthritis – tolerating the uncertainty. Social Science and Medicine 9: 97–104

Weinstein N D 1982 Unrealistic optimism about future life events. Journal of Personality and Social Psychology 39: 806–20

Zigmond A, Snaith R P 1983 The hospital anxiety and depression scale. Psychiatry Scandinavian 67: 361–370

FURTHER READING

Ajzen I, Fishbein M 1980 Understanding attitudes and predicting social behaviour. Prentice Hall, Englewood Cliffs NJ

Laborde J M, Powers M J 1985 Life satisfaction, health control, orientation and illness related factors in persons with osteoarthritis. Research in Nursing and Health 8: 183–190

GLOSSARY

* *Control*
  The individual believes that they can affect their own outcome.
* *Locus of control*
  The place where control resides, for example:
  Internal locus of control is where a person believes that their own actions can influence events.
  External locus of control is where a person believes that events are not within individual control but are governed by chance, fate or other people.
* *Learned helplessness*
  The individual does not believe that his or her own actions will influence events due to past unsuccessful experiences to influence outcomes.
* *Health belief model*
  Here behaviour is dependent on the value an individual places on the outcome of engaging in a particular behaviour.

6

Body image and sexuality

Jackie Prady, Angela Vale, Juliet Hill

The aim of this chapter is to provide an insight into the effects that rheumatic disease has on body image and the expression of sexuality in all its dimensions. Although it aims to dispel the view that sexuality is solely the physical act of sexual intercourse, issues such as comfortable sexual intercourse, parenting and contraception are discussed. After reading this chapter you should be able to:

- **Describe the complex nature of sexuality**
- **Discuss the effects of altered body image on the expression of sexuality**
- **Discuss why sexuality is an aspect of patient care that is often neglected by nurses**
- **Interpret how your personal values, background and beliefs influence your ability to address this emotive aspect of patient care**
- **Discuss practical aspects of sexual intercourse with patients**
- **Summarise the methods of contraception available to the rheumatic patient and their partner**
- **Outline the problems of pregnancy and parenting.**

Sexuality is more than just the act of sexual intercourse and much more than people's genitalia. It is an integral part of the whole person. People are sexual in every way all of the time, and to a large extent, our sexuality determines who we are and is an integral factor in the uniqueness of every person (Savage 1990, Stuart & Sundeen 1979). Hogan (1980) considers that sexuality is the quality of being human, all that we are as men and women encompassing the most intimate of feelings and the deepest longings of the heart to find meaningful relationships.

Jones (1994) has stated that an individual's expression of sexuality is influenced by a number of factors including their:

- Background
- Accumulated life experiences
- Values of the society in which they have been brought up
- Their attitudes, personality and views
- The attitude of others.

BODY IMAGE

Society largely determines what is 'normal' and this picture of normality will be the only one that is accepted by many (Drench 1994). Our society is preoccupied with physical attractiveness. Emphasis placed on physical beauty and perfection predisposes the disabled or disfigured person to stigmatisation (Chandani et al 1989). This may effect not only how the individual is viewed by society, but also how the individual views themselves and their perceptions of the way in which others view them.

Jones (1994) suggests that body image has three aspects:

1. The body ideal – what we aspire to. This is strongly influenced by the society in which we live and the cultures within that society, all forms of media and within that context, what we personally want to reflect to others.
2. The body reality – what nature actually gave us.
3. Body presentation – how we choose to present our body to the rest of society. It is the way that we express our individuality.

Body image is a very vulnerable part of our make-up (Price 1990). Illness or injury that distorts the body structure may alter the individual's image of the body. It may also interfere with the entire self image including interrupting social and vocational roles that may ultimately affect the individual's self esteem (Webb 1985, Drench 1994).

Self concept

Self concept develops as part of our personality and results from how we think that others view us. It involves notions about femininity, masculinity, physical prowess, endurance and capabilities (Drench 1994). Body image is closely linked to self concept as it is the part that involves attitudes and experiences pertaining to the body.

Self esteem

Self esteem is how a person values himself or herself. The loss of a job that afforded status can alter a person's perception of the way that others value them and how they value themselves. Self esteem combined with self worth is the basis from which man functions. If people feel well, they feel positive about themselves. They have the energy to invest in life and in relationships, and give the impression of health and vigour to other people, who may see them as attractive and worthwhile. However, the impression given may be radically altered for a person experiencing the effects of a progressive degenerative disease such as RA (Webb 1985, Webb 1987).

SEXUALITY IN HEALTH CARE

In 1975 the World Health Organisation identified the need for sexuality to be included in health care. It saw three basic elements in the concept of sexual health:

1. The capacity to enjoy and control sexual and reproductive behaviour in accordance with social and personal ethics.
2. Freedom from fear, shame, guilt, misconceptions and other psychological factors that inhibit sexual response and impair sexual relationships.
3. Freedom from organic disorders, diseases and deficiencies that may interfere with either sexual or reproductive function or both.

Judged by these criteria, all aspects of sexuality should be a basic human right for every individual regardless of their abilities, disabilities and state of health. In reality, practice in health care frequently falls short of the WHO criteria and sexuality and sexual problems are not dealt with as well as they should be in many areas.

Roper, Logan and Tierney (1980) included the expression of sexuality as one of the activities of daily living in their model of nursing care. They also noted that although doctors and nurses were beginning to acknowledge that illness and hospitalisation could cause sex-related problems, they were still reticent about discussing them openly with patients. Patients with RA often experienced marital and sexual problems, but were frequently left to deal with them by themselves, receiving very little help from professional health care workers (Smith 1994). Many factors may contribute to this lack of sexual support and these include:

- The personal views and bias of medical and nursing staff

- The belief systems of the patients
- Society's views of sex, sexuality and disabled people
- Lack of counselling skills amongst healthcare professionals
- Practical and organisational difficulties.

Despite this apparent recognition by some caring professionals, sexuality is still a neglected subject (Savage 1989, Smith 1994). In 1994 Smith pointed out that since her previous research in 1981, little or no progress has been made. Nurses are still avoiding the topic of sexuality and are not helping their patients to overcome the problem of the impact of disability on their expression of their sexuality.

It has been suggested that one reason why some nurses do not broach the subject of sexuality with their patients is because they feel vulnerable and potentially at risk of sexual harassment (Lawler 1991). The image of female nurses as 'golden-hearted sex objects' and male nurses as 'homosexuals' (Savage 1989) which is sometimes portrayed by the media is unhelpful.

However, nurses should be providing holistic care for their patients and it could be argued that by neglecting the area of sexuality they are in breach of their Code of Professional Conduct as set out by the United Kingdom Central Council (1992). This clearly states that all nurses should at all times 'safeguard and promote the interests of individual patients and clients'.

Male and female sexuality

The dominant Victorian medical view was that women did not need or enjoy sexual activity. The majority of women were not very much troubled with sexual feelings and to have intercourse with their husbands was an act of duty rather than one of pleasure. Even by the late 1970s, it was suggested that evidence concerning the nature of female sexuality had made very little impact on medical ideology and practice. For many doctors, the basic paradigm for understanding the sexual nature of women was a crude and often distorted Freudian model (Doyal & Pennell 1979). According to Williams and Wood (1982), the literature indicates that disability has a greater impact on the sexuality of men than of women. However, they believe that this is a reflection of covert sexism on the part of a number of the investigators and highlight this by a quote from the literature:

'In the female, the problem of sex has not been studied as extensively as in the man. In a woman the problem is not so traumatic. She plays a passive role in sexual relations usually' (Singh & Magner 1975).

This encapsulates the attitude that reduces sex and sexuality to the act of intercourse, excluding important factors such as childbirth, gestation and menstruation.

Overall, fertility, the coital act and the physical attributes that are associated with 'having sex' have largely defined female sexuality.

Sex and disability

Disabled people tend to be perceived by the general public to be 'asexual', and their need for sexual fulfilment regarded as inappropriate, or even unthinkable (Hahn 1981). Work carried out in the 1980s suggested that this belief was also held by many caring professionals who were excessively puritanical in their outlook. The majority tended to give no consideration to the sexual needs of their clients. However, it was noted that while during the preceding decade there had been some improvement and the sexual needs and difficulties of the disabled were being given some attention, there were still many exceptions (Carolan 1984a).

Dawson-Shepherd, a disabled person herself, acknowledged in 1984 the beginning of an increased awareness that sexuality did exist despite disability. This must have been encouraging, as disabled people need to be given choices, opportunities and support in this most fundamentally important aspect of their lives (Carolan 1984a).

Attitudes

For a person to be aware of another's sexuality, they must be aware of and recognise their own sexuality (Savage 1990). It is important for nurses to explore their own attitudes, as those who have never considered their own sexuality are unlikely to realise that their patients may experience problems with theirs. In this event they may not even consider that disability and disease have any bearing on the expression of sexuality (Jones 1994). Some nurses have preconceived ideas in relation to their patient's ability, desire and need for sexual fulfilment.

The attitude of others within the disabled community is also a factor that either enables patients to discuss their own sexual problems or feel that they should be hidden. Nurses and society at large often have negative attitudes towards older people and their sexuality, dismissing the idea that older people ever had or still do have a sex life (Webb 1987, Jones 1994). Although sexual functioning usually diminishes with age, sexuality remains important to many older people (Jones 1994).

The sexual orientation or preference of the patient is an issue that creates problems for some health professionals, usually due to their own belief systems. Sexual orientation refers to an individual's tastes or preferences in sexual partners. This can be:

- Heterosexual – preference for a partner of the opposite sex, ('hetero' meaning different)
- Homosexual – preference for a partner of the same sex ('homo' meaning same)
- Bisexual – a choice of both kinds of partner, although there may be a preference for one or the other (Gross 1992).

A person's sexual preference should be respected and nursing and medical staff need to be able to discuss these issues with the patient in a professional and non-judgmental manner.

To do this effectively nurses need to recognise their own personal values and attitudes if they are to help patients overcome problems with their sexuality.

It is also important to be aware of the social and cultural influences that effect their own and their patients' sexuality (Savage 1989). For example, some religions not only continue to ban contraception and homosexuality, but also consider some positions for coitus to be abnormal (Webb 1985, Jones 1994).

Society today is supposedly more sexually aware. However, even in this enlightened age sex remains a taboo subject. Nurses have an important role in indicating to patients that sex is not taboo (Smith 1994). Annon (1976) addresses this in his model and suggests that when nurses give information regarding sexuality the delivery is as important as the content. All information should be accurate and be delivered in a sensitive manner (Smith 1994).

If nurses are to help patients, it is important that they enter the client's 'frame of reference'. Everyone views the world in a unique way, and it is therefore vital that nurses try to see the world, their body image and their sexuality as the patient does, non-judgmentally and without moralising even if it does not comply with their own personal bias and belief systems.

NURSE EDUCATION

In order to deal adequately with the problems arising from sexuality, nurses must be:

- Intuitive
- Open minded
- Aware of their own feelings.

However in addition to this they require a high standard of knowledge and an awareness of organisations that are able to help with any problems that the client may encounter. This can only be achieved by educating nurses to enable them to deal with these issues. However, there is not a long tradition of nurses as counsellors, nor do nurses necessarily see themselves as fitting into this role. They appear to feel far more able to give information and advice than to handle feelings and confrontation (Burnard 1992). Sexual counselling is a very specialised area, and nurses cannot be expected to carry it out without further education and proper training. Whilst nurse education acknowledges the unease that may be experienced by patients, little attention is paid to the unease experienced by nurses who deal with the most intimate aspects of patient care (Savage 1989). This unease may even lead them to avoid the patient altogether. In general, nurses are not taught how to help patients with their sexuality and as a result may experience discomfort and embarrassment when confronted with a patient expressing their problems (Andrew & Andrew 1991).

CONFIDENTIALITY

Privacy is a rare commodity in the busy hospital environment, but if patients are to share intimate details they must be treated as individuals with dignity and respect; therefore privacy is paramount. Privacy can be a particular problem in the ward area but confidentiality is extremely important. Time and a private place should be made available for patients to talk openly with no fear of being overheard by other patients, staff or visitors.

For those seen in outpatient clinics, privacy may be easier to achieve but these patients are often seen by a different professional at each consultation which makes the subject more difficult for the patient to broach. A clinical nurse specialist practising from a private consultation room and who builds a rapport with patients through continuity of care, should feel able to discuss the topic of sexuality as part of the package of care.

PATIENT EDUCATION

Sexual education is a delicate subject and needs to be dealt with sensitively and with discretion. Information should be given to the patient when they ask for it as most people find it difficult to discuss the intimate details of their sexual lives. If the request is ignored they may not feel able to broach the subject again. From the professional viewpoint, information on sexuality should be an accepted part of the care package.

Patients who do not seek information should be offered it when the nurse feels that the time is right for the patient and themselves. This can be done as part of routine activities, for instance when carrying out an articular index (Hill 1991). If the hips, hands or knees are painful on movement or to pressure it is natural to ask 'does this cause you a problem when you make love?' During an explanation of Sjögren's syndrome it is easy to mention that it can cause the vagina to become dry which can naturally lead to the question 'have you found this at all?' If the answer is yes then it should be followed up by asking if it causes a problem with love making. These types of question tell the patient that the nurse is happy to discuss the topic without placing any undue pressure on the patient.

Another important aspect is to assess whether to involve the patient's partner and if so, whether the nurse has the knowledge to cope with counselling or teaching two people. Nurses should recognise that if they do not feel knowledgeable, comfortable or capable of offering advice they can suggest to the patient that they could be referred to somebody more qualified to deal with their problem (Glover 1982).

Other sources of information

It is very important that nurses are aware of the:

- Boundaries of their knowledge
- The scope of their abilities
- How and where to get backup for themselves and their patients.

Further advice and written information is available from the Association to Aid Sexual and Personal Relationships of the Disabled (SPOD). SPOD was set up in 1973 by the National Fund for Research into Crippling Diseases in order to study and advise on sexual problems experienced by disabled people in the United Kingdom (Carolan 1984b). They supply a wide range of literature and advisory leaflets on all aspects of sexuality. The Arthritis and Rheumatism Council (ARC) and Arthritis Care also produce leaflets that cover many aspects of arthritis, including problems related to body image, sexuality and parenting.

This material should be readily available on wards and in outpatient clinics. Information in this form may be all that the patient requires and further intervention by the nurse may not be necessary. However, the nurse needs to be familiar with the effect that illness and disability may have on the patient's sexuality and watch for verbal and non verbal signals that indicate the patient may require additional help.

ASSESSMENT

The sections on the nursing assessment sheet relating to patients' expression of sexuality are often left blank, or read 'likes to wear make-up' or 'shaves on alternate days'. However, Roper et al (1980) have urged the assessor to seek the answers to the following questions:

- How does he/she express sexuality?
- What factors influence his/her expression of sexuality?
- What does he/she know about expressing sexuality?
- What does he/she feel about expressing sexuality?
- What difficulties does he/she have in expressing sexuality?

When asked about expressing sexuality, most people think directly of the sexual act or acts, and this may be an entirely inappropriate concern for a person who is ill. As the expression of human sexuality and body image are virtually inseparable, in health and illness (Price 1990), it may also be appropriate to include questions regarding:

- How the patient sees their own body image
- How their disease has affected their image of themselves
- How their disease has affected their quality of life.

The timing of assessments

Smith (1994) suggests that sexuality should be treated like any other problem and should be addressed as part of a routine assessment on ward admission. However, this may not be the most appropriate time. The patient may not have had enough time to develop a relationship with the nurse to the point where they feel that they can put their trust in him/her. Annon (1976) who has devised a model for helping people with sexual difficulties acknowledges this. People often feel embarrassed about their sexual problems and may need permission to ventilate their feelings and worries. He suggests that the patient will need time and evidence that the nurse is willing to listen and suggests that the subject should be raised when it is felt appropriate, which may be later on in the admission. If the nurse raises the subject of the patient's sexuality too early, the patient may feel under pressure to answer questions that cause them a great deal of embarrassment.

Unfortunately, many patients will only express their problem when it has reached crisis point (Smith 1994). This is particularly so of those with rheumatic disease, who tend to be exceptionally stoical and uncomplaining. Many patients come into hospital with a 'flare' in their arthritis and are in a state of crisis. They are at their lowest ebb and their sexual problems and body image are generally low on their agenda, their primary concern being the pain of the 'flare'. This is illustrated by Maslow's hierarchy of need (Maslow 1970). In this theory Maslow asserts that basic needs must be met before the person can consider satisfying their less essential wants (Fig. 6.1). Only when the symptoms of the flare subside and they are able to mobilise and carry out basic activities of daily living do other problems take precedence. They begin to think about their experience and worry about issues such as:

- What caused the flare?
- Will I be able to cope with relationships?
- Will I manage financially?
- How will my family cope?
- Will I manage on a day to day basis with my disabilities?
- Will my joints become disfigured?
- What will I look like?
- Will other people find me attractive?

Patients often feel depressed even if they are not actually clinically depressed, they are often low in mood, tearful and in need of support and help. It is therefore important that the nurse is sensitive to the patient's difficulties in expressing their feelings and to the delicacy of the subject. Patients who are met by a judgmental attitude or embarrassment on the part of the nurse, are unlikely to raise the subject again (Smith 1994).

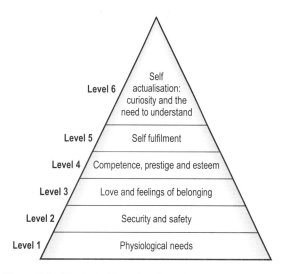

Figure 6.1 Maslow's hierarchy of needs.

THE EFFECTS OF RHEUMATIC DISEASE

Effects on relationships

Smith (1994) suggests that most problems tend to occur if the arthritis develops after the relationship has started, indicating that when the arthritis is there from the start, both partners may know what they potentially have to cope with. Even so, because of the unpredictability of RA some problems may not have been anticipated and once RA has taken a significant hold on the patient, the impact is intense (Le Gallez 1993). This study highlighted a number of indicators that influence the outcome of relationships, including:

- The patient's ability to adjust to the disease
- Their acceptance of the physical limitations that it imposed
- The amount of support that the partner was prepared to give
- The partner's acknowledgement of the existence of the patient's disease.

Locker (1983) pointed out that even when support and care is given willingly, problems may still occur. This is more likely to happen if the patient has previously been proud of their independence and been care giver rather than care receiver.

Le Gallez (1993) found that both the women and the men adjusted reasonably easily to their role of care giver. However, problems sometimes occurred when men were in need of care. Some were unable to accept this and saw it as a threat to their perceived role as head of the family. Ultimately, their ego was damaged which resulted in a loss of self esteem.

A job gives a person status and feelings of self worth and can raise self esteem. It may also influence how a person considers others value him in society (Webb 1987, Savage 1987). There is the suggestion that present day society values only those who can contribute to the economy and without a job people become classless (Jones 1994). The disabling nature of the more serious rheumatic diseases often results in the patient having to change their job and it is not uncommon for a patient to give up work completely within ten years of developing the disease (Chesson 1984). Women appear to adjust more easily to stopping work than men, many of whom express fears of uselessness and feelings of inadequacy if they have to cease paid employment (Le Gallez 1993).

If there are work related problems, the Redeployment Officer (RDO) may be able to help. After referral to the social work department, the RDO can visit patients in hospital or the patient can visit the RDO in their local job centre. Although it may not prove possible to find suitable alternative employment in the same field, if their present employment is causing damage to their joints a change in career may help the patient's condition.

If the disease progresses additional problems may be encountered. The well partner may also have to alter their working pattern or stop work altogether in order to take on the responsibilities of the home (Le Gallez 1993). This renders them both 'classless' in the eye of society and can ultimately erode the self esteem of both the patient and the carer. Total dependence on their partner may mean that the patient has not only got to come to terms with being a burden to someone else, but the consequences of their illness is seriously affecting the quality of their partner's life (Locker 1983). Many marriages break down under the strain of one partner becoming totally dependent on the other, most commonly when the wife has become disabled. There is evidence that for men it is not the care, but the housekeeping and caring for the children that causes the majority of problems as these are not considered part of the natural role of the male (Greengross 1976, Le Gallez 1993). Whatever their gender, the patient's self esteem is likely to be affected when they realise that they are unable to contribute to the running of the home or to achieve even the simplest of goals due to their disabilities (Chesson 1984, Smith 1994).

Case study 6.1   Alteration in body image for a wife and mother

Mrs White is a 35-year-old woman who has a clear picture of her own body image and sexuality. She has a husband, three small children and a job. She loves clothes, jewellery especially rings, and enjoys cooking and entertaining and is happy with her life. She wakes one day with pain and swelling in the smaller joints of her feet and hands. She ignores them and hopes they will go away. They do not, so she goes to her doctor who diagnoses her as having rheumatoid arthritis and refers her to a consultant rheumatologist, but the appointment is a number of months hence. Within weeks the pain gets worse and the joints swell. Work, family relationships, cleaning and keeping the home tidy, cooking and all aspects of daily life, including sexual intercourse become more difficult and anxiety sets in. A new way of life starts and an alteration in body image begins.

Social implications

Many patients tell nurses that they have not been out of their own home environment for months. Some

have not managed to either go upstairs or downstairs and have altered their way of life to accommodate their disabilities. Many no longer have the hobbies that they had prior to their rheumatic disease, gardening, dancing, socialising; even reading a book can become difficult because they cannot hold it. For some, their medications prevent them taking alcohol, so men who have previously had social contact in the 'pub' can become isolated. This can have an impact on self esteem.

It can be argued that social limitations could be due to the disease or the change in body image. In practice it is likely to be a combination of the two. A damaged body image can significantly harm a person's whole identity. However, when reality can no longer be denied depression associated with loss and grief frequently occurs (Drench 1994). Depression can lead to the loss of energy and lack of motivation. When this is in addition to the pain and fatigue commonly experienced in rheumatic disease the cumulative effect can result in avoidance of social activities. Cohen (1991) suggests that patients with chronic illness or disability tend to 'withdraw from life', breaking off contact with friends and show less interest in going out or entertaining. This can lead to increasing isolation, which makes it difficult for the patient to develop new relationships. Existing friendships may also be threatened as other people may find it difficult to cope with their newly, or progressively worsening disabled friend. Although for most patients some sort of social activity will be possible, their pain, exhaustion and discomfort may hinder enjoyment. They may also be conscious of restricting what should be an enjoyable time for their friends and families and avoid activities of which they are capable, resulting in further isolation (Lee & Moll 1987). Patients with rheumatoid disease are often unable to make plans for the week ahead as they never know when a flare will occur. They may make plans and then 'let friends down' because of their pain and stiffness. Constant pain is an extremely demotivating and depressing condition for both the sufferer and their friends.

Dining out also has its difficulties. Many patients feel embarrassed eating in restaurants because they have difficulty holding cutlery and people stare and may even comment. Rheumatoid patients do not need pity; they need understanding and help to maintain their own independence and dignity.

EXPRESSING SEXUALITY

It is acknowledged that a chronic disabling condition, such as rheumatoid arthritis, may result in the patient experiencing a decrease in sexual desire and ability to express sexual love through bodily movement (Cochrane 1984, Smith 1994). This can be due to:

• Reduced mobility
• Lack of manual dexterity
• Pain and discomfort
• Reduced general well-being.

There may also be a great deal of uncertainty as to the future and because of this the patient may experience anxiety, fear and depression all of which contribute to the lack of desire. Loss of independence may result in a change in role for both the patient and their partner, which may affect how they view one another sexually. For example, a wife who takes on the role of care giver may no longer view herself as a wife and lover (Webb 1987).

Personal appearance

The patient's self esteem can be affected if deformities alter their body causing worries that others will no longer find them attractive (Smith 1994). RA commonly affects the small joints of the hand. If the patient's condition deteriorates, the hands can become deformed and holding small objects such as a make-up brush becomes impossible. For those wishing to wear make-up this can be a devastating blow and the help of the occupational therapist should be sought to find ways of overcoming the difficulty. If patients are unable to present themselves to society in the way that they feel most comfortable it affects their confidence and self worth leading to feelings of low self esteem (Smith 1994).

RA is an extremely cruel disease and also a very 'open' one. It is there for the whole world to see. Ulnar deviation can make holding cutlery difficult, so eating out can become embarrassing. The hands are always on show, even when holding a conversation; for most people they are an aid to speech. Osteoarthritis (OA) of the knees causes varus or valgus deformities and muscle wasting which many find visually distressing. Patients can overcome these problems by wearing long skirts or trousers.

Physical body changes may be met by strong resistance, especially when they devalue self esteem. The patient may try to remain 'normal' and maintain an unchanged lifestyle. For example, they may refuse to wear resting splints on their wrists and hands because they consider them unsightly and they draw attention to their illness. The result can be more wear and tear on the joints and ultimately more deformity and loss of function.

The psychological impact of rheumatic disease on the young must not be disregarded. This may be more severe for those who are first afflicted in their teens than those whose disease starts at an earlier age as very young children tend to accept disability. However, adolescents and older teenagers may experience particular difficulties in establishing a satisfactory self image, believing themselves to be unattractive, unlikely to find a sexual partner and likely to be unable to express physical love as they would wish. The nurse should be aware of this and pay particular attention to this group.

Touch

Although they may not wish to or may not be able to have sexual intercourse, there is often an increase in the need for love, reassurance and physical closeness for both the patient and their partner. The patient may worry that they will not be able to demonstrate this because of the symptoms of their disease (Chesson 1984). The patient's partner may be inhibited from showing any physical love by the anxiety of causing their loved one pain (Smith 1994). For the patient, even a hug may be too painful to give or to receive. The action of hugging may be impossible to perform because of joint stiffness or disorganisation of the shoulder or elbow joints, reducing movement. Kissing may be a painful experience if the temporomandibular joints are affected (Cochrane 1984). Potentially, anticipation of pain may colour entirely pain-free periods of the patient's life, for both the patient and their partner resulting in even strong emotional bonds weakening under the stress (Lee & Moll 1987, Cochrane 1984, Smith 1994).

The hands are an important, if not the ultimate tool of touch. Patients with hand involvement will be less inclined to touch their partner and less willing to be touched themselves. When the small joints are swollen and painful, even holding hands can be traumatic. Therapeutic touch can be used to the benefit of many patients, especially if they are disfigured, alone and lacking human contact. Massage helps to overcome problems of body image (see Ch. 13). Touching is a natural and literal reaching out of one human being to another, but some cultures find it difficult to show their warmth through touch. The problem with touch is circular. When there is little physical touching in a culture it begins to take on a mysterious connotation and hence it is mistrusted and little used. Yet when touching occurs it is usually experienced as perfectly natural and not at all discontinuous with the flow of communication between those involved (Mearns & Thorne 1988).

Sexual intercourse

For some patients the act of sexual intercourse can be painful and physically difficult. This may be due to psychological problems that are addressed elsewhere in the chapter, or the physical problems that arise from rheumatic diseases. These include:

- Joint or muscle pain
- Joint stiffness
- Reduced range of movement
- Fatigue
- Anaemia
- Loss of tactile sensation
- Dry vagina due to Sjögren's syndrome
- Drug therapy
- Reduction in libido.

When we then add the psychological problems, the list appears endless. However, it should not be assumed that people with rheumatic disease are unable to have pleasurable sexual intercourse. Many patients have no problems at all and even those with the most severe disability can overcome difficulties. As is the ethos of nursing, each patient should be treated as an individual.

Providing practical verbal and written advice can help patients and their partners to enjoy sexual intercourse and it also gives them the 'permission' to try different techniques that many seek.

Planning sexual intercourse

Although spontaneous unplanned intercourse is often pleasurable, the limitations caused by disease symptoms may mean that the time that intercourse takes place needs to be planned. At first sight this seems cold and calculating, but it should be viewed in a positive light. Patients and their partners should be reminded that the anticipation of planning ahead could heighten rather than diminish their pleasure!

Although many people have intercourse either last thing at night or on waking in the morning, these are not always the best times for someone with a disease such as RA. The joints are often less mobile and stiff in the morning, and by the end of the day patients can be very fatigued. The middle of the day tends to be favoured by many.

If pain is a problem, planning intercourse when non-steroidal anti-inflammatory drugs are at their most effective can be helpful. Alternatively, an analgesic taken about half an hour before intercourse reduces pain.

Some limbering up exercises followed by a warm shower or bath that will also help the patient to relax can relieve joint stiffness. Gentle massage can act as a form of pain relief and this can be incorporated into foreplay and be pleasurable for both patient and partner.

Positioning

There are many positions in which intercourse is possible and no matter which joints are affected there is usually at least one that couples find pleasurable. The conventional position in which the man lays on top and the woman is underneath with her legs spread may not be suitable for someone with arthritis. For instance if the woman is the patient and has hip involvement which prohibits abduction a side-lying (Fig. 6.2a) or standing (Fig. 6.2b) position may be more suitable. If the male has shoulder or elbow involvement he may be better lying on his back with his partner sitting or lying over him (Fig. 6.2c). Painful joints or those with reduced or fixed range of movement may need to be supported by pillows or cushions.

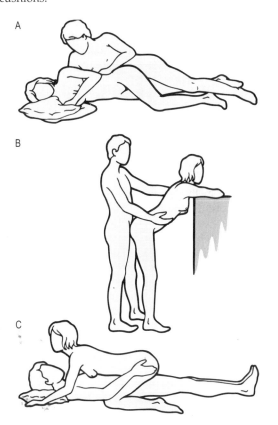

Figure 6.2 Alternative positions for sexual intercourse. (A) Side lying position. (B) Standing position. (C) Woman on top.

A number of patients undergo prosthetic surgery of the hip (see Ch. 14) and need advice regarding when and how sexual intercourse can be resumed. Genital intercourse is not usually recommended during the first six weeks post operatively. Cochrane (1984) recommends that the side-lying position is adopted for the following six weeks as this will avoid the adduction and internal rotation of the prosthesis and so avoid dislocation.

Sex aids

Not everyone feels comfortable with the idea of using sex aids, but for those who do they can be a valuable asset to foreplay. Vibrators can give pleasure to both the disabled and able bodied partner. They are particularly helpful for those with impaired, painful hands.

Vibrators are available in a wide variety of shapes, sizes and powers and can be useful for increasing stimulation of the:

- Penis
- Vagina
- Clitoris.

SPOD produces a catalogue of sex aids and simply offering this to a patient may make them feel that using mechanical sexual stimulation is both permissible and acceptable.

Sexual satisfaction does not necessarily rely on penetration. Other ways of giving and receiving sexual pleasure include:

- Kissing and cuddling
- Oral sex
- Masturbation.

Even these methods can cause discomfort. Oral sex may be painful if the patient has temporomandibular involvement or unpleasant with the reduced salivary production of Sjögren's syndrome. Masturbation may prove difficult if they have reduced manual dexterity. Although masturbation can provide a satisfying alternative or addition to sexual intercourse, it attracts more than its fair share of taboos, myths and smutty jokes. Patients need to be made aware that it is an acceptable and harmless form of sexual pleasure.

Vaginal dryness

Vaginal dryness can cause painful intercourse for both the woman and her male partner. A secondary condition that often occurs in rheumatoid arthritis is Sjögren's. Venables (1985) describes this syndrome as a group of diseases characterised by common pathological features, namely:

- Inflammation
- Destruction of exocrine glands.

The salivary and lachrymal glands are principally involved giving rise to dry eyes and a dry mouth, though other exocrine glands including those of the pancreas, sweat glands and mucus secreting glands of the bowel, bronchial tree and vagina may be affected. Although many patients are given artificial tear eye drops and artificial saliva sprays, very few women with RA are given any advice regarding their vaginal dryness. Lubricants such as KY jelly are available from pharmacies and their use can ensure painless sexual intercourse. The use of oils and other lotions are not recommended as they may give rise to infection.

It is generally assumed that people know how to get help or can actually 'work things out' for themselves. This is not always the case and nurses should not shy away from their responsibilities in the area of providing practical sexual advice, or if they do not have confidence in their abilities, make sure that patients are referred to another professional.

Drugs and sexual intercourse

Some drugs are known to have an effect on sexual function (Table 6.1) but this varies from person to person and is also dose dependent. Those listed do not always induce sexual dysfunction, sometimes they can cure it. For example, lack of arousal in the clinically depressed patient is sometimes resolved by the introduction of tricyclic antidepressants, on the other hand these drugs can also induce problems.

If particular drugs are necessary to the patient, it may not be possible to eliminate the side effects. In these cases the nurse should discuss the side effects with the patient and suggest alternative ways of love and giving and receiving sexual pleasure.

PARENTING

It is not only the patient's isolation that is a problem when developing relationships and expressing sexuality, but the attitudes of the general public towards disabled people and their sexuality. Sexual fulfilment for a disabled person is not always considered appropriate and for some of the general public, the concept of a disabled person being a parent may be hard to accept. Problems in relation to parenting begin in pregnancy, often created by the responses of others who assume that disability and pregnancy do not go together and the ability of a disabled person to become a parent is often questioned (Campling 1981, Hahn 1981).

Table 6.1   Drugs that affect sexual function

Drug	Effect on:		
	Desire	Arousal	Orgasm
Alcohol	Initially increased, later reduced	Reduced	Much reduced
Analgesics			
Opiates	Reduced	Reduced	Reduced
Non opiates	Reduced	Reduced	Retarded ejaculation
Antihypertensives			Failure or retrograde ejaculation
Anticholinergics	Often reduced	Erectile impotence	Reduced
Antidepressants	Often reduced	Reduced	Reduced MAOIs give retarded ejaculation
Antihistamines	Often reduced	Reduced lubrication	
Beta blockers	Reduced	Erectile impotence	
Cimetidine		Some erectile dysfunction	
Diuretics		Erectile impotence common, some reduction of lubrication	
Hormones			
Contraceptive pill	Variable	Variable	Variable
Androgen	Raised (in androgen-deficient male – rare)	Raised (in androgen-deficient male – rare)	Raised
Oestrogen		Increased vaginal lubrication in oestrogen-deficient female	
Anti-androgens		Reduces both desire and performance in nearly all cases	
Tranquilizers			
Minor (benzodiazepines)	Reduced	Reduced	Reduced
Major (phenothiazides)	Reduced	Delayed ejaculation in male	Reduced

When contemplating parenthood, a person with systemic rheumatic disease has to take into account his or her ability to care for children (Cochrane 1984). Some problems that may be encountered have already been described in relation to any loving relationship that involves hugging and cuddles as a demonstration of love. The progressive nature of a disease such as RA can be inhibiting. The mother may encounter difficulties caring for her child and may have to give up her role as carer if her disabilities increase. This may lead to a great deal of emotional distress for both the mother and the child, especially if the child is too young to understand. It is not only the mother who experiences problems in parenting; for men with rheumatic disease fulfilling a parental role can also problematic (Box 6.2). They may be unable to share in activities with their children and have to hand over their parental role to someone else, possibly leading to them experience loss of self esteem and self worth (Locker 1983). Family dynamics are changed and illness may result in the patient being unable to fulfil their usual role. Other family members may have to take on additional responsibilities and the patient's need for rest imposes limitations on other family members (Blau & Blau 1991).

Case study 6.2   The middle-aged husband and father

Jim is a 50-year-old man, ex-Navy, with a previously well paid job. He has a wife and two sons, one 21 and the other 19. He developed RA and it was acutely progressive, requiring many joint replacements and a series of medications that did not control the illness. He felt that he was unable to do the things that other fathers did with their sons who were avid sports players. A trip to the 'pub' meant lemonade because of his medications. The idea of being a grandparent and being able to play with small children was impossible for Jim to reconcile. He feels deeply hurt at not being able to be, in his opinion, a true father to his sons and a true husband to his wife.

This is an extreme example, but anybody who has nursed rheumatoid patients can probably identify with any number of their patients either male or female.

There are multitudes of factors that may influence a patient's decision to get married and have children. For example, it is commonly believed that RA is hereditary and patients fear that the disease will be passed to their offspring. In fact, the risks are just as great for children of healthy parents as for those with parents who have RA (Cochrane 1984, Smith 1994).

As well as being able physically to care for their children, the patient also has to consider whether they will be able to support their family financially, especially in view of the possibility that both partners may be unable to work in the future (Cochrane 1984). The patient might worry that their children may suffer as a result of them having a disabled parent. However, there is little researched evidence to support this view. Le Gallez (1993) found that for 75% of the children in her study, the effect had been far from detrimental and that living with a sick parent had brought them closer together as a family. Even so, 25% of the children in the study expressed resentment, anger and guilt, all of which was directed at the sick parent.

Pregnancy and arthritis

For those who decide they want a child and who take drugs for their arthritis, it is essential for the safety of the foetus that they plan their pregnancy. Some drugs are teratogenic (Le Gallez 1988) and others such as methotrexate, which is given for RA, psoriatic arthritis and myositis, needs to be stopped a number of months prior to conception (see Table 12.3). Low to moderate doses of corticosteroids are generally safe and effective.

When managing pregnant patients with rheumatic diseases, it is especially important to individualise their drug therapy with careful assessment of the disease activity, severity and risk to the foetus (Soscia & Zurier 1992).

Pregnant women with arthritis may undergo additional difficulties compared to healthy women. They may experience more backache if they have ankylosing spondylitis or exacerbated pain in the knees and ankles as they gain weight. However for those with RA, pregnancy can bring welcome but temporary relief from their symptoms. This phenomenon was described by Hench in 1949. He remarked that during pregnancy RA 'finds it difficult to progress, or indeed to do otherwise than beat a hasty retreat'. Unfortunately the symptoms return within 8 months of giving birth and the nurse should ensure that the parents are aware of this. Although the majority of rheumatic diseases pose no threat to the unborn child, conception is unwise during active phases of systemic lupus erythematosus.

Antenatal aspects

Fatigue is quite normal during pregnancy but for women with rheumatic disease who already suffer from fatigue the effect is additive. Extra rest is important and teaching the principles of energy conservation should be a priority. Tiredness may also be brought about by the anaemia that often accompanies RA and iron and vitamin supplements will need to be taken.

A healthy diet is important to rheumatic patients (see Ch. 10) but this is particularly so during pregnancy. About 300 extra calories a day are needed during pregnancy and 500 extra calories are required during lactation (Richardson 1992). It is important to advise the patient that excess weight post partum will cause extra stress on already damaged lower limbs and so this needs to be avoided.

The birth

Rheumatic diseases do not usually pose significant problems during labour or at delivery. Sometimes involvement of the hips means that the woman has difficulty or is unable to abduct her hips to give birth vaginally. The anaesthetist may encounter difficulty administering spinal anaesthetics to those patients with spinal problems. If a general anaesthetic is required patients with RA who have cervical spine involvement should wear a cervical collar to prevent hyperextension causing injury to the spinal cord.

Caring for the child

Caring for babies and children is difficult and tiring even for a healthy woman. For those with an energy depleting, painful disease it is doubly so. Patients will need a lot of support and advice during this time. It may be necessary to provide extra help in the form of a home help to ease the situation. If the mother has shoulder or elbow involvement, cuddling and feeding her baby may be difficult. If the elbow joint is weak a hinged elbow brace may provide additional support. If the upper limbs are painful, a TENS unit worn whilst feeding or nursing can sometimes bring relief. Some women find physical contact is easier to achieve in comfort if they lie on a bed supported by pillows with the baby at their side.

Breast or bottle?

One of the earliest decisions the mother must make is whether to breast or to bottle feed. There are pros and cons for both methods. Breast feeding is not contraindicated in the rheumatic diseases, but mothers need to be aware that any drugs they take will pass into the breast milk. Most health professionals advocate breast feeding, even if it is only for a short period of time as the baby receives some immunity from the mother. Breast feeding also has the advantage of being less work in terms of bottle washing and sterilisation and it is also cheaper.

However bottle feeding is advantageous in that partner, family or friends can do the feeds! For patients with painful hands or reduced dexterity, teats can be rather fiddly to clean and of course it is essential that they are scrupulously clean.

The best method of feeding is that with which the mother is most comfortable and on which the baby thrives.

Contraception

Family planning is an important decision whether a couple is healthy or not. If one or both partners have a rheumatic disease the timing and spacing of pregnancies is crucial. The opportunity to discuss pregnancy and family planning often arises when patients begin disease modifying drug therapy. Drugs such as sulphasalazine reduce the sperm count and patients need to be informed about this. It is then natural to follow this up with questions about family planning. Fertile women who are considering cytotoxic drugs should be counselled about the reliability of their preferred method of contraception and the consequences to the foetus if they become pregnant.

Those patients who wish to avoid pregnancy may experience a great deal of anxiety at the prospect of an unwanted pregnancy and potential problems with contraception may add to this anxiety. There are a growing number of methods of birth control (Fig. 6.3), some are more reliable than others. They fall into six categories:

- Hormonal contraception
- Intra-uterine devices
- Barrier methods
- Spermicides
- Natural methods
- Sterilisation.

Hormonal contraception

Second to sterilisation, hormonal contraception is the most effective method of fertility control and arthritis does not exclude its use. However it should be noted that the effectiveness might be slightly reduced if the

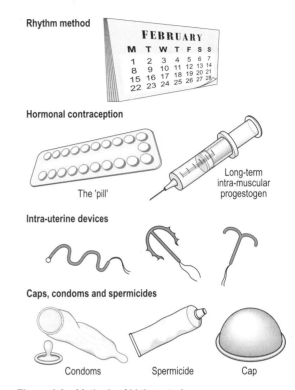

Figure 6.3 Methods of birth control.

patient is taking non-steroidal anti-inflammatory drugs (Smith 1994). Hormonal contraceptives come in two forms:

1. A combination of oestrogen and a progestogen, which is the most effective preparation.
2. Progestogen only.

The latter have a higher failure rate and consequently are usually given when oestrogens are contraindicated. Both types of contraception come in the form of a 'pill', but progestogen can be given by deep intramuscular injection in a form that is effective for 12 weeks. This drug is sometimes given as a long term contraceptive for women who are unable to use other methods. Patients should be made aware that there is a risk of infertility and irregular periods for up to a year following cessation of progestogen treatment. Some patients also experience heavier and more frequent periods.

Intra-uterine devices (IUD)

IUDs are commonly called the 'coil'. They are usually made of inert plastic and some have a copper coating. IUDs are highly effective and once in place rarely cause the patient any further concern. They are not recommended for nulliparous women because of the increased risk of pelvic sepsis and ensuing infertility. IUDs sometimes causes menorrhagia, which can pose particular problems for those women with RA who are prone to anaemia. Coils have to be changed by a doctor at approximately 2-yearly intervals.

Barrier methods

Condoms and diaphragms are barrier methods of birth control. Both are non-invasive methods which do not interfere with the chemistry of the body.

Condoms or sheaths are available for both males and females and can be bought from pharmacies and supermarkets. They are effective if used properly, but for patients with painful hands or decreased manual dexterity, the male condom in particular can be difficult to put on. If this is the case then the able-bodied partner may need to assist.

Diaphragms fit over the cervix and need to be applied prior to intercourse. A doctor should check them for correct fit at regular intervals. For women with painful or non-dextrous hands they can be difficult to use and the help of the partner may be necessary.

Barrier methods should be used in conjunction with spermicidal creams.

Natural methods

The two common natural methods of contraception are:

- The rhythm method
- Coitus interruptus.

These are the most unreliable methods of contraception.

The rhythm method relies on the so called 'safe period' to have intercourse. This is based on predicting when the egg will be present by recording the woman's daily temperature. Sexual intercourse needs to be avoided for approximately 10 days of each menstrual cycle. It is a little more reliable if spermicides are also used.

In coitus interruptus, also known as the withdrawal method, the man has to withdraw his penis before he ejaculates. This is extremely unreliable.

Sterilisation

Male or female sterilisation is a relatively simple operation that is very difficult to reverse. Therefore careful consideration by both partners is needed before proceeding. Providing the patient is completely happy that it will not alter their sexuality, it does not interfere with the pleasure of sexual intercourse. Indeed for many couples, the certainty that pregnancy

---

Action points for practice:

1. Describe the nature of self image and how illness and disease may influence it.

2. Write a case history of a patient with severe rheumatoid arthritis and describe what effect it has had on their sexuality.

3. A 45-year-old patient with systemic lupus erythematosus asks advice about contraception. What advice can you give her?

4. From your own experience write about a situation in which a patient has expressed problems with their sexuality. Reflect on your practice and then consider:

- Any clues that may have been missed
- Responses to the patient from yourself and other staff
- Your feelings at the time
- Contrast the available resources and the help that the patient received.

4. Mrs Smith is a 34-year-old woman who has had RA for 3 years. She has one 5-year-old child. Her RA is very aggressive and has caused deformities of her hands and feet. She has synovitis at the metacarpophalangeal joints which means she is unable to wear her wedding ring, a very important symbol of her love. She finds playing with her child difficult and very tiring. She used to like socialising and would wear smart clothes and beautiful high-heeled shoes, which is now no longer possible. She has a loving husband who is 36 years old but she fears he may, in her words, 'stray'. She no longer feels attractive. Pain and hip involvement make sexual intercourse painful and she feels that her relationship is, along with her health, deteriorating.

- Describe how you would feel about discussing her problems
- How will you deal with your feelings?
- If you feel embarrassed, how can you overcome this?
- Who do you think can help you to deal with this situation?

will be avoided enhances rather than detracts from the experience.

Chronically ill patients and their families require an understanding, accepting professional who is willing to give the additional time necessary to explore sexual attitudes and family interactions. The nurse should be able to accept the healthy aspects of sexual activity so that non-harmful means of aiding performance can be encouraged. Within this context the psychological limits and unique family relationship must be considered (Blau & Blau 1991).

Sexuality is complex and multidimensional and must be addressed by the nurse in a holistic fashion. To achieve this it is crucial to make the distinction between the patient's physical sexual needs and their need to enjoy love and non-sexual relationships. This was succinctly described by Freud in 1936, who said 'sex is something we do, sexuality is something we are'.

REFERENCE

Andrew C, Andrew H 1991 Sexuality and the dying patient. Journal of District Nursing 8–10 (November)

Annon J S 1976 The PLISSIT model: a proposed conceptual scheme for behavioural treatment of sexual problems. Journal of Sex Education Therapy 2(2): 1–15

Blau S P, Blau B 1991 Sexuality and family life. In: Spiera H, Oreskes I (eds) Rheumatology for the health care professional. Warren H Green, USA

Burnard P 1992 Counselling: a guide to practice in nursing. Butterworth Heinemann, UK

Campling J 1981 Images of ourselves. Routledge & Kegan Paul, London

Carolan C 1984a Sex and disability. Nursing Times 80: 28–30

Carolan C 1984b Bridging the gap. Nursing Times 80: 49–50

Chandani A T, Mass F, McKenna K T 1989 Attitudes of university students towards the sexuality of physically disabled people. British Journal of Occupational Therapy 52(6): 233–236

Chesson S 1984 Social and emotional aspects of rheumatoid arthritis. Nursing 31: 914–915

Cochrane M 1984 Sex and disability: immaculate infection. Nursing Times 80: 31–32

Cohen M 1991 Sexuality and family life. In: Spiera H, Oreskes I (eds) Rheumatology for the health care professional. Warren H Green, USA

Dawson-Shepherd R 1984 Why the carpet is no longer big enough. Nursing Times 80: 33–34

Doyal L, Pennell I 1979 The political economy of health. Pluto Press, London

Drench M E 1994 Changes in body image secondary to disease and injury. Rehabilitation Nursing 19(1): 31–35

Freud A 1936 The ego and mechanisms of defence. Hogarth Press, London

Glover J 1982 Psychosexual counselling. Nursing 35: 1509–1512

Greengross W 1976 Entitled to love. Malby Press, London

Gross R D 1992 Psychology – the science of mind and behaviour. Hodder & Stoughton, London, p 675

Hahn H 1981 The social component of sexuality and disability: some problems and proposals. Sexuality and Disability 4(4): 220–233

Hill J 1991 Assessing rheumatic disease. Nursing Times 87(4): 33–35

Hogan R 1980 Human sexuality – a nursing perspective. Appleton Century Crafts, New York

Jones H 1994 Mores and morals. Sexuality, older people. Nursing Times 90(47): 55–58

Lawler 1991 Behind the screens. Nursing somology and the problem of the body. Churchill Livingstone, London

Lee M V, Moll J M H 1987 Nursing care of the rheumatic patient – principles and practice. Croom Helm, London

Le Gallez P 1993 Rheumatoid arthritis: effects on the family. Nursing Standard 7(39): 30–34

Le Gallez 1988 Teratogenesis and drugs for rheumatic disease. Nursing Times 84(27): 41–44

Locker D 1983 Disability and disadvantage – the consequences of chronic illness. Tavistock Publications, London

Maslow A 1970 Motivation and personality. Harper & Row, New York

Mearns D, Thorne B 1988 Person-centred counselling in action. Sage Publications, London, pp 69–70

Price B 1990 Body image – nursing concepts and care. Prentice Hall, New York

Richardson A 1992 Rheumatoid arthritis in pregnancy. Nursing Standard 6(45): 25–28

Roper N, Logan W W, Tierney A J 1980 The elements of nursing. Churchill Livingstone, Edinburgh

Savage J 1987 Nursing gender and sexuality. Heinemann Nursing, London

Savage J 1989 Sexuality an uninvited guest. Nursing Times 85(5): 26–28

Savage J 1990 Sexuality and nursing care – setting the scene. Nursing Standard 4(37): 24–25

Singh S J, Magner T 1975 Sex and self: the spinal cord injured. Rehabilitation Literature 36(1): 2–10.

Smith P 1994 Rheumatoid arthritis and sexual relationships. Rheumatology in Practice, Winter:12–13

Soscia P N, Zurier R B 1992 Drug therapy of rheumatic diseases during pregnancy. Bulletin on the Rheumatic Diseases 41(2): 1–3

Stuart G W, Sundeen S J 1979 Principles and practice of psychiatric nursing. Mosby, St Louis

Smith P J 1994 Rheumatoid arthritis and sexual relationships. Rheumatology in Practice, Winter: 12–13

United Kingdom Central Council for Nursing, Midwifery and Health Visiting 1992 Code of professional conduct. United Kingdom Central Council, London

Venables P 1985 Sjögren's syndrome. In: Collected reports on the rheumatic diseases. Arthritis and Rheumatism Council for Research, UK, p 93

Webb C 1985 Gynaecological nursing – a compromising situation. Journal of Advanced Nursing 18: 47–54

Webb C 1987 Sexuality, nursing and health. John Wiley, Chichester

Williams G H, Wood P H N 1982 Sex and disablement: what is the problem and whose problem is it? International Rehabilitation Medicine 4: 89–96

FURTHER READING

Blake D J, Weaver W, Maisiak R, Alarcon G S, Brown S 1990 A curriculum in clinical sexuality for arthritis health care professionals. Psychosomatics 31(2): 189–191
Gamel C, David B D, Hengeveld 1993 Nurses' provision of teaching and counselling on sexuality: a review of the literature. Journal of Advanced Nursing 18(8): 1219–1227
Gibson H B 1992 The emotional and sexual lives of older people: a manual for professionals. Chapman Hall, London
Katzin L 1990 Chronic illness and sexuality. American Journal of Nursing 90(1): 54–59
Redfern S 1991 Sexuality and arthritis. Nursing 4(44): 17–19
Salter M 1988 Altered body image : the nurse's role. John Wiley, Chichester

7

The social implications of rheumatic disease

Sarah Ryan

This chapter explores the effect that living with a rheumatological disease has on social relationships, the family unit, changes in role at home and in the workplace. The chapter concludes with a section on pregnancy. After reading this chapter you should be able to:

- **Describe the implications for the family unit of living with a rheumatological condition**
- **Discuss the function of social support**
- **Understand both the advantages and disadvantages of social support**
- **Describe the advantages of a telephone helpline service**
- **Describe the role of the nurse in supporting and educating both the patient and family members**
- **Understand how rheumatological conditions can affect a person's ability to work**
- **Discuss the implications of rheumatic disease for pregnancy.**

Rheumatological conditions have a global impact on the well-being of an individual and their family. Although many of the symptoms of chronic disease are physical in presentation, for example pain, stiffness and synovitis, the reality of illness for the patient is the restraints it places on valued aspects of everyday life. These include the ability and option of remaining active and contributing both socially and in employment. A person may find it impossible to continue with activities, such as engaging in sports, that bring meaning to their life and this will require a major adjustment in lifestyle. Living with RA has been described as 'the tightrope between freedom and a life sentence' (Maycock 1988). Not surprisingly this exacts a heavy psychological toll on some patients. Yelin et al (1987) suggest that one half to two thirds of persons with RA experience:

- Losses in social relationships
- Disrupted leisure activities
- Limitation in work activities
- Transportation problems.

THE FAMILY

The family is a dynamic social unit that undergoes many changes in the course of life and fulfils many functions that are essential for physical, psychological and social well-being (Box 7.1). It is within the family that an individual is able to share thoughts and be themselves, benefiting from an environment of mutual trust and respect. The family unit can be an area of retreat which acts as a protective framework from the strains of everyday life. It is often in the family where ties or relationships are cemented, and the individual has concerns and cares for their partner and children.

Box 7.1 Functions of the family

- Emotional support such as love and affection
- Sexual well-being
- Physical assistance with everyday tasks such as personal hygiene
- Recreational activities and social commitments.

The family has a paramount role when one of its members is faced with chronic illness such as arthritis (Bury & Anderson 1988). The social support offered from within the family unit influences the individual's response to illness and also has a major bearing on subsequent outcomes such as compliance with treatment and rehabilitation. This is especially true as the repercussions for family members are considerable. They have to cope with the social, emotional and financial impact of the disease not only on the affected family member, but on the family unit as a whole.

The effect on the family

The family will be affected in one of three ways (Affleck 1988):

1. The arthritis brings the family unit closer together.
2. The family experiences minimal alteration in role responsibility or division of labour.
   > is a negative effect on relationships with
   y members as a consequence of the illness.

Prior to the illness, different family members will have adopted certain responsibilities for the various functions outlined in Box 7.1. Members will be comfortable with their present roles as they will have been negotiated within the unit, and accepted largely from choice and desirability. Roles will also have been influenced by cultural norms, women often undertaking responsible for the domestic management of the unit. The onset of a rheumatological condition such as RA in one of its members will cause the family to look at itself and alter role responsibility within it. This can cause great disruption especially as the patient's emotional reaction to the illness may lead to feelings of helplessness. This can place great stress on the whole unit as other family members may find it difficult to adapt to new roles such as carrying out domestic tasks. It will be a time of great adjustment. Family members must learn when to give and when to withhold help, as being over-supportive or providing support at the wrong time may produce negative outcomes (Revenson 1990).

The effect on social contact

The affects of arthritis can place significant restrictions on social contact (Box 7.2). In an attempt to minimise this, the patient may become expert at disguising the pain, fatigue and other symptoms of the condition to the outside world. This will be more difficult within the family unit, where members will recognise alterations in habits and mood. Unless the family has received information, education and guidance from the nurse, about the nature of the condition and its manifestations, this can prove very bewildering and relationships can be placed under great strain. For example, if the family is not aware of the importance of pacing activities in conditions such as RA and systemic lupus erythematosus, a patient's resting time may be perceived by family members as lazy and wasteful. Similarly, a patient with RA can experience a vast daily variation in the severity of symptoms, such as stiffness. Unless the implications of the condition have been discussed with a health care worker, family members may find this difficult to comprehend.

Box 7.2 Factors affecting social contact

- Impairment of mobility
- Pain, stiffness and fatigue
- Symptom control
- Time required for treatment interventions such as exercise
- Emotional status
- Self esteem.

Limitation in family role functioning

It has been shown that a reduction in the extent to which the family functions as a unit is associated with diminished well-being as measured by life satisfaction and depressive symptoms (Reisine et al 1987). Activities within the family unit can be divided into two main areas (Gove 1984):

1. Instrumental activities – cooking, cleaning, financial management and shopping.
2. Nurturing activities – making family arrangements, maintaining family ties, looking after family members and listening to others.

It is the latter category that is often highly valued by both the individual and the family (Reisine 1995).

A rheumatological condition such as rheumatoid arthritis or osteoarthritis can impact negatively on both instrumental and nurturing function. Yelin et al (1987) describe the most affected areas being:

- Shopping
- Cleaning
- Maintaining family ties.

The severity of the illness can also be influential. Women with severe RA are able to undertake a significantly smaller proportion of household tasks compared with those with mild arthritis, or those unaffected by the disease (Allaire et al 1991, Allaire 1992).

In women with RA, the level of involvement in each role is dependent on both the woman's situation and her age. Younger women generally carry out more roles than those who are retired or who have raised children. Women with children tend to have significant levels of involvement with their families that decrease during active phases of their condition. Eventually temporary changes in role responsibility evolve into a redistribution of duties, some shared, others delegated and some former activities are foregone. Women who work outside the house tend to push themselves at work and then retire early to bed (Shaul 1995).

Sources of physical and emotional support most frequently cited by patients include family and friends. Frequently, patients with RA are able to discuss their situation more openly with a friend, because friends can offer empathy without having to take full responsibility for the consequences (Bury & Anderson 1988).

Due to the complexity of chronic illness many patients will have difficulty understanding what is happening and may experience feelings of denial, hostility and fear. However they may not voice concerns to their partner for fear of burdening them with emotional pressures when they may already feel they are burdening the family with physical limitations. This is part of the problem of discovering meaning, both in terms of practical consequences and in terms of the wider significance of the disease as a crippling condition (Bury & Anderson 1988). The depth of impact depends not on the degree of disability but on how well each patient is able to adjust to the disease and accept the physical limitations it imposes (le Gallez 1993).

Isolation

Arthritis does not only affect household activities, it can also limit social activity leading to social isolation. This can be very destructive and often causes depression. Families frequently become isolated but do not seek outside help, possibly because our culture encourages family emotions to be kept within the family (Broome 1989). From childhood, social attitudes emphasise the containment rather than the expression of emotion. Discussion outside the family can be interpreted as betraying the family. Equally, there can be a lack of awareness as to which agency to approach for help.

Effects on the spouse and marriage

Living with a rheumatological condition can cause considerable stress on the healthy partner, as the partner with the illness faces a complex set of illness-related demands including:

- Pain
- In some cases disability
- Uncertainty about disease progression
- Frequent medical care.

Family cohesiveness has been found to be a significant factor in influencing pain perception, disability and psychological functioning in patients with RA and fibromyalgia (Nicassio & Radojevic 1993). The importance of the family role in patient outcome was illustrated in a study of the benefits of behavioural intervention to minimise pain in patients with RA. The intervention incorporating family support was more effective in reducing pain than the intervention with the patient alone (Radojevic et al 1992).

The extent to which partners are prepared to acknowledge the existence of illness and provide support is more important than the level of disability in influencing patient well-being. Families with a severely disabled member often cope better than families with fewer disabilities (le Gallez 1993). Spouses of patients with RA can have poor perception of the disability, pain and stiffness their partners live with (Phelan et al 1994). These negative perceptions have been shown to lessen by attendance at an education programme aimed at improving knowledge about the condition. The spouse may report greater and longer lasting distress than the patient, causing anxiety and depression, which can have a negative effect both within the home and the workplace (Flor et al 1987). However, work by Revenson and Majerovitz (1991) found that the level of depressive symptoms in the healthy spouse was no greater than that found in community samples.

Role alteration

The disabling effect of arthritis can herald a change in the role of both the patient and the partner. This change of role is recognised by the majority of female patients but by only a minority of male patients. Men largely accept the role of caring for their female partner. However, whilst the female partner is as willing as the male to accept the responsibility of caring, some male patients are unable to accept this offer, viewing it as a threat to their perceived role as head of the house and family provider (le Gallez 1993).

Communication within the family unit is essential. It is not unusual for there to be conflict, especially between feelings of over protectiveness on one hand and anger and resentment at the disruption of their lives on the other. In a study into the lived experience of RA, one female patient stated 'he was bewildered he did not know whether to answer back or try and console me' (Ryan 1996). It will take time for all members to adjust to the new situation that the family finds itself in. When carrying out an assessment on the patient it is of vital importance that the rheumatology nurse assesses the patient's social circumstances. The family may have certain limitations in insight which adversely affect communication links. If so, the nurse can include this in the care management plan and provide the intervention required to improve communication and understanding.

The effect of marriage

Many studies have demonstrated that married people have fewer health problems and a lower mortality rate than those who are single, divorced, separated or widowed (Reisine 1993). It has been suggested that the benefits of marriage are due to having a more supportive social network. One study of patients with RA supports this theory. Married women perceived better access to help with instrumental tasks, experienced more physical affection and had greater feelings of being needed by others compared with those who were not married (Manne & Zautra 1989).

Although considerable data supports the notion that marriage constitutes a special social tie that confers health protection to those who are married, negative aspects of the marital relationship can affect coping and psychological adjustment. High levels of spouse criticism are directly related to maladaptive coping behaviour (Reisine 1995).

Sexual relationships

In a study by Ryan et al (1996), almost 70% of patients living with inflammatory arthritis attributed inhibitions in their sexual relationships directly to their arthritis. Factors contributing to this included:

- Pain
- Joint function
- Medications.

The nurse was cited as the most appropriate person to provide support in this area. However, if the nurse is to take on this role she must be given adequate training and preparation. Only then will the nurse feel able to include it in the assessment stage and plan interventions that match identified need. This area is discussed further in Chapter 6.

The future

Central to the experience of illness is the uncertainty and worries about prognosis of variable and fluctuating disorders such as rheumatoid arthritis (Weiner 1975). Patients with rheumatoid arthritis are often unduly pessimistic about their future and are frequently inaccurate in their perceptions of their illness (Hewlett 1994). Negative beliefs whether well founded or not, may affect a person's ability to cope and to learn positive methods of living with their illness. If they are convinced of a negative future, they may lose faith in prescribed treatments and inadvertently cause more pain and other manifestations of the condition, by ignoring advice relating to analgesia taking, exercise, pacing activities and so on.

The nurse must find time to ascertain what most concerns the patient about their condition and perception of the future. Being admitted to hospital can be a bewildering and frightening experience. As one participant stated: 'being on the ward and seeing all these people with twisted joints or using wheelchairs, you do wonder if that is going to happen to me' (Ryan 1996). Talking through fears may help the patient to see them as more manageable. If the fear is of something specific, for example a reduction in mobility, the nurse can discuss remedies such as:

- Exercise regimes
- Suitable footwear
- The possibility of surgical intervention.

Active involvement in care can be used as a coping strategy and the nurse must endeavour to inform fully on all aspects, so choices can be made and alternatives offered. The patient needs to feel in control of the situation through knowledge and through full participation. Consistency is important; being given conflicting information by members of the health care team will only heighten feelings of anxiety. Fear is a natural expression of concern, but intervention is required if it prevents the patient from taking action that is in their best interest (Pigg et al 1985). Knowledge and involvement will breed hope. If hope is threatened a spiral of decline can occur involving depression and isolation.

The effect on children

Nearly three quarters of children living with a parent who had RA have been found to be afraid of developing the disease, but did not communicate this fear to their parents (le Gallez 1993). Silences such as this within the family unit makes the support and education of all family members an essential role of the nurse (see Ch. 15).

It has also been found that the self esteem of adolescent children living with a parent having arthritis was lower than that of children living with healthy parents, but comparable to that of children living with a parent suffering depression. Greater family and peer support did not effect their self esteem in any positive way (Hirsch & Reishch 1985). For adolescents whose parents had arthritis, involvement of friends with their family presents more opportunities for friends to see the disability, and so to view the whole family in a negative light. In this way the parent's physical disability might adversely affect the adolescent's ability to draw on friendship for support (Revenson 1993). However this was not substantiated by other work (le Gallez 1993) that showed that 75% of children living with a parent with RA experienced either a minimal impact on their lives or that it had brought them closer together as a family. These children expressed deep concern and displayed a nurturing attitude towards the ill parent. The 25% of children

who felt living with a parent with arthritis was detrimental, could be divided in to two groups:

1. Those whose parents were unable to accept the pain and physical limitations.
2. Those children who resented the fact that a parent was ill and as a result showed little consideration or compassion for them.

SOCIAL SUPPORT

Social support refers to the process by which interpersonal relationships promote:

- Physical;
- Psychological;
- Social;
- Emotional well-being.

The functions of social support are shown in Box 7.3. The need for this support is especially heightened at the time of chronic illness, where the affects on an individual invade all domains of life. The person will often experience anger, resentment and grief at their new situation. The degree and type of support offered is probably one of the most important factors in determining how both the individual and the family unit accept the disease.

Box 7.3 Functions of social support

- Expressing positive affect
- Encouraging communication of feelings
- Providing information and advice
- Validating beliefs, emotions and actions
- Enhancing psychological well-being
- Providing material aid.

In coping with arthritis patients are helped by three factors (Affleck et al 1988). These are:

1. Being given the opportunity to express feelings and concerns.
2. Receiving encouragement, hope and optimism.
3. Receiving advice and information.

Mechanisms of support

There are two common models for support:

- The stress buffering model (Cohen & Wills 1985) which states that support acts as a protector at a time of crisis.
- The direct effect model (Revenson 1993) which states that support is beneficial regardless of the stress experienced; that support can enhance well-being at all times and not just in the face of chronic illness.

The validity of these models has been tested in patients with RA, using pain as the stressor. It was found that irrespective of the level of pain experienced, greater support was related to reduced levels of depression and that this correlation prevailed after six months (Brown et al 1989). This work supports the direct effect model.

Regardless of disability, greater levels of social support are also associated with an increased level of self esteem and lower reported depression levels (Fitzpatrick et al 1988). This is not surprising as patients living with a rheumatological condition experience a fluctuating pattern of symptoms and progression. The knowledge that support is available constantly and not just at times of acute activity must contribute to general well-being.

The stress buffering model might be more appropriately applied to individuals experiencing acute illness, such as appendicitis, where support will be required for a limited time.

The benefits of social support

Social support has numerous benefits:

- Patients with arthritis who received support from family and friends exhibit greater self esteem (Fitzpatrick et al 1988); psychological adjustment (Affleck et al 1988; life satisfaction (Burckhardt 1985); and report less depression (Revenson & Majerovitz 1991).
- Involvement of the family in patient care increases sensitivity to the perception of functional disability, pain and stiffness experienced by the patient. Maycock (1988) refers to a young person, newly diagnosed with RA, who complained that because the arthritis was not visible the family could not comprehend the severity of the illness.
- Social support increases the motivation to partake in instrumental action and reduces the emotional stress that may impede other coping efforts so increasing patient's adherence to treatment (Cohen 1988). For example, if the family accepts the need for exercise it can be incorporated in the family routine.
- Support may encourage the performance of positive health behaviour, thus preventing or minimising illness and the reporting of symptoms (Cohen 1988).
- Patients with arthritis who have a greater number of close friends and relations report fewer activity losses and make activity modifications (Katz 1995).
- Social support may be important in predicting health outcomes in patients with RA. Both unmarried men and married women with a poor social support

network, predict greater impairment and depression (Revenson 1993).

Negative aspects of social support

Social support is not beneficial in all circumstances and negative effects can occur:

- Patients may resent their need for support and reject it when it is offered, viewing its acceptance as reducing self autonomy and reinforcing the concept of powerlessness.
- The family may become over protective, encouraging the patient to constantly rest rather than partake in exercise. This will have negative consequences causing increased pain, stiffness and muscle wasting.
- Patients can become over dependent on the family, adopting disability as a way of life, and ceasing to be an active participant in care management. In effect the patient withdraws into a childlike condition, allowing everything to be done for them in a paternalistic environment.
- Patients may be less likely to seek help if they feel they are not able to return the support, causing a reduction in self esteem.
- Support from some family members can become a form of social control in the relationship that limits patient participant in self management (Rook 1990).

Effectiveness of support

The balance between the recipient's support needs and the amount of support offered influences the effectiveness of support. For example, a newly diagnosed patient with inflammatory arthritis will require information about how to self manage the condition in a supportive educational partnership with the nurse. It would certainly be inappropriate at this stage in a person's condition to discuss surgical intervention. This would not be addressing the patient's perceived needs. If the nurse is underpinning her practice with the therapeutic care philosophy described in Chapter 1, and providing care that has both meaning and relevance for the patient, the nurse will engage in a partnership with the patient and their significant others to draw up a plan of care that is appropriate to the individual's situation (Fig. 7.1).

THE TELEPHONE HELPLINE

The telephone can be invaluable, for instance patients with osteoarthritis who received biweekly telephone contact for six months have reported increased levels

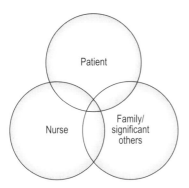

Figure 7.1   The care partnership.

of perceived support and less pain (Weinberger et al 1989).

Many rheumatology nurses are involved in operating a telephone helpline service for patients. This ensures that there is a designated point of contact for the patients should they need advice regarding any aspect of their condition. This is reassuring for the patient and their family as they know they can easily access and communicate with a professional involved in their care. A 12-month audit of a helpline demonstrated that patients' most frequent needs include advice on:

- Drug therapy
- Pain control
- How to cope with a flare
- Benefit entitlements.

The nurse is able to provide advice directly to the individual concerned and coordinate further action if it is required. A patient with a swollen joint may require aspiration and injection to relieve the inflammation, and this can be arranged quickly by liaison with the appropriate member of the rheumatology team. It may be the nurse herself that will conduct this procedure, so providing comprehensive care for the patient, and reinforcing the relationship of trust that will have developed during the communication period.

The telephone helpline can also provide direct access for other members of the team involved in the patient's medical and nursing care. A general practitioner for example may ring to question whether gold injections should be discontinued due to the presence of haematuria. The advice by the nurse to continue will prevent treatment being stopped unnecessarily. It will also enable a consistency to care management to develop between members of the primary and secondary health care team. This will reinforce communication links and promote a greater appreciation of the

different roles of these two groups, who are both key providers in the patients care.

SUPPORT GROUPS

Some patients become members of support groups in order to obtain both an additional source of support and as a means of obtaining more information about living with their condition. This can empower the patient and the family on many different aspects of their condition, for instance the purpose of drug therapy. Support groups can also be active in raising public awareness of the problems faced by people living with arthritis. For some patients it prevents isolation and provides a regular point of contact with a group of people living with similar difficulties and limitations in lifestyle. Those attending the group and who are coping well, may serve as role models and motivators for those members who are coping less well. It is important that the facilitator of the group maintains a positive attitude, with the emphasis on education and support. If this is not done, the group could be used unconstructively as a forum for complaints and no longer serve its members in a positive way.

The role of the nurse

Practitioners can work towards a number of goals (Revenson 1993). These include:

- Teaching patients how to develop and maintain family ties
- Teaching patients how to recognise and accept the help and emotional encouragement provided by family members
- Improving family member skills for determining the patient support needs and offering help
- Facilitating positive appraisals of support.

When is support most beneficial?

Different types and levels of support will be needed at different stages of the illness. After diagnosis and commencement of therapy, a patient with inflammatory arthritis will expect that the condition will be controlled and that they can return to the pattern of life they enjoyed prior to the illness. However, if the treatment is not effective and the disease remains active, the patient will experience increased pain and stiffness, and their ability to carry out activities of daily living independently will reduce. It is at this stage that a patient may experience feelings of anxiety, despondency and depression. Whereas, in the initial phase the role of the nurse may have centred around the provision of information, a negative response to treatment will necessitate a change in care provision to emotional support, guidance and motivation. Conditions such as RA with its fluctuating pattern of symptoms, will require the nurse to be receptive to the patient's needs at various stages of the illness and match the support required with the patient's identified needs. The types of support the nurse can provide are described in Box 7.4.

Box 7.4 Types of support the nurse can provide

- Emotional: providing the opportunity for discussing feelings about the condition
- Instrumental: arranging for the occupational therapist to carry out an assessment of the home environment
- Informational: providing self management information on how to cope with a flare of the condition.

THE THERAPEUTIC RELATIONSHIP

The nurse will need to enter into a therapeutic relationship with the patient as described in Chapter 1, and spend time relating and communicating with them on a personal level. This will allow care to be planned that has meaning and relevance for the patient. The patient will be able to identify with the care programme and to become an active participant in it, promoting a worthy relationship between patient and nurse, seeking common goals and objectives. Once a problem, such as unrelenting pain has been identified, the nurse and the patient will need to agree on the necessary interventions to minimise the problem. This will involve ascertaining the patient's lay beliefs. Exercise may be recommended, but a patient who doubts its efficacy is unlikely to persist if there are no immediate benefits.

The care management plan will require regular evaluation. This may be a weekly occurrence whilst the patient learns to implement self management techniques such as pacing activities. As the patient and the family begin to develop effective coping skills the evaluation will be needed less frequently.

Experiencing frequent flares will be stressful to both the patient and their family. As social support needs change, carers must learn when to give and when to withhold help as providing too much support or providing it at the wrong time, may produce negative outcomes like reduced autonomy and self worth. Attempts at achieving the necessary balance of support can be difficult because individuals do not know automatically how to provide support that does not demean the recipient (Coyne et al 1988). This is why it is so important to involve family members and

significant others in all aspects of care planning so that information and subsequent understanding can be shared. This will enable the family to function as a unit rather than in isolated parts.

THE EFFECT ON ROLE

The most difficult task the nurse faces is helping the patient and their family to recognise that roles and relationships have changed (Pigg et al 1985). The nurse needs to assist patients to communicate their feelings about the change in lifestyle that their condition has caused. The individual can often feel afraid and lost if they see their traditional role being eroded. If a person is unable to return to paid employment, the despondency this causes the individual will have repercussions within the family, especially if the healthy partner has to increase their working activity for financial reasons. The nurse needs to encourage and support the patient and assist them to explore ways in which their skills can be used positively and constructively. This may include referral to the disability employment officer for advice on retraining, active involvement on a committee of a support group, or assisting with teaching of junior staff at the hospital. In America patients with a musculoskeletal condition assist junior staff to learn more about examination, by volunteering themselves as a 'live model'. This serves to increase patient satisfaction as the individual feels they are still able to make a worthwhile contribution to society.

The nurse will need to assess family reactions to the illness at the time of patient assessment. This should be done by the use of open-ended questions such as:

'How did your family react to your illness?'

or

'How do the family support you?'

The response may reveal limitations in insight that can be addressed by providing information or family counselling. It may be useful for the family members to meet others in a similar situation and the nurse can facilitate this.

Sharing feelings

The nurse needs to encourage the patient to share their feelings. Sometimes the patient feels unable to do this within the home situation due to the emotional pressure it places on family members. The nurse can act as an emotional support and work through the patient's feelings with them. If the patient reveals signs of clinical depression a referral to the psychiatrist for appropriate management might be necessary. However, for the vast majority of patients coming to terms with living with a chronic illness, the nurse will be able to provide adequate support. By knowing the patient through a therapeutic relationship, the patient will feel able to trust the nurse and share their feelings openly.

Family insight

To be able to support the patient the family needs a similar knowledge base and understanding as the patient. Family members who do not believe that a person's disease is a major or serious problem may be unable to support measures such as rest or pacing activities that will change the family's lifestyle. Unless it is explained to them and they are included in the family discussions, children may not understand the reason that their father can no longer play sport with them. A family with unrealistic expectations places an unnecessary burden on the patient, especially if they believe that all will be well if only the patient works hard enough.

WORK

The experience of chronic illness always operates simultaneously at two levels; biological functioning and cultural competence. Society often defines a person by their occupation, and the status associated with particular work effects self esteem.

The impact of musculoskeletal condition on employment is of concern to:

• The individual, who faces the loss of income as well as role alteration
• Family members, who may alter their own employment, sometimes by leaving the workforce to provide care or by entering the workforce to compensate for the lost income
• Society, that must meet the cost of benefit payments.

Several studies have evaluated the relationship between the type of work undertaken and the extent to which the disease impairs the ability to carry out that work; work disability (Yelin et al 1987). In the work characteristic model it is the interaction between the impairment caused by the disease and the job requirement that affects the work disability rate. If an individual, employed in a job that requires manual dexterity, develops hand and wrist synovitis, they may no longer be able to carry on in that particular job. Equally if an individual has RA and needs to leave work for regular monitoring of treatment, the proba-bility of ceasing employment is increased if the job offers no flexibility.

Persons with a musculoskeletal condition are more likely to stop working if they (Yelin et al 1995):

• Are older
• Are female
• Have fewer years in education
• Have pain and comorbidity
• Have experienced limitation in function.

In Great Britain work loss due to back disorders has doubled in 5 years, accounting for 52.6 million days lost from work in 1988–1989 and for one-seventh of all sickness invalidity benefit payments. Back disability is growing faster than any other form of disability (Frymoyer & Cats-Baril 1991).

In the United States 57% of people with a musculoskeletal condition were not working and 64–72% of people with RA were unemployed (Pincus et al 1989, Yelin & Callahan 1995).

The intrusiveness of RA is greatest in the areas of active recreation, work and health. The degree of interference with active recreation and work is equivalent to that found in individuals with multiple sclerosis (Devins et al 1993). Furthermore the intrusiveness of RA increases as physical function worsens (Devins et al 1992).

Most patients with RA stop work within 10 years of developing the disease (Meenan et al 1981, le Gallez 1993). As the condition most commonly affects individuals in their third and fourth decade of life, patients may face many years without being able to work. It is of particular importance that the individual concerned and their family are given time to adjust to this radical change in their lifestyle. It is also important that the person believes their limitations to be real, rather than accepting the judgement of someone else, such as the doctor. This will prevent them aimlessly wondering whether they could have returned to work and prevent wishful thinking which can be viewed as a negative coping strategy (Newman 1993).

During this difficult stage, substantial counselling and support should be made available to both the patient and their family to help them adjust. Boredom and a sense of uselessness needs to be faced, and alternative interests found. This is particularly important for men, who often have a poor support network (le Gallez 1993). Unemployment will affect self perception, lead to an alteration of role and have financial implications. The nurse must be proactive in this area, referring patients to the appropriate agencies, for example social worker for advice on benefits, whilst at the same time providing the family with guidance and support.

PREGNANCY

An individual's decision about whether or not to have children is likely to be influenced by:

- How the women is coping with the condition
- Disease activity
- Drug therapy
- Practical support
- Family finances.

Preconception counselling and education are vital to ensure that prospective parents are given the necessary information regarding their disease to enable them to make a fully informed decision.

Preconception advice

Patients planning a family should be encouraged to seek advice from the rheumatology team. Women with RA often need to achieve disease suppression to increase their chance of conceiving. Decisions regarding the withdrawal of potentially toxic drug therapy, need to be made in good time, since many drugs can affect the vulnerable stage of embryogenesis. Women should discontinue teratogenic agents such as methotrexate, azathioprine and cyclophosphamide at least 6 months before attempting conception. Ideally all drug therapy should be avoided during pregnancy and lactation. The implications of taking the most frequently prescribed medication in arthritis are shown in Figure 12.3.

Antenatal care

In RA 75% of women experience some remission of their condition during pregnancy, but often return to disease status comparable with their pre-pregnant state within 8 months of giving birth.

The effect of pregnancy is less predictable in systemic lupus erythematosus. If the patient has renal involvement close monitoring will be required, as deteriorating renal function is also associated with toxaemia.

In ankylosing spondylitis 80% of patients may experience a worsening of symptoms or no alteration in their condition during pregnancy (le Gallez 1988).

During the antenatal phase the nurse will need to provide:

- Advice on pacing activities. Fatigue is quite normal in pregnancy but may be compounded by disease activity so there must be a balance between rest and activity. Good quality sleep, gentle exercises such as swimming and early maternity leave are all important (Richardson 1992).

- Advice on coping with pain. This should include relaxation techniques, the application of hot and cold therapy and the use of diversion techniques. The occupational therapist may also be involved at this stage to offer advice on joint protection and the suitability of proposed baby equipment.
- Advice on diet. An additional 300 calories a day will be needed during pregnancy and an extra 500 calories a day during lactation.

Management of labour and delivery

Hip involvement in musculoskeletal disorders may limit thigh abduction or pelvic measurements. If a caesarean section is indicated and the patient has cervical spine disease a cervical collar will be required to prevent hyperextension.

Postnatal care

The support of the community rheumatology sister and the health visitor will be essential in providing both physical and psychological support. If the mother has physical limitations and is unable to lift the baby, their advice will be required and alternative methods found such as supporting the baby on a pillow across the knees, or lying on the bed to provide physical contact.

Breast feeding is not contraindicated, but all drugs taken by a nursing mother will pass into the breast milk. The actual amount of drug passing to the baby will depend on the maternal rates of:

- Absorption
- Metabolism
- Distribution
- Elimination.

Women who develop an exacerbation of rheumatoid arthritis post partum will need to recommence their suppressive drug therapy and individual advice from the rheumatology nurse will be required if the mother is breast feeding. Due to the demands placed on lifestyle by a new baby, it may be necessary to plan a specific time for sexual activity (see Ch. 6).

Patients living with a rheumatological condition will find it has a vast impact on their social life and the family unit and the social support offered needs to match their needs. In this area the rheumatology nurse can be proactive; supporting, guiding, motivating, informing and involving the patient and their significant others in all areas of care management. This will ensure that the family unit works in unison, sharing the same knowledge base and treatment objectives.

> **Action points for practice:**
>
> 1. List the functions of the family unit.
>
> 2. Plan a teaching session for colleagues to illustrate the effects on the family, when one of its members has arthritis.
>
> 3. Look at ways of involving the family more fully in care planning.
>
> 4. Design a poster informing patients where they can receive advice regarding employment and benefit entitlements.
>
> 5. Provide a handout for family members explaining the ways in which the family can provide positive support.
>
> 6. Provide information for patients on the local support groups in the area.

REFERENCES

Affleck G, Fifield J, Pfeiffer C, Tennen H 1988 Social support and psychological adjustment to rheumatoid arthritis. Arthritis Care and Research 1: 71–77

Allaire S H 1992 Employment and work disability in women with rheumatoid arthritis. The Journal of Applied Rehabilitation and Counselling 23: 44–50

Allaire S H, Anderson J J, Meenan R F 1991 The impact of rheumatoid arthritis on the household performance of women. Arthritis and Rheumatism 34: 669–678

Broome A 1989 Health psychology processes and applications. Chapman and Hall, London.

Brown E K, Nicassio P M, Wallston K A 1989 Social support and depression in rheumatoid arthritis; a one year prospective study. Journal of Applied Social Psychology 19: 1164–1181.

Burckhardt C S 1985 The impact of arthritis on quality of life. Nursing Research 34: 11–16

Bury M, Anderson R 1988 Living with chronic illness. The experience of patients and their families. Unwin Hyman, London.

Cohen S, Wills T A 1985 Stress social support and the buffering hypothesis. Psychological Bulletin 98: 310–357

Cohen S 1988 Psychological models of the role of social support in the aetiology of physical disease. Health Psychology 7: 269–297

Coyne J C, Lehman D, Wartman C B 1988 The other side of support, emotional over-involvement and miscarried helping. In : Gottlieb B H (ed) social support, formats processes and effects. Sage Publications, Newbury Park CA, pp 305–330

Devins G M, Edworthy S M, Guthrie N G, Martin L 1992 Illness intrusiveness in rheumatoid arthritis, differential impact on depressive symptoms over the adult lifespan. Journal of Rheumatology 19: 709–715

Devins G M, Edworthy S M, Klein G M, Mandin H, Paul L C, Seland T P 1993 Differences in illness intrusiveness across rheumatoid arthritis, end stage renal disease and multiple sclerosis. Journal of Neurology and Mental Disorders 181: 377–381

Fitzpatrick R, Lamb R, Newman S, Shipley M 1988 Social relationships and psychological well-being in rheumatoid arthritis. Social Science and Medicine 27: 399–403

Flor H, Scholz O B, Turk D C 1987 Impact of chronic pain on the spouse; marital, emotional and physical consequences. Journal of Psychosomatic Research 31: 63–71

Frymoyer J W, Cats-Baril W L 1991 An overview of the incidence and costs of low back pain. Orthopaedic Clinical North America 22: 261–271

Gove W R 1984 Gender differences in mental and physical illness. The effect of fixed roles and nurturant roles. Social Science Medicine 19: 77–84

Hewlett S 1994 Patients' views of changing disability. Nursing Standard 8(31): 25–29

Hirsch B J, Reishch T 1985. Social networks and developmental psychopathology, a comparison of adolescent children, of a depressed, arthritic or normal parent. Journal of Abnormal Psychology 94: 272–281

Katz P, 1995 The impact of rheumatoid arthritis on life activities. Arthritis Care and Research 8(4): 272–278

le Gallez P 1988 Teratogenesis and drugs for rheumatic disease. Nursing Times 84(27): 41–44

le Gallez P 1993. Rheumatoid arthritis effects on the family. Nursing Standard 7(39): 30–34

Manne S L, Zautra A J 1989 Spouse criticism and support: their association with coping and psychological adjustment among people with rheumatoid arthritis. Journal Personal Social Psychology 56: 608–617

Maycock J 1988 the image of rheumatic disease. In Salter M (ed). Altered body image. The nurse's role. J Wiley, New York

Meenan R F, Espstein V W, Newitt M, Yelin E H 1981 The impact of chronic diseases, a socio-medical profile of rheumatoid arthritis. Arthritis and Rheumatism 24(3): 544–548

Newman S P 1993 Coping with rheumatoid arthritis. Leader in Annals of the Rheumatic Diseases 52: 553–554

Nicassio P M, Radojevic V 1993 Models of family functioning and their contribution to patient outcome in chronic pain. Motivation Emotion 17: 295–316

Phelan M, Campbell A, Byrne J, Hough Y, Hunt J, Lynch M 1994 The effect of an education programme on the perception of arthritis by spouses of patients with rheumatoid arthritis. Scandinavian Journal of Rheumatology, Suppl 74.

Pigg J S, Caniff R, Driscoll P W 1985 Rheumatology nursing. A problem orientated approach. John Wiley, New York.

Pincus T, Burkhausen R, Mitchell J 1989. Substantial work disability and earning losses in individuals less than 65 years with osteoarthritis: comparisons with rheumatoid arthritis. Journal of Clinical Epidemiology 42(5): 449–457

Radojenic V, Nicassio P M, Weisman M H 1992 Behavioural interventions, with and without family support for rheumatoid arthritis. Behavioural Therapy 23: 13–30

Reisine S 1993 Marital status and social support in rheumatoid arthritis. Arthritis and Rheumatism 36: 589–592

Reisine S 1995. Arthritis and the family. Arthritis Care and Research 8(4): 265–271

Reisine S, Goodenow C, Grady K E 1987 The impact of rheumatoid arthritis on the homemaker. Social Science Medicine 25: 89–95

Revenson T A 1990 Social support processes among chronically ill elders; patient and provider perspective. In: Giles H, Coupland N and Wiemann J (ed). Communication, health and the elderly. University of Manchester Press, Manchester, pp 92–113

Revenson T A 1993 The role of social support. In: Newman S, Shipley M (ed). Psychological aspects of rheumatic diseases. Baillière's clinical rheumatology 7(2): 377–396

Revenson T A, Majerovitz D M 1991 The effects of illness on the spouse: social resources as stress buffers. Arthritis Care and Research 4: 63–72

Richardson A 1992 Rheumatoid arthritis in pregnancy. Nursing Standard 6(45): 25–29

Rook K 1990 Social networks as a source of social control in older adults' lives. In : Giles H, Coupland N, Weimann J M (eds). Communication, health and the elderly. University of Manchester Press, Manchester, pp 45–63

Ryan S 1996 Living with rheumatoid arthritis: a phenomenological exploration. Nursing Standard 10(41): 34–37

Ryan S 1996 Does inflammatory arthritis affect sexuality? British Journal of Rheumatology (Suppl 2) 35: 19

Shaul M 1995 From early twinges to mastery. The process of adjustment in living with rheumatoid arthritis. Arthritis Care and Research 8(4): 290–297

Yelin E, Henke C, Esptein W 1987 Work dynamics of the person with rheumatoid arthritis. Arthritis and Rheumatism 30: 507–512

Yelin E, Callahan L 1995 The economic cost and social and psychological impact of musculoskeletal conditions. Arthritis and Rheumatism 38: 1351–1362

Weiner C E 1975 The burden of rheumatoid arthritis: tolerating the uncertainty. Social Science and Medicine 9: 97–104

Weinberger M, Bootier P, Katz B P, Tierney W M 1989 Can the provision of information to patients with osteoarthritis improve functional status? A randomised controlled trial. Arthritis and Rheumatism 32: 1577–1583

FURTHER READING

Newman S, Fitzpatrick R, Revenson T, Skevington S, Williams G 1996. Understanding rheumatoid arthritis. Routledge London.

Yelin E 1995. Musculoskeletal conditions and employment. Arthritis Care and Research 8(4): 311–317

8

Pain and stiffness

Jackie Hill

Pain and stiffness are two of the most disabling symptoms of rheumatic disease. The aim of this chapter is to help the nurse to understand these symptoms, the effect they have on their patients and the various treatments available to minimise these effects. After reading this chapter you will be able to:

- Understand the meaning to the patient of pain and stiffness
- Determine some of the causes of pain and stiffness
- Demonstrate knowledge of the nociceptor sensory system
- Describe influences that effect the perception of pain
- Discuss the use of assessment tools
- Select appropriate treatments for each individual.

PAIN

For patients with rheumatic disease, pain can be a life-changing experience that makes each day a challenge. Liebeskind & Melzack 1987 made the profound statement 'Freedom from pain should be a basic human right limited only by our knowledge to achieve it'. Unfortunately our knowledge in this area is limited, but thankfully increasing.

Pain is subjective and unlike some other symptoms, such as swelling and redness, it cannot be seen only observed. In humans, pain is experienced emotionally and is primarily demonstrated behaviourally (Harvey 1987). To be fully understood, it should be separated into its perception and the reaction to it (Pigg et al 1985).

Pain is one of the most discomforting symptoms of rheumatic disease (Bradley 1993a), and is the primary reason that many seek medical advice (Symmons & Bankhead 1994). In research carried out by Parker et al (1988), patients with rheumatoid arthritis (RA) said that pain was their most important symptom. It has also been found that the patient's current experience of pain is likely to predict their subsequent pain and disability, and it makes a major contribution to both physician and patient assessment of general health status (Kazis et al 1983). Pain is usually perceived as being unpleasant, and the relief of pain and the provision of comfort are considered as two of the main functions of the nurse (Maycock 1984). This makes it incumbent on nurses to increase their knowledge of pain and its management.

DEFINITIONS OF PAIN

Although pain is a common symptom that everyone will experience at sometime in their life, it is a difficult sensation to elucidate. Pigg et al (1985) have likened it to love, a feeling most people understand but have difficulty explaining!

Pain is a complex phenomenon, which does not occur in isolation. It is an emotional, sensory and physiological event, which no two people experience in the same way. This makes it impossible to quantify in absolute terms. However, some authors have formulated definitions of pain, which are commonly used. One of the earlier definitions by Merskey (1973), considers pain to be:

'An event which occurs in the mind but always refers to events experienced by the body.'

This definition acknowledges that pain is both emotional and physical.

The International Association for the Study of Pain has produced a interpretation which expands on this definition:

'Pain is an unpleasant sensory and emotional experience associated with actual or potential tissue damage, or described in terms of such damage'.

They then added these notes:

'Pain is always subjective. Each individual learns the application of the word through experience related to injury in early life. It is unquestionably a sensation in a part of the body but is also always unpleasant and therefore always an emotional experience. Many people report pain in the absence of tissue damage or any likely pathophysiological cause; usually this happens for psychological reasons. There is no way to distinguish their experience from that due to tissue damage, if we take the subjective report' (Merskey 1979).

Within the realms of nursing, the most accepted meaning is suggested by McCaffery (1983):

'Pain is whatever the experiencing person says it is, existing whenever he says it does'.

This definition accepts that pain is an individual, emotional and subjective experience which makes the patient the authority on their pain, and their impressions on frequency and intensity must be believed.

PAIN THRESHOLD

'All pain is real, how much you suffer from it is a question of attitude' (Skevington 1993). Nurses often refer to the patient's 'pain threshold', suggesting that it is high or low. For instance, those patients who are stoic are said to have a high threshold, those who complain frequently have a low threshold. It is believed that gender, culture and upbringing have an important bearing on tolerance to pain. Skevington (1993) suggests that it is important to make a distinction between the presence of pain and the reporting of pain. In order to do this she has identified three discreet levels of pain threshold:

1. Sensation threshold – lowest level at which anything is felt (warmth, tingling, itching).
2. Pain perception threshold – lowest level at which pain is felt.
3. Pain tolerance level – point at which pain becomes unbearable.

Sensation threshold is thought to be physiologically determined, and its perception appears to be universal and cross-cultural. This is in contrast to the pain perception threshold, and the pain tolerance level, which vary according to cultural group and acceptable societal norms. Surgical procedures such as circumcision are endured without any apparent pain following ritual preparation in some cultures. Sargent (1984) has cited this as evidence of cultural influence on pain perception.

When caring for patients in pain, their culture, beliefs about expressing or inhibiting such expression, should be explored as part of the nursing assessment.

THE PURPOSE OF PAIN

The primary purpose of the pain perception apparatus is protection of the organism (Harvey 1987). Pain tells us that there is something wrong with our body. For instance someone with appendicitis will feel pain due to the inflammation of his or her appendix. Once the appendix has been removed, the system will return to normal and become pain free. It also protects us from harming ourselves; notice how quickly a very hot item is dropped, usually before the pain from the burn is actually felt.

Although pain can arise because of a noxious stimuli, it should also be noted that some patients endure chronic pain in the absence of any organic pathology, these are termed *somatoform* pain disorders.

THE NOCICEPTOR SENSORY SYSTEM

Pain receptors

The sensation that we know as pain is brought about by the excitation of receptors in the nociceptive sensory system known as nociceptors. However, pain should not be equated with nociception alone as it can arise in its absence. Conversely, nociception may be present without the sensation of pain (Jones 1997).

Two types of pain receptors have been identified:

1. Mechano nociceptors
2. Polymodal nociceptors.

Mechano nociceptors are activated by pinching or heavy pressure and *polymodal nociceptors* by heat, cold and pain producing chemicals. The intensity of the stimulus determines the frequency of nerve impulses (frequency coding), and this is an important element in the severity of pain perception (Campbell 1995).

Nociceptors are attached to fibres projecting to the dorsal horn of the spinal cord. Two different types of sensory fibres are responsible for signalling different qualities of pain. These are:

• A delta – small myelinated fibre
• C fibre – smaller unmyelinated fibres.

A delta mediated pain is pricking or sharp and well localised. This is also called first pain. By comparison, C fibre pain, known as second pain, feels dull, burning or throbbing and is poorly localised. Although some pain is easy to determine in these terms, many people with rheumatic disease have difficulty discriminating between the two types.

Transmission of pain to the brain

Nociceptors are sensory neurones, which carry impulses to the central nervous system. All sensory nerves enter the spinal cord via the dorsal (posterior) horn (Fig. 8.1). From here, they cross over the spinal cord to the opposite anterior horn where they ascend the spinothalamic tract to the medulla, thalamus and

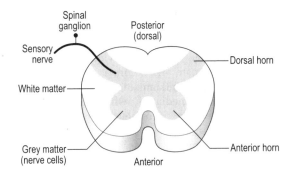

Figure 8.1   Sensory nerve entering the dorsal horn.

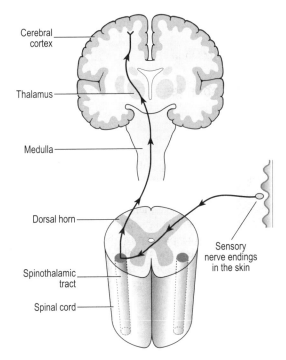

Figure 8.2   Sensory nerve pathway to the cerebral cortex.

on to the cerebral cortex for interpretation and action (Fig. 8.2). Simultaneously, impulses are carried from the thalamus to the limbic system, which is associated with basic emotions such as pleasure, fear, anxiety and anger. Impulses arising in the cerebral cortex are also carried to the thalamus and limbic system, modifying their responses (Gallop 1983).

PAIN GENERATION

Pain can be classified according to its cause, such as inflammation, spasm and irritation of the serous membrane (Morgan 1993). Pressure, intense heat, surgery and ischaemia have also been cited (Davis 1993). In the rheumatic diseases, inflammation is particularly prevalent and causes pain through hyperalgesia. Hyperalgesia causes previously non-painful stimuli to cause pain and occurs as a result of nociceptor sensitisation. Inflammation damages cells and releases chemical mediators, which include bradykinin, histamine, and prostaglandins, which cause chemical sensitisation.

Pain in the rheumatic diseases is essentially caused by inflammation, pressure or mechanical disorganisation. Pigg et al (1985) has suggested that the causes of pain in the rheumatic diseases can be placed into several discreet categories, which include:

• Physical changes
• Biological
• Chemical irritation.

Physical changes

Disease activity

Many rheumatic diseases cause physical changes within and around joints. The joint capsule, periosteum, blood vessels and deep subcutaneous fascia are well supplied with nerves capable of carrying pain signals, and these structures are the most sensitive to pain. Muscle, fat and synovial membranes are less receptive and compact bone and articular cartilage are insensitive. However, the pain from rheumatic diseases is often deeply located and widely dispersed around the joints and often bears little relationship to the tissue affected, be it periosteum, ligament or fascia (Pigg et al 1985).

Pressure

Pressure is known to cause pain. Within the context of rheumatic diseases, inflammatory effusion and synovial hypertrophy exert increased pressure on the joint capsule and on any exposed bone within it. Pressure at the site of attachment of capsule to sensitive bone can also cause pain. Increased venous pressure, caused by hyperaemia induced by inflammation, is an additional stressor.

Some patients report that the pain in their joints changes with the weather, but there is no consistent evidence of a causal link (Redelmeier & Tversky 1996). However, it has been found that pressure changes in the joint capsule lag behind the changes in atmospheric pressure which accompany changing weather (Hill 1966). This leads to the capsule being either distended or compressed which results in the stimula-

tion of the mechano sensory fibres. As intra articular pressure is already raised in the damaged joint, the changes in barometric pressure cause increased pain (Kantor 1987).

Obesity can be an additional problem, as the excess weight puts further pressure on the diseased joints.

Mechanical damage

Mechanical damage within the joint usually occurs as a result of long term aggressive disease from both RA and osteoarthritis (OA). The loss of cartilage and erosion of bone leaves the joint disorganised and misaligned. Although the cartilage itself is insensitive to pain, its loss leaves the bone surfaces exposed and unprotected, allowing them to come into contact. In this situation, pain tends to occur on movement and when the patient is weight bearing.

Small overgrowths of bone can cause pain both within the joint capsule, and such diverse sites as the heel or spine. They sometimes press on nerve roots, causing excruciating, severe pain.

A further source of pain is fractures. These can sometimes develop in subchondral bone in RA, and are common in osteoporosis.

Biological causes

Biological causes of pain are those which involve microbial agents. These acute infections are known collectively as 'septic arthritis'. The most common septic arthritis is gonococcal arthritis, but this is less destructive and less serious than that caused by the staphylococcus (Mahowald 1993). The inflammation and pressure within the joint cause pain whatever the bacterium involved. Once the causative agent has been eliminated the pain will cease. If appropriate treatment is started early in acute gonococcal or streptococcal infections, pain will subside in about 2 weeks, but it may take longer in staphylococcal and Gram-negative infections. In joints with previous disease, or when joint damage has occurred due to the infection, pain can become chronic.

Chemical origins

Gout, calcium pyrophosphate dihydrate deposition disease and apatite crystal disease are examples of chemically induced pain.

The pain during acute attacks of these crystal deposition diseases can be excruciating, even light pressure, such as that from a bed sheet can be unbearable. Sydney Smith, the great wit described his pain during a particularly acute attack as 'feeling as though I am walking on my eyeballs'.

Inflammation and pressure once again cause the pain.

TYPES OF PAIN

It is important to make a distinction between the different types of pain, as interventions that can be used to bring relief differ. Pain is usually classified according to its cause and duration, namely:

- Acute
- Chronic.

Whilst acute pain may serve as an indicator of the presence of disease, chronic pain rarely serves any biological function but causes a great deal of human suffering, is financially costly to the individual, society and the state.

Acute pain

There are five main features of acute pain:

1. It happens suddenly
2. There is an identifiable cause
3. Healing takes place
4. Its duration is short
5. It has a predictable end.

Infections, injury, or surgery usually cause acute pain. Common everyday examples, which can affect us all, are tonsillitis, fractured limbs or hernia repair. Although the majority of patients with rheumatic disease experience chronic pain, there are instances when their arthritis concurrently causes acute pain. For instance, if they develop septic arthritis, bursitis, tenosynovitis or if they experience a flare. In these circumstances, the patients appear well able to differentiate between chronic pain and acute pain. They often return to clinic saying 'this pain is different from my usual arthritis pain'. Nurses should always take care to listen to their patients and investigate the patient's symptoms; after all, they are the experts.

Some patients with rheumatic diseases undergo surgery for the relief of pain and improvement of function (see Ch. 14). Postoperative pain is classed as acute pain as it fits the above criteria. Anecdotally, some patients who have endured severe, disabling, chronic pain do not perceive their postoperative pain to be as severe as those who have not had this experience.

Iatrogenic pain

Iatrogenic, when referring to illness or symptoms, is defined in the Collins' English Dictionary as 'induced in a patient as the result of a physician's words or actions'. There is no mention of any problems being inflicted by nurses! Unfortunately, nurses do inflict pain on their patients. Sometimes it is unavoidable but at other times it is not. Lifting or moving a patient can be painful, as can taking a blood sample or administering an intra-articular injection. Thankfully, the pain we knowingly inflict is usually of short duration, but this does not obviate the use of all means possible to reduce or eliminate iatrogenic pain.

Chronic pain

Chronic pain is usually defined as that which lasts for 6 months or longer. McCaffery (1983) makes three further classifications:

1. *Limited pain* – This is when there is a known and existing pathology, which is time limited, although the pain may go on for months or years. Examples are carcinoma, which is limited by death, or slow healing injuries such as burns or repetitive strain injury.

2. *Intermittent pain* – Here the patient has pain free periods. The pathology may by understood, but this is not always the case. Examples are migraine or back pain.

3. *Persistent pain* – also called 'chronic benign pain'. This is a rather unfortunate term as it implies that the pain tends to be mild and insignificant, but as Boas (1976) exclaims 'Chronic pain certainly is not benign'. Perhaps a better term for its use in rheumatology is *'chronic non-malignant pain'*. This is pain due to non-life threatening causes, which is not responsive to currently available methods of pain relief and may continue for the remainder of the patient's life (McCaffery & Beebe 1989). This is the category that applies to many of those with RA and OA.

Chronic non-malignant pain has been described as a 'downward spiral' by Everatt (1995), which emphasises the feelings of hopelessness that some people experience when they can see no end to their pain. Perhaps for the purpose of nursing, the less pessimistic model of the 'vicious circle' should be envisaged, as this can be intercepted at some point, and the pain therefore moderated or alleviated (Fig. 8.3). Chronic non-malignant pain brings particular problems. The longer patients have their pain, the less able they seem to tolerate it. Patients sometimes become desperate for relief, using inappropriate drugs and techniques. Increasing passivity and dependency can occur, and worried spouses, family and friends can unwittingly support this. Health professionals can become '

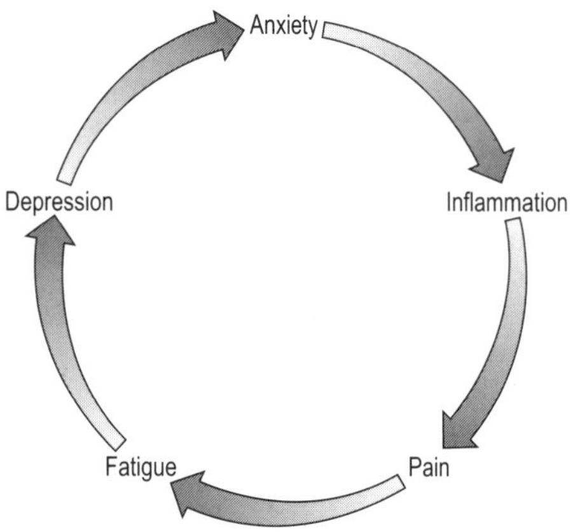

Figure 8.3 Pain circle.

trated at their inability to diminish pain, and tend to accuse patients of exaggerating its severity.

FACTORS WHICH INFLUENCE PAIN

Two people with the same medical diagnosis may report different levels of pain and exhibit different behaviours during pain (Lewis 1978). This illustrates that the intensity of the pain experience cannot simply be equated with tissue damage or the severity of disease (Bellamy & Bradley 1996). The lack of correlation has been acknowledged by Melzack & Wall (1988), who state that 'there are still too many instances where a one to one relationship does not occur to ignore them'. The inference is that other factors must be implicated. In his extensive review of pain and pain control, Weisenberger (1977) considered the following factors to be influential in the pain experience:

- The circumstances in which pain occurs
- Socialisation
- Past experience
- Personality and mood of the person in pain
- The meaning or significance of the pain to that person.

There is also widespread agreement that anxiety exacerbates pain (Skevington 1993).

Donovan (1989) has identified a number of beliefs about pain. They are that pain is:

- A punishment
- A warning that something is wrong
- An emotion (therefore separating psychogenic from somatic aspects of pain)
- Neurotransmission
- A challenge to science
- A complex interaction between mind and body.

We all have our own ideology of pain and so if optimum alleviation is to occur, it is important for nurses to examine their own beliefs as well as those of the patient and their caregivers. For instance, a nurse who does not believe there is merit in aromatherapy for the treatment of pain is unlikely to practise its use, thereby reducing the chances of a successful outcome for some patients.

The attitude of nurses is crucial to pain control, and a number of studies into post operative pain serve to underline this (Davies 1988, Lloyd 1994). Nurses frequently underestimate the patient's pain (Seers 1989); the level of pain experienced by the patient cannot be 'read by the nurse' (Jacques 1992).

THE GATE CONTROL THEORY

There was a young woman from Keele,
Who said, although pain is not real,
When I'm pricked with a pin and it punctures my skin,
I dislike what I fancy I feel.

This ditty demonstrates the enigma of pain. The basic elements of the traditional pain pathways (Fig. 8.2) fail to account for a variety of clinical phenomena. For instance, phantom limb pain, and the absence of pain from major sporting and wartime injuries. Patients and health professionals alike owe much to Melzack & Wall (1965, 1988) for their pioneering work on the 'Gate Control Theory'. This was the first attempt to incorporate physiological and psychological mechanisms into a feasible theory, and although it remains unproven, it underpins many of the pain relieving techniques used by nurses.

The site of control

The grey matter of the dorsal horn in the spinal cord is capped by the *substantia gelatinosa*, which is thought to be the site of control. The theory postulates a 'gate' between the peripheral and higher centres of the central nervous system. When the gate is closed, impulses cannot gain access to the brain. When the gate is open, impulses have free access to the spinal cord and ascend to the brain where the feeling of pain is perceived.

Opening and closing the gate

Gate closure can be achieved by a number of methods (Gallop 1983). They include:

- Increasing large diameter fibre activity, for example by skin stimulation

- Increasing brain stem activity, for instance by distraction from the painful sensation
- Altering thalamic activity by reducing anxiety
- Altering cortical function by changing the significance of painful sensations.

Two important features of gate control are:

1. *Substance P* – an excitatory neurone transmitter, which is released by nociceptor afferent (sensory) neurones at the substantia gelatinosa.
2. *A beta fibres* – thick, heavily myelinated fibres which release inhibitory neurotransmitters at the substantia gelatinosa.

The gate is closed when the input of A beta fibres is greater than the input of the A delta and C fibres (nociceptive input), and open when nociceptive input exceeds A beta input.

It is thought that A beta stimulation can be achieved by gentle massage or rubbing, or by the application of heat or cold. It has been suggested that the reason why many patients with rheumatic disease find rocking chairs comfortable, is that the rhythmic rocking of the chair stimulates a barrage of impulses which inhibit nociceptive transmission (Wyke 1981).

A number of other factors at other sites are also though to be implicated in gate control. For instance, McCaffery & Beebe (1989) suggest that feelings of confidence and control cause inhibitory signals from the cerebral cortex, which help to close the gate.

Endogenous opioids

The first evidence to support the presence of endogenous analgesia pathways was published in the late 1960s (Reynolds, 1969), and Hughes et al (1975) isolated the first endogenous opiate substances shortly after. Endogenous opiates are naturally produced by the body and have properties similar to morphine. They are thought to be neuromodulators, which close the gate by inhibiting the release of substance P. Acupuncture and low frequency transcutaneous electrical nerve stimulation (TENS) increase the production of endogenous opiates.

ASSESSMENT OF PAIN

Pain is a complex phenomenon and so there is no single method of assessment that encapsulates the experience. The most comprehensive assessment will include both:

- Measurement of the pain
- Observation of the expression of pain.

Pain measurement

When measuring pain, a number of factors need to be recorded. These include its:

- Onset
- Intensity
- Location
- Frequency.

Pain is a subjective phenomenon that can only be assessed by the person experiencing it. Patients who are able to do this will need to be taught pain measurement techniques and their recording systems. However, if patients are incapable of recording their own pain, for instance immediately following surgery, the nurse should undertake this task.

Assessment tools

There are a number of commonly used pain assessment tools and these are discussed in Chapter 4. Consideration should be given as to the most appropriate tool to use at a given time. For instance, those patients who are seen in the outpatient clinic at monthly or two monthly intervals could use a simple daily diary card. This usually consists of a 5 point numerical scale with space to record optional analgesic intake. Patients should be encouraged to record any activity that exacerbates their pain, and any therapy, or activity, which relieves it (Fig. 8.4).

Those patients who are hospitalised because of a 'flare' in their RA will require a multidimensional approach and the use of a body map or the McGill Pain Questionnaire (MPQ) may be appropriate (see Ch. 4). The latter is a comprehensive assessment that includes verbal scales that evaluate sensory, emotional and the intensity dimensions of pain (Melzack 1975). There is also a short form MPQ which is less time consuming for the patient to complete, and may be more suitable for patients who are very ill or fatigued (Melzack 1987).

Frequency of measurement

The appropriate timing and frequency of assessment depends on the circumstances, and should be assessed individually for each patient. Assessment should be made whenever the patient and the nurse feel it is appropriate, and this can vary within a 24 hour period, depending on the efficacy of intervention.

A patient who has been admitted to a ward with septic arthritis may need to assess their pain hourly in the first instance. As they begin to improve and their

---

Pain diary

Please fill in the diary each day.
Record the worst pain that you feel
by circling one of the numbers.

1 = no pain
2 = mild pain
3 = moderate pain
4 = severe pain
5 = very severe pain

Please write down any activity that causes or increases your pain,
and anything that relieves it.

Please write down the number of painkillers that you take every day.

Date	Pain Circle one of these numbers	What causes your pain? What relieves your pain?	Number of pain killers
	1 2 3 4 5		
	1 2 3 4 5		
	1 2 3 4 5		
	1 2 3 4 5		
	1 2 3 4 5		
	1 2 3 4 5		
	1 2 3 4 5		
	1 2 3 4 5		
	1 2 3 4 5		
	1 2 3 4 5		
	1 2 3 4 5		
	1 2 3 4 5		

Figure 8.4 Pain diary.

pain decreases, frequency of assessment will gradually diminish until discharge.

Pain assessment should not be regarded as a single encounter between the patient and nurse; it has far wider implications. Firstly, the collaborative, two way communication that is the essence of pain assessment can help to build a strong nurse/patient relationship. Secondly, discussions can also be used as an educational opportunity. By recording their pain and their ability to control it, patients become more confident in their self management and coping skills, which can in itself help to reduce their pain.

Expressing pain

When someone is in pain they communicate it:

- Verbally
- Bodily.

Pe~ le with chronic rheumatic disease often experi-
~ome degree of pain for years on end. As they
~o their disease, many patients learn to control

both their verbal and bodily expressions either as one of their coping strategies, or in the belief that other people find it unacceptable and 'get tired of hearing complaints'. This lack of expression can be misleading, and may be one of the reasons that the literature records that nurses constantly underestimate their patients' pain (Seers 1989).

Encouraging patients to discuss their pain experience will help to indicate its presence more accurately. In a study by Jacox (1979), patients who were being interviewed about their pain began by denying any pain or discomfort at the start of the interview. However, after 10 or 15 minutes encouragement, they admitted to a minimum of mild discomfort.

In addition, visual observation is essential, as many patients do not like to complain verbally. Formal video recorded assessments have shown that observing pain behaviour is a reliable method of assessing pain (Bradley 1993b). Research has been undertaken on pain behaviours associated with both OA (Keefe et al 1987) and RA (McDaniel et al 1986).

Behaviours adopted by patients with OA are:

- Guarding
- Active rubbing
- Unloading joints
- Rigidity
- Joint flexing.

Those with RA shared some of these characteristics, and use the following methods:

- Guarding
- Bracing
- Grimacing
- Sighing
- Rigidity
- Passive rubbing
- Active rubbing.

These behaviours and facial expressions should be watched for and noted as they can signal the presence of unvocalised pain.

The most potent assessment techniques available to the nurse are shown in Fig. 8.5!

MANAGEMENT OF PAIN

When discussing pain, a patient with RA related how she had been told by her General Practitioner 'you've had everything that there is for your pain, you've had all the drugs and now you'll have to get used to it. Go home and learn to live with it'. She described her feelings of devastation, fear and isolation. It is a misconception that those who have intractable pain get used

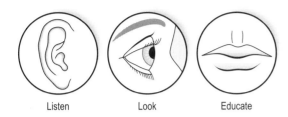

Listen   Look   Educate

Figure 8.5   Potent assessment techniques.

to it. It is more likely that they will become more fearful of it, as their anxiety about their inability to control it and cope with it increases. However, it is important that patients realise that the responsibility for pain control lies partly with them. Nurses and other health professionals should help them to set realistic goals, in the realisation that complete relief may not be possible. Care should incorporate coping techniques as well as pharmacological and complementary therapies.

There are a number of factors to consider when caring for patients in pain. These include:

- Environment
- Equipment
- Handling and positioning
- Patients' expectations
- Pain relief measures.

Environment

Wherever the patient in pain is cared for, the environment can play an important role in pain exacerbation or its diminution.

The patient's home

The home environment is where patients spend most of their time, and therefore it should be adapted in such a way as to cause as little discomfort as possible. Devices such as extended tap handles and jar openers should be provided where necessary, and chairs and sofas need to be easy to access, be comfortable and appropriate. Many patients cause themselves pain when carrying out their personal hygiene and dressing. The occupational therapist will be able to help these patients to eliminate unnecessary pain (see Ch. 11). Splints can help to relieve pain or prevent its appearance and a referral to the physiotherapist can pay dividends.

Pain may cause sleeping difficulties exacerbating fatigue, which in turn makes it harder for the patient to control their pain. This is discussed in Chapter 9.

Hospital ward

Atmosphere. When patients are admitted to hospital, they enter an alien environment that makes them nervous and anxious. They are afraid that staff will not understand their physical problems, such as slowness of movement and reduced dexterity. Patients are frequently reliant on their drug therapies to control pain and these are often taken away from them on admission, and then given to them at inappropriate times. When discussing admission, a patient stated 'I'm better at home, I have my own routine. When I'm at home I can take my pain killers when I need them, and when I need them, I really do need them' These kinds of anxieties need to be addressed, as they only serve to increase the patient's pain.

The atmosphere of the ward can significantly affect the patient's pain. Hurried movement increases their pain and so patients with rheumatic disease require a relaxed and unhurried ward ambience. Periods of rest throughout the day are important to help to restore the energy that will help patients to deal with their pain.

Peaceful, restorative sleep is unhappily not associated with many hospital environments! Hospital wards can be busy, noisy places, particularly if they are mixed speciality medical and surgical wards. Every attempt must be made to provide the patient with a quiet atmosphere in which to sleep. Patients often describe their pain as feeling worse at night. Unfortunately, the dark, quiet nights which we endeavour to provide, are the conditions which restrict sensory information, leaving the 'gate' open and allowing pain to be more readily perceived. Techniques such as distraction and guided imagery can be used to provide the sensory stimulation to close the 'gate' and help to reduce pain. Other methods are discussed in Chapter 9.

Equipment

All wards admitting rheumatic patients should be specially adapted for their needs. Chairs, beds and lifting equipment should be designed to enable the patient to maintain their independence without causing them pain or putting stress on their joints. Washing and bathing facilities should be appropriate and bedside lockers need to be easy to access.

Handling and positioning

When a person has deformed, painful joints and limited mobility, a great deal of skill is required to handle and lift them without inflicting further pain. Each patient requires a slightly different technique, and it is important to listen to the patient, who will know which areas of his or her body is least likely to hurt.

Teaching the patient to place the joints in the most comfortable and least harmful positions and use resting and sleeping splints, will help to alleviate and palliate pain. Good posture helps to keep joints in alignment, and so reduces the chances of placing extra stress on inflamed joints. Patients need to be encouraged to assess the way that they stand, sit, lay and walk and carry.

PAIN RELIEF MEASURES

Relieving or palliating physical and psychological pain is one of the primary functions of the rheumatology nurse. As the causes of pain are so diverse, it is incumbent on nurses to equip themselves with a battery of interventions and skills. The most commonly used treatments are:

- Drug therapy
- Physiotherapy
- Transcutaneous electrical nerve stimulation
- Heat/cold
- Patient education
- Patient's own remedies.

Drug therapy

Pharmacology plays an important role in pain control and the drugs used are discussed in more depth in Chapter 12. The most common medications are:

- Simple and compound analgesics
- Non-steroidal anti-inflammatory drugs (NSAIDs)
- Steroids
- Antidepressants.

Analgesics

Analgesics are usually classified as non-opioid or opioid drugs.

Non-opioids. Simple analgesics such as paracetamol work by blocking the synthesis and secretion of prostaglandins, thereby preventing nociceptor sensitisation (Speight 1987). These drugs are quite mild and usually prescribed at a maximum dose of 8×500 mg tablets a day. Perhaps the most commonly prescribed analgesic for rheumatic diseases is a compound analgesic, co-proxamol. This is a combination of dextropropoxyphene and paracetamol. Again the maximum dose is two tablets, four times a day.

Opioids. Opioid analgesics are potent drugs that ` by fitting into the opioid receptors of the brain inal cord. Controversy surrounds their use

in non-malignant pain, as side effects and dependence is said to occur in most patients (Justins 1996). They are used following surgery, and occasionally and with great caution, when rheumatic pain is very severe.

Different analgesics suit different patients at different times. The way in which drugs are used is probably more important than which drug is prescribed (McCaffery & Beebe 1989).

When treating the rheumatic patient, analgesics are rarely prescribed alone. In RA, they are usually prescribed in addition to a non-steroidal anti-inflammatory drug and a slow acting anti-rheumatic drug. In OA, they are the first drugs of choice, but as the disease progresses and the pain increases, they are often combined with a non-steroidal anti-inflammatory drug.

When given in combination, analgesics are at the discretion of the patient. They should be informed of the maximum dose and advised to take them before the pain gets severe. This means that if they are in a flare, it may be necessary to take the maximum dose on a regular basis, but if pain is mild, an occasional ingestion will suffice.

Analgesics can also be taken prophylactically, to prevent predictable pain in chronic disease. A good example is taking analgesics half an hour before sexual activity. Many analgesics are quickly absorbed and have a short half-life. For the quickest effect, they can be taken on an empty stomach, but this is contraindicated if the patient is using aspirin based analgesics, as these are gastric irritants.

If patients habitually need the maximum dose, or are overdosing on their analgesics, this is an indicator that they are not working as they are intended. In these cases, pain should be assessed using an appropriate chart, and new drugs and therapies initiated.

Non-steroidal anti-inflammatory drugs

The anti-inflammatory drugs are one of the mainstays of drug therapy in the rheumatic diseases (see Ch. 12). They are in the form of tablets, suppositories, gels and creams. Tablets and suppositories are taken as a regular regimen, gels and creams are used as necessary. They can take effect extremely quickly, reducing pain and joint stiffness. They also have an antipyretic effect. Efficacy usually increases as the levels of drug in the plasma rise and steady state is reached.

Tablets should always be taken with or after food, as this reduces the chance of gastric irritation. Many patients take their first non-steroidal anti-inflammatory drug of the day as soon as they wake up. If they are in hospital, this means that they will need an early morning snack with which to take them.

Steroids

Steroids are commonly administered via the following routes:

- Oral
- Intramuscular
- Intra-articular
- Intravenous.

When used at the right time, via the correct route and in the correct dose, steroids can be very effective at reducing pain and stiffness (see Ch. 12). One of the most common applications is intra-articular treatment to a single or small number of inflamed joints. This treatment can have a dramatic effect on pain. In a recent study, triamcinolone hexacetonide was shown to bring about greater sustained pain relief in rheumatoid knees than hydrocortisone succinate or triamcinolone acetonide (Blyth et al 1994). Although nurses cannot prescribe these drugs, they can suggest their use and administer them after appropriate training. In the UK, guidelines have been published by the Rheumatology Nursing Forum and are available from the Royal College of Nursing (Appendix 3). Many patients are fearful of steroid therapy, worrying about the side effects such as gastric ulceration and weight gain. Discussion with the patient of their beliefs, and education, can help to alleviate these worries.

Antidepressants

Depression is known to affect the perception of pain and if the patient is depressed, antidepressants can help. Amitriptyline is an antidepressant that is used in the rheumatic diseases as a pain modulator. It is usually taken at night, which helps the patient to sleep. Having slept, they feel less tired and more able to cope with their pain.

Self administration of drugs

Some rheumatology wards have incorporated self administration schemes into their ward practice. Following her research, Bird (1990) concluded 'Self administration of drugs would appear to be a more appropriate method than the conventional system for selected hospital patients.' Rheumatic patients are certainly in this category. They need to be able to take their drugs both prn, prophylactically, and if indicated, with or directly following food. This becomes very difficult if patients have to wait to be given their drugs by the nurse.

Physiotherapy

Pain relief is a multidisciplinary process and liaison with the physiotherapist is imperative. Physiotherapy can help to control pain in a number of arthritic conditions, including RA, OA and back pain (Minor & Sanford 1993). The Clinical Standards Advisory Group (1994) has published an epidemiological review of low back pain. It highlights the necessity for active rehabilitation within the first 6 weeks of onset, which helps to prevent long-term pain and disability.

Osteoarthritis of the patelofemoral compartment of the knee has been shown to be an important cause of knee pain (McAlindon et al 1992). The medial application of tape to this area has been shown to reduce pain in this condition (Cushnaghan 1993).

Referring patients to the physiotherapist at an early stage in their disease may help to prevent malalignment and so prevent pain from occurring.

Transcutaneous electrical nerve stimulation (TENS)

Electrical stimulation is not a new idea. Electric eels were used by the Romans to relieve arthritis pain as early as 46 AD. The Victorians went on to produce galvanic stimulation machines. Present day machines are called TENS. This is a noninvasive therapy, in which electrical current is applied via electrodes placed on the skin. There are two types of TENS, which work in distinctly different ways (Davis 1994):

- High frequency.
- Low frequency.

High frequency TENS (15–150 Hz) works by stimulating A fibre activity which closes the gate, inhibiting the transmission of pain sensations to the brain via the C fibres.

Low frequency TENS (2 Hz) works by increasing the production of endogenous opiates. TENS is felt by the patient as a buzzing, tingling or vibrating sensation, but it does not appear to cause many side effects. Skin irritation has been reported by some patients, usually associated with the electrode, gel or tape application (Richardson 1985). TENS helps some patients with arthritis (Lewis et al 1984), but by no means all. It is worth trying on particularly painful joints and it has the advantage to the patient of being self-administered. The application, contraindications and effectiveness are discussed in more depth elsewhere (Hayes 1996).

Heat and cold

Patients often feel that warming a joint reduces their pain, and many patients report global improvement following heat treatments. Heat is thought to contribute to pain relief in several ways. They include:

• Increasing pain threshold
• Increasing blood flow
• Washing out pain producing metabolites
• Decreasing muscle guarding.

Two types of heat are used to reduce pain:

1. Superficial heat
2. Deep heat.

As the name implies, superficial heat only penetrates the skin to a depth of a few millimetres. Its effects are thought to occur through reflex vascular and neural responses. Common ways of applying superficial heat are:

• Hot packs
• Heat lamps
• Warm baths/showers
• Wax baths.

Heat is usually applied for about 20 minutes. It is an easy treatment for the nurse to apply, and convenient, cheap and safe for the patient to use at home.

Deep heat is usually administered by a physiotherapist using:

• Ultrasound
• Short wave diathermy

It works in the same way as superficial heat, but penetrates deeper, reaching muscles and connective tissue.

Contraindications to the application of heat are discussed by Hayes (1996).

Cold

Some patients feel quicker and longer lasting pain relief by the local application of cold to their joints. This can be provided by:

• Ice packs
• Cold packs
• Iced water
• Vapocoolant sprays.

Applications of cold decreases three of the symptoms of arthritic disease, namely:

1. Pain
2. Swelling
3. Inflammation.

Pain relief is brought about by slowing or blocking nerve conduction or releasing endorphins. Reduction of swelling is through vasoconstriction, and the reduction of inflammation is aided by blocking the release of histamine.

Cold is particularly effective for acutely inflamed joints, close to the skin surface. It is also an effective therapy for, tendonitis and bursitis. Side effects include:

• Ice burns
• Hypersensitivity
• Joint stiffness.

Cold should not be used on patients with impaired peripheral circulation.

Patient education

Patient education is the keystone of successful treatment and this is discussed in Chapter 15. The foundation of many patient education programmes is grounded in self-efficacy theory. The term self efficacy refers to the belief that one can manage a specific challenging situation (Bandura 1977). Teaching patients about their disease and treatments has been shown to bring beneficial effects (Hill 1995), and a number of studies have shown that patient education can help to bring pain relief to those with rheumatic disease (Lorig et al 1987).

Pain behaviour is related to belief in self-efficacy, rather than being solely accounted for by disease activity (Buescher et al 1991). Depression has been shown to effect pain perception (Wolfe & Hawley 1993), but anxiety and depression occur as a result of pain rather than being the cause of it (Smedstad et al 1995).

Teaching patients about their disease helps to relieve anxiety and lift depression, which helps to relieve their pain (Hill 1991a). Verbal education should always be backed up by written information, and an example of a patient information sheet on pain control is shown in Appendix 2.

Patients' own remedies

Expectations regarding outcome are also important. The patient's beliefs must be taken into account. If someone believes that a treatment will help, then it has more chance of being successful. If patients expect to feel pain, or do not expect a treatment to work, their expectations tend to be fulfilled. Once expectations are formed, it is hard to change them. Providing they are not harmful, incorporate the patient's own remedies into the treatment plan.

COMPLEMENTARY THERAPIES

As well as conventional treatments for pain relief, nurses have access to an array of techniques to complement these therapies. They include:

- Massage
- Relaxation
- Therapeutic touch
- Aromatherapy
- Reiki
- Reflexology
- Visualisation
- Guided imagery.

Many of these therapies are discussed in Chapter 13. All treatments must be with the agreement of the patient, and many of these therapies can be undertaken safely by the patient or carer at home. For instance, someone who is close to the patient can undertake simple massage, or essential oils can be used in the bath.

JOINT STIFFNESS

Stiffness is a major problem for those with rheumatic disease. It can alter the quality of their lives and ability to function normally (Brown et al 1987). Although it is often worst first thing in the morning when it is known as 'morning stiffness', it can occur at other times of day, usually following rest when it is termed 'inactivity stiffness' (Hill 1991b). When patients with rheumatic diseases are admitted to a ward, consideration will need to be given to the effect that their stiffness has on their mobility. An unhurried atmosphere is essential and they will need extra time to limber up and mobilise in the mornings. Washing and dressing will take longer and they may require an early hydrotherapy treatment or a warm bath or shower before other patients.

DEFINITIONS OF STIFFNESS

Stiffness is a very complex sensation and so has proved a remarkably difficult symptom to define. Steinberg (1978) described it as 'shorthand for a general increase in musculoskeletal symptoms'. The Dictionary of the Rheumatic Diseases (1982) defines early morning stiffness as 'the subjective complaint of localised or generalised lack of easy mobility of the joints upon arising'.

For those experiencing stiffness it is often defined by its affects. These terms include:

- Immobility
- Limitation of movement
- Resistance to movement
- Tightness.

CAUSES OF STIFFNESS

In the rheumatic diseases, joint stiffness is usually caused by:

- Inflammation
- Soft tissue thickening
- Changes to the articular surfaces of the bones
- Loss of mechanical integrity
- Environmental factors.

Inflammation causes tissue swelling or oedema that leads to an increase in the amount of synovial fluid within the joint. This causes the feeling of tightness, that many patients complain of. Baker's or popliteal cysts (see page 56) are also a common problem. They occur at the knee and are a common cause of stiffness and tightness. Roughening of the articular surface can increase friction within the joint, which limits movement. This is often described by the patient as the sensation of 'stiffness'.

Muscle stiffness

Most people are affected by muscular stiffness at some time, perhaps as a result of unaccustomed exercise or following an extra vigorous exercise routine. Most muscle stiffness resolves spontaneously after a few days. Patients with rheumatic disease are not exempt from this type of stiffness and unfortunately when it happens, it may be more pronounced and of longer duration (Pigg et al 1985).

The relationship between pain and stiffness

Stiffness can be perceived in the absence of pain, but for patients with rheumatic disease, it is often accompanied by pain. A study that investigated morning stiffness qualitatively and quantitatively showed that 40% of patients with RA and non-inflammatory conditions mentioned pain as often as stiffness as descriptors (Hazes et al 1993). This finding concurred with that of Rhind et al (1987), who found that out of 100 patients interviewed, 68 indicated that limited movement was accompanied by pain.

Stiffness can also be a symptom of pain. If this is the case, then treating the pain will help the stiffness.

Association of stiffness and disease activity

Although stiffness is unpleasant at any time, morning stiffness is of particular significance in inflammatory arthritis, and a significant indicator of disease activity in RA. For many years the duration rather than the severity of morning stiffness has been used as a measure of disease activity. Although the duration of morning stiffness is placed at the head of the most recent criteria for the classification of RA (Arnett et al 1988), this rational has recently been questioned by Hazes et al (1993). In their study, the severity of morning stiffness was found to be a better discriminator between active and inactive RA. From the patient's viewpoint, it is usually the duration of morning stiffness, rather than its severity that has the most profound effect. Prolonged morning stiffness creates many practical problems that stem from limited and slow movement and reduction in grip strength. These include:

• Getting out of bed
• Washing/bathing
• Dressing
• Preparing food
• Eating food
• Driving.

These difficulties are compounded if the patient is a young mother who has to care for a baby or is trying to get the children off to school.

MEASURING STIFFNESS

A measurement of the duration and severity of stiffness will help the nurse to assess the patient's problems and formulate a meaningful care plan. Sequential readings will help to evaluate the effects of any treatments.

Objective measurement of stiffness has been attempted, but for practical purposes, stiffness measurement relies upon the patient's subjective assessment. Unfortunately, some patients have great difficulty dissociating their stiffness from their pain and the nurse needs to take the time to explain the difference. Another area that causes confusion is that patients often have morning stiffness, which is followed by inactivity stiffness if they rest or sit for prolonged periods. This may then be proceeded by evening stiffness. The type of stiffness the patient is required to note will depend on why it is being recorded. A thorough explanation to the patient of what is required and why it is needed will help accurate measurement.

The most sensible way to record morning stiffness is on a daily diary card similar to that used to record pain (Fig. 8.4). If the patient completes it each day, they will get into the habit of noting:

• Duration of stiffness
• Severity
• Location

• What if anything causes stiffness
• Treatments that are helpful.

The stiffness diary card can then be used as a teaching aid as well as an assessment tool.

RELIEVING STIFFNESS

Many of the treatments that relieve pain also relieve stiffness. They include:

• Drug therapy
• Exercise
• Hydrotherapy
• Splinting
• Heat
• Massage
• Patient education.

Drug therapy

Anti-inflammatory drugs reduce stiffness by decreasing inflammation. Indomethacin, which can be given as a suppository in the evening, is particularly effective for morning stiffness. If the cause of joint stiffness is an excess of synovial fluid, this can be aspirated and when inflammation is also present, an intra-articular injection of steroid may be efficacious.

When patients are in pain they often tense their muscles, which causes stiffness and further pain. Analgesics will help the stiffness by reducing the pain that is causing the stiffness.

If the morning stiffness is caused by disease activity, the introduction of disease modifying drugs will help to alleviate it over time.

Exercise

Morning stiffness can be prolonged for those with active RA. There are a number of activities that patients can undertake that will ease their morning stiffness:

• Gentle limbering up movements before getting out of bed
• A daily exercise regime
• Gentle range of motion exercises before going to bed.

In addition to these methods, inactivity stiffness can be relieved by:

• Frequent changes of position
• Frequent gentle stretching movements
• Range of movement exercises.

Patients need to get into a routine of exercising, but they often find this difficult as in addition to their stiffness, they may be in pain, feel debilitated and fatigued. The best way to ensure that patients undertake exercise is to make sure that they believe that what they do will make a difference. The exercise regime should not be too long, and when possible it should be incorporated it into their daily routine. The nurse's role is to encourage, guide and enable the patient. Once they begin to notice the benefits, they will become more confident in their own self efficacy ability, which will foster their willingness to carry out their exercise programme.

Splinting

Splinting tends to bring greater relief from pain than from morning stiffness. However, splints do help to reduce inflammation and consequently this can help to alleviate stiffness. For instance, a resting or night splint may help to relieve pain and morning stiffness.

The elastic or stretch glove is a type of soft splint that is worn specifically to reduce morning stiffness. They work by gently compressing the hand and providing neutral warmth, and there is some research to show that they are effective (Erlich & DiPiero 1971). However, for those patients with carpal tunnel syndrome, they should be provided with caution as they can exacerbate paraesthesia.

Heat

Heat can be very comforting and relaxing and this may well help to alleviate stiffness. For patients who are hospitalised, prolonged morning stiffness can be lessened by hydrotherapy. This should be scheduled as early as possible and prior to their exercise regime. If hydrotherapy is not available, or when the patient is at home, a warm bath or shower taken first thing in the morning helps to alleviate or moderate their morning stiffness. Local applications of superficial heat as discussed on pages 147–148 are cheap and easy to apply both in hospital and at home. Stiff hands and feet can be placed into warm water, and the addition of flexing and stretching movements will make them feel more flexible. Contrast baths consist of dipping the hands or feet alternately into warm and cool water. This technique works for some people, but should be avoided if the patient suffers from circulatory problems or Raynaud's phenomenon.

Massage

Massage can help to reduce stiffness and its application is discussed in Chapter 13. Gentle stroking massage has been advocated to reduce oedema and stiffness (Pigg et al 1985). Patients can carry this out for themselves if the area is accessible, but it is more relaxing when undertaken by a carer or friend.

Patient education

The patient's knowledge of the causes of their stiffness and the treatments available to relieve it should be assessed and whenever possible relatives and carers should also be included. Patients may be unaware of the association between lengthening morning stiffness and increasing disease activity. It is important that they and their significant others are taught to discriminate between the differing causes of stiffness so that they can choose the most effective treatments to manage it.

The effective management of pain and stiffness are major challenges to both nurses and patients alike. Patients place the alleviation of pain and stiffness high on their list of priorities, and it is incumbent on nurses to try to meet their aspirations as far as it is possible. To be successful, nurses require a high degree of knowledge and skill to enable their patients to cope with these debilitating symptoms. Uncontrolled, chronic pain leads to loss of grace and dignity in any human being. It can be destructive to both the person who feels it and to those who witness it; this includes family, friends and health professionals alike. Elimination of pain is rarely achievable in the rheumatic diseases, but moderation to a level which is acceptable to the patient must be.

Action points for practice:

- Describe the nociceptor receptor system, and discuss its effects on the perception of pain.
- Keep a reflective diary whilst working in a situation when you are nursing a patient in pain. Note the critical incidents that occur and demonstrate how your knowledge of pain affects your ability to care for the patient.
- Write a case history of a patient with severe RA. Discuss the tools used to assess their pain and stiffness and the treatments used to alleviate their symptoms.
- Write a list of the causes of pain and stiffness. In the opposite column, write a list of all the possible treatments. Include complementary therapies and the patient's own remedies.

REFERENCES

Arnett F C, Edworthy S M, Bloch D A et al 1988 The American rheumatism association 1987 revised criteria for the classification of rheumatoid arthritis. Arthritis and Rheumatism 31: 315–324

Bandura A 1977 Self-efficacy: toward a unifying theory of behavioral change. Psychological Review 84: 191–215

Bellamy N, Bradley L A 1996 Workshop on chronic pain, pain control and patient outcomes in rheumatoid arthritis and osteoarthritis. Arthritis and Rheumatism 39(3): 357–362

Bird C 1990 A prescription for self help. Nursing Times 86(43): 52–55

Boas R A 1976 Chronic benign pain. Pain 2: 1119–1125

Blyth T, Hunter J A, Stirling A 1994 Pain relief in the rheumatoid knee after steroid injection; a single-blind comparison of hydrocortisone succinate, and triamcinolone acetonide or hexacetonide. British Journal of Rheumatology 33: 461–463

Bradley L A 1993a The challenges of pain in arthritis. Arthritis Care and Research 6: 169–170

Bradley L A 1993b Pain measurement in arthritis. Arthritis Care and Research 6: 178–186

Brown G M M, Dare C M, Smith P R, Meyers O L 1987 Important problems identified by patients with chronic arthritis. South African Medical Journal 72: 126–128

Buescher K L, Johnston J A, Parker J C et al 1991 Relationship of self-efficacy to pain behavior. Journal of Rheumatology 18(7):968–972

Campbell J 1995 Making sense of pain management. Nursing Times 91(27): 34–35

Clinical Standard Advisory Group 1994 Epidemiology review: the epidemiology and cost of back pain. HMSO, London

Cushnaghan J 1993 Tackling pain. Nursing Times 89(22): 32–34

Davis P S 1994 Reducing pain. In: Davis P S (ed) Nursing the orthopaedic patient. Churchill Livingstone, Edinburgh, ch 7, p 133

Davis P 1993 Opening up the gate control theory. Nursing Standard 7(45): 25–27

Davis P A 1988 Changing nursing practice for more effective control of post operative pain through a staff initiated education programme. Nurse Education Today 8: 325–331

Dictionary of the Rheumatic Diseases (1982) Signs and symptoms. American Rheumatism Association, Atlanta

Donovan M I 1989 An historical view of pain management. Cancer Nursing 12(4): 257–261

Erlich G E, DiPiero A M 1971 Stretch gloves: nocturnal use to ameliorate morning stiffness in the arthritic hand. Archives of Physical Medicine and Rehabilitation 51: 479–480

Everatt R 1995 Pain management. Nursing Times 91(10): 40–41

Gallop S M 1983 Patient teaching: pain and pain control. In: Wilson-Barnett J (ed) Patient teaching. Churchill Livingstone, Edinburgh, ch10, p178

Harvey A 1987 Neurophysiology of rheumatic pain. Baillière's Clinical Rheumatology, 1(1): 1–26

Hayes K W 1996 Physical modalities. In:Wegener S T (ed) Clinical Care in the Rheumatic Diseases. American College of Rheumatology, Atlanta, ch13, p 79–82

Hazes J M W, Hayton R, Silman A J 1993 A reevaluation of the symptom of morning stiffness. Journal of Rheumatology 20(7): 1138–1142

Hill D F 1966 Climate and arthritis. In: Hollander J L (ed) Arthritis and Allied Conditions, 7th edn, Leo Febiger, Philadelphia, p589–596

Hill J 1995 Patient education in rheumatic diseases. Nursing Standard 9(25): 25–28

Hill J 1991a Caring and curing. Nursing Times 87(45): 29–31

Hill J 1991b Assessing rheumatic disease. Nursing Times 87(4): 33–35

Hughes J, Smith T W, Kosterlitz H W et al 1975 Identification of two related pena peptides from the brain with potent opiate antagonist activity. Nature 258: 577–579

Jacox A 1979 Assessing pain. American Journal of Nursing 79: 895–900

Jacques A 1992 Do you believe I'm in pain? Professional Nurse 249–251

Jones A K P 1997 Pain and its perception. Topical Reviews, Arthritis and Rheumatism Council, Chesterfield

Justins D M 1996 Management strategies for chronic pain. Annals of the Rheumatic Diseases 55: 588–596

Kantor T G 1987 Chemical mediators and treatment of pain in rheumatic disease. Baillière's Clinical Rheumatology, 1(1): 57–70

Kazis L E, Meenan R F, Anderson J J 1983 Pain in the rheumatic diseases: investigation of a key health status component. Arthritis and Rheumatism 26(8): 1017–1022

Keefe F J, Caldwell D S, Queen K et al 1987 Osteoarthritic knee pain: a behavioral analysis. Pain 28: 309–321

Lewis D, Lewis L, Sturrock R 1984 Transcutaneous electrical nerve stimulation in osteoarthritis: a therapeutic alternative? Annals of the Rheumatic Diseases 43: 47–49

Lewis G 1978 The peace of pain in human experience. Journal of Medical Ethics 4: 122–125

Liebeskind J C, Melzack R 1987 The international pain foundation: meeting a need for education in pain management (editorial). Pain 30: 1–2

Lloyd G 1994 Nurses' attitudes towards management of pain. Nursing Times 90(43): 40–43

Lorig K, Konkol L, Gonzalez V 1987 Arthritis patient education: a review of the literature. Patient Education and Counselling 10: 207–252

McAlindon T E, Snow S, Cooper C, Dieppe P A 1992 Radiographic patterns of osteoarthritis of the knee joint in the community: the importance of the patellofemoral joint. Annals of the Rheumatic Diseases 51: 844–849

McCaffrey M 1983 Nursing the patient in pain, 2nd edn. Harper & Row, London

McCaffery M, Beebe A 1989 Pain. Clinical manual for nursing practice. C V Moseby, St Louis

McDaniel L K, Anderson K O, Bradley L A et al 1986 Development of an observation method for assessing pain behavior in rheumatoid arthritis patients. Pain 24: 165–184

Mahowald M 1993 Infectious arthritis: bacterial agents. In: Schumacher H R, Klippel J H, Koopman W J (eds) Primer on the rheumatic diseases, 10th edn. Arthritis Foundation, Atlanta, p192–197

Maycock J 1984 Pain – a different approach. Nursing 31: 924–925

Melzack R 1987 The short form McGill pain questionnaire. Pain 30: 191–197

Melzack R 1975 The McGill pain questionnaire: major properties and scoring systems. Pain 1: 277–299

Melzack R, Wall P D 1988 The challenge of pain, 2nd edn. Penguin, Harmondsworth

Melzack R, Wall P D 1965 Pain mechanisms: a new theory. Science 150: 971–978

Merskey H 1973 The perception and measurement of pain. Journal of Psychosomatic Research 17: 251–255

Merskey H 1979 Pain terms: a list with definitions and notes on usage recommended by the IASP subcommittee on taxonomy. Pain 6: 249–252

Minor M A, Sanford M K 1993 Physical interventions in the management of pain in arthritis: an overview for research and practice. Arthritis Care and Research 6: 197–206

Morgan J M 1993 An introduction of pathology. Campion Press, Edinburgh

Parker J, Frank R, Beck N et al 1988 Pain in rheumatoid arthritis: relationship to demographic, medical and psychological factors. Journal of Rheumatology 15(3): 433

Pigg J S, Driscoll P W, Caniff R 1985 Pain. In: Rheumatology nursing a problem-oriented approach. John Wiley, New York, ch 5, p 107

Redelmeier D A, Tversky A 1996 On the belief that arthritis pain is influenced by the weather. Proceedings of the National Academy of Sciences of the United States of America 93(7): 2895–2896

Reynolds D V 1969 Surgery in the rat during electrical analgesia induced by focal brain stimulation. Science 164: 444–445

Rhind V M, Unsworth A, Haslock I 1987 Assessment of stiffness in rheumatology: the use of rating scales. British Journal of Rheumatology 26: 126–130

Richardson C 1985 Plugged in to pain control. Nursing Mirror 160(5): 6–8

Sargent C 1984 Between death and shame: dimensions of pain in Bariba culture. Social Science and Medicine 19(12): 1299–1304

Seers K 1989 Assessing pain. Nursing Standard 15(3): 32–34

Skevington S M 1993 The experience and management of pain in rheumatological disorders. Baillière's Clinical Rheumatology 7(2): 319–335

Smedstad L M, Vaglum P, Kvien T K M, Moum T 1995 The relationship between self reported pain and sociodemographic variables, anxiety and depressive symptoms in rheumatoid arthritis. Journal of Rheumatology 22(3): 514–520

Speight T M 1987 Avery's drug treatment. Churchill Livingstone, Edinburgh

Steinberg A D 1978 On morning stiffness. Journal of Rheumatology 5(1): 3–6

Symmons D, Bankhead C 1994 Health care needs assessment for musculoskeletal diseases: the first step – estimating the number of incidents and prevalent cases. Arthritis and Rheumatism Council, Chesterfield

Weisenberger M 1977 Pain and pain control. Psychological Bulletin 84(5): 1008–1044

Wolfe F, Hawley D J 1993 The relationship between clinical activity and depression in rheumatoid arthritis. Journal of Rheumatology 20(12): 2032–2037

Wyke B 1981 The neurology of joints: a review of general principles. Clinics in Rheumatic Diseases 7(1): 223–239

FURTHER READING

Lehmann J F 1982 Therapeutic heat and cold, 3rd edn. Williams & Wilkins, Baltimore

McCaffery 1983 Nursing the patient in pain. Harper & Row, London

McCaffery M, Beebe A 1994 Pain. Clinical manual for nurses. C V Moseby, St Louis

Melzack R 1996 The challenge of pain. Penguin Press, London

9

Fatigue and sleep

Christine E. White

The aims of this chapter are to provide the nurse with an understanding of the relationship between fatigue and sleep in the rheumatic diseases, and to identify the role of the nurse in its management. After reading this chapter you should be able to:

- Define fatigue and identify its causes
- Discuss the effects of rheumatic disease on fatigue
- Advise patients on how to minimise the effects of fatigue
- Define sleep and the benefits of restorative sleep
- Advise patients on ways to achieve a restful night's sleep.

FATIGUE

Fatigue is a major debilitating problem for patients with rheumatic illness and it is particularly associated with active disease. It can interfere with the patient's ability to function adequately and cope with every day tasks. Consequently, it may lead to a reduction in work output, a predisposition to personal injury and cause an incremental loss of usable time which cumulates in:

- Irritability with self and with others
- Frustration due to inability to complete a task
- An overwhelming sense of helplessness and hopelessness
- Strained relationships with friends and family members due to lack of understanding of the nature and severity of fatigue
- Lack of personal control.

Fatigue can also lead to an inability to contribute to many aspects of normal family life. For instance, the fulfilment of the individual's role within the family may change and the ensuing financial consequences can be considerable.

To manage their generalised fatigue, patients must recognise it as part of their disease and learn what causes it and what may help to alleviate it.

Peripheral and central muscle fatigue

It is important to differentiate between *weakness* and *fatigue*.

Weakness is defined as 'an inability to produce the expected or desired force' whilst fatigue is defined 'as an inability to maintain the desired or expected force' (Edwards 1981). A further distinction is usually made between central and peripheral fatigue (Table 9.1).

Central fatigue is when the impairment is located in the central nervous system. That is the lack of central drive, which may be of either a voluntary or non-voluntary type, due for example to poor motivation or the effects of anaemia.

Peripheral fatigue is when impairment is located in either the peripheral nerve, or contractile apparatus of the muscle. A voluntary muscular contraction involves a complex series of events. Weakness and fatigue can occur as a result of impairment at one or several links in the hierarchical neuromuscular chain, which links

Table 9.1 Central and peripheral fatigue (adapted from Edward's Hierarchical chain of command (1981))

	Site of fatigue	Cause of fatigue
Central	Brain	• Pain • Fear of pain • Anaemia • Poor motivation • Effects of drugs • Lack of energy due to disease activity (e.g. RA) • Psychological aspects including: depression, anxiety, stress, boredom, responsibility and conflict • Environmental factors including: social, surroundings, noise, light and climate • Inadequate sleep or rest • Inadequate nutrition and obesity • Illness including: drug therapy, physiological imbalance and surgery
	Spinal column	Myelopathy e.g. RA neck
Peripheral	Peripheral nerve	Entrapment neuropathy Peripheral neuropathy (e.g. in RA) Radiculopathy
	Neuromuscular junction	Penicillamine induced myasthenia
	Muscle cell membrane	Steroid atrophy Disuse atrophy
	Transverse tubular system	Reflex inhibition atrophy RA associated myositis
	Calcium release	Other drugs (Simvestatin) Inactivity
	Actin-myosin activation	Exercise Work
	Myofibrillar cross bridge-formation	
	Force generation	

• All of the rheumatic problems will cause the central effect through increased perception of effort.

functions in the central nervous system to this contractile machinery.

Fatigue or dysfunction may result from defects in any of the commands in the chain of hierarchical physiological steps required to produce voluntary skeletal muscle contractions (Edwards 1981). Patients with rheumatoid arthritis (RA) are highly susceptible to peripheral dysfunction which includes:

- Entrapment neuropathy
- Metabolic muscle wasting including steroid myopathy
- Intragenic muscle wasting
- Peripheral neuropathy
- Drug induced myasthenia.

Central dysfunction may also occur through pain or fear of pain.

Other definitions and classifications of fatigue

Definitions of generalised fatigue

Generalised fatigue is also known as 'whole body fatigue'. Fatigue has been defined by a number of authors. Smith Pigg et al (1985) describes it as 'a subjective complaint of weariness, exhaustion or lassitude, frequently associated with irritability, inefficiency, and decreased capacity for work'; whilst Piper (1991) states that it is 'an overwhelming sustained sense of exhaus-

tion and decreased capacity for physical and mental work'.

Classifications of fatigue

There are four classifications of fatigue:

1. Acute fatigue
2. Chronic fatigue
3. Subjective fatigue
4. Objective fatigue.

Acute fatigue is primarily induced by an excessive use of an organ or bodily system, and is usually of short duration and relieved by rest, sleep or a change in situation (Crosby 1991).

Chronic fatigue is persistent, cumulative, not eliminated by rest and is usually associated with illness. Pronounced day to day fatigue may, eventually lead to chronic fatigue (Crosby 1991).

It is important to differentiate between fatigue which is chronic in nature and chronic fatigue syndrome. To qualify for the diagnosis of chronic fatigue syndrome a person must have debilitating fatigue that has lasted for more than 6 months and no other medical or psychiatric condition that produces similar symptoms (Crosby 1991).

A comparison of the distinguishing characteristics of acute and chronic fatigue is shown in Table 9.2.

Table 9.2 Acute and chronic fatigue – distinguishing characteristics (adapted from Piper (1988))

Characteristics	Acute fatigue	Chronic fatigue
Purpose/Function	Protective	Unknown, may no longer be protective
Population at risk	Anybody	Primarily those suffering from some form of disease
Aetiology	Usually identifiable	May not be identifiable
	Usually involves a single mechanism or cause	Usually multiple causes
	Often experienced in relation to some form of activity or exertion	Often in experience with no relationship to activity or exertion
Perception	Normal	Abnormal
	Expected with specific activities	Excessive in comparison and disproportionate to past experience
	Primarily localised to specific body part or system	Generalised, physical and mental
	Pleasant or unpleasant	Unpleasant
Time to onset	Rapid	Insidious, gradual
		Cumulative
Duration	Short	Persistent
		More than one month
Method of relief	Usually alleviated by a good night's sleep, adequate rest, proper diet, exercise programme, or stress management techniques	Relief only partial or temporary with any method
		A combination of approaches may be needed
	Resolves quickly	Does not resolve quickly
Impact on activities of daily living and quality of life	Minimal	Major

Subjective fatigue is defined in Dorland's Medical Dictionary as 'perceptual, pertaining to or perceived only by the affected individual'.

Objective fatigue is perceptible externally and may be physiological, biochemical or behavioural.

Symptoms of fatigue

The word 'fatigue' is used to describe a wide variety of signs and symptoms related to the failure to sustain some form of physical activity. It is a common experience in everyday life which limits our activities and horizons (Holder-Powell & Jones 1990). In any healthy individual, fatigue may result from strenuous exercise, a busy day at work or emotional tension. Rest, relaxation or a change in activity usually brings relief. Both the fatigue and ensuring recovery period are normal experiences. Healthy people rarely consider fatigue as a serious problem because the condition is temporary and relief measures are effective (Tack 1990). However, the symptoms of fatigue described by Hashimoto et al (1975) are clearly felt by those afflicted and include:

- Decrease of attention
- Slow and impaired perception
- Impairment of thinking
- Decrease of motivation
- Decrease of performance speed
- Decrease of accuracy and an increase of errors
- Decrease of performance capability for physical and mental activity.

They also state that:

'In a tired condition the subjective sensation of fatigue predominates. We feel not only tired or dull in bodily parts and clumsy in motion, but we also feel hampered and inhibited in doing either physical or mental work. Our activities are reduced until at last we are forced to give up. This sensation of fatigue is not unpleasant when we are able to rest, but it is painful when rest is not permitted. Through experience we have learned that the sensations of fatigue have a protective function, similar to those of hunger and thirst which forces us to avoid further stress, and allow recovery to take place'.

Persons who are affected by fatigue exhibit the following symptoms:

- A general weakness in drive
- Loss of initiative
- A tendency to depression which is associated with unmotivated worries
- Increased irritability and intolerance
- Occasional unsociable behaviour.

Factors related to fatigue and the rheumatic diseases

Although all rheumatic conditions can be implicated in fatigue, there is a particularly strong association with:

- RA
- Systemic lupus erythematosus
- Fibromyalgia
- Myositis.

Common causes of fatigue

There are a number of factors which cause fatigue in the rheumatic diseases. Some are directly associated with the diseases and their symptoms, such as disease activity and pain. Others are due to subsidiary circumstances, for instance employment and environment.

Disease activity

Patients presenting with active inflammatory joint diseases generally feel unwell and tired and have painful, swollen joints. They also exhibit an increase in the duration of their morning stiffness and a reduced grip strength. Laboratory investigations show an increase in the acute phase response, a fall in haemoglobin level and an increase in the platelet count (see Ch. 3). The combined effects of active disease lead to:

- Pain
- Depression
- Increasing fatigue.

Once treatment aimed at controlling the disease becomes effective, the fatigue should in theory, be substantially reduced. However, this does not always happen due to a number of other factors which can significantly affect function. One common contributor is cardiorespiratory unfitness.

Pain

Pain is a common feature of rheumatic disease and three of the more common causes are:

1. Inflammation
2. Mechanical defects caused by joint destruction
3. Over stressing affected muscles.

Patients complain that pain induces excess fatigue and that fatigue makes it more difficult to cope with pain. Many endure constant or chronic pain (see Ch. 8), and this is very fatiguing.

Other factors pertaining to pain which affect fatigue include:

- Intensity of pain
- Nature of the pain
- Duration of pain
- Fear of pain
- Location of pain
- Patient expectations
- Pain management

If pain is managed effectively, it may help to increase the patient's activity which will lead to a reduction in the peripheral element of fatigue that results from deconditioning and disuse atrophy. Consideration must also be given to the effects of pain control medication as these may also cause drowsiness (see Ch. 12). Where possible alternate pain control such as a TENS machine or heat and cold may be tried. These methods are discussed in Chapter 8.

Anaemia

Anaemia is an important indicator of disease activity in rheumatic disease and may add to the patients disability by causing or increasing fatigue. The anaemia associated with systemic disease activity is an identifiable cause of fatigue brought about by the perception of increased effort. Appropriate treatment of anaemia can significantly reduce fatigue (Turnbull 1987).

Muscle atrophy

Many rheumatic diseases result in muscle atrophy (wasting). This can be brought about either as a direct result of the disease and its treatment, or as a result of disuse. When a muscle is atrophied, the remaining muscles are required to work harder in order to compensate, which reduces endurance and as a consequence, fatigue occurs more rapidly. In addition, muscles do not adapt, but remain the size and strength that is appropriate for the patient's ideal body weight (Newham et al 1983). Consequently, if the body weight is excessive, they are under greater stress than normal (Holder-Powell & Jones 1990).

Physical activity

Disorder in the structure and function of the musculoskeletal system leads to physical limitation and the inability to exercise. These disruptions include inflammation of the:

- Tendons
- Joints
- Muscles.

Regardless of the underlying cause, a dysfunctioning musculoskeletal system will have a direct effect on motor function thereby impairing the amount of physical activity performed. Increased physical activity can be a cause of fatigue in most individuals. However, people with arthritis require extra energy simply to undertake normal activity and as a result, the amount of activity required to cause fatigue is much less than in a healthy person (Smith Pigg et al 1985). For instance, mechanical defects of the lower limbs caused by arthritis, requires the patient to expend extra effort to mobilise; even walking short distances can be extremely fatiguing.

A frequent explanation by patients is that since they developed RA, they need to exert twice the effort and expend twice the energy in order to accomplish the same task (Crosby 1991).

After a period of immobility, most rheumatoid patients initially find exercise exhausting. This is due in part to unfamiliar sensations and inadequate cardiovascular and autonomic responses. These patients fatigue more easily after a period of inactivity and many, due to the nature of their disease, are forced to be less active (Holder-Powell & Jones 1990).

Medication

Medications can be implicated in fatigue. Some cause drowsiness and others simply exacerbate the feeling of fatigue. These include:

- Analgesics
- Anticonvulsants
- Antidepressants
- Tranquillisers
- Hypnotics
- Antihistamines
- Beta-blockers
- Diabetic drugs
- Diuretics
- Hypotensives
- Muscle relaxants
- Cytotoxic agents.

Steroid induced atrophy causes peripheral fatigue. This requires a greater expenditure of energy in order to maintain physical activity, which increases central fatigue. Medication such as steroids and cyclosporin can cause electrolyte imbalance, which can also cause fatigue.

Nutrition

There are many problems which can make it difficult for the rheumatic patient to maintain adequate nutrition, but adequate nutrition is essential in the alleviation of fatigue (see Ch.10).

1. The systemic nature of many rheumatic diseases causes an increase in energy expenditure for basic cellular function. For instance, low grade fever will raise basal metabolic rate incurring an increased intake of nutrients.

2. The painful nature of rheumatic diseases can lead to anorexia, due to the effects of disease on the person's physical or psychological functioning.

3. Treatments such as non-steroidal anti-inflammatory drugs may cause gastric side effects, and penicillamine, intramuscular gold and oral steroids can bring about changes in taste or cause mouth ulcers.

4. Local pain in the temporomandibular joint may cause difficulty with chewing.

5. Patients with scleroderma often find swallowing problematical.

6. Sjögren's syndrome, associated with reduced tear formation and reduced salivary flow, induces a dry mouth which can also lead to difficulty in swallowing.

7. Constipation is a side effect of some medications and this can cause loss of appetite.

It should be noted that alcohol and caffeine intake can also contribute to fatigue.

Psychological aspects

Irritability, intolerance and unsociable behaviour are all behaviours associated with fatigue. Patients with rheumatic disease are often depressed due to:

- Chronicity of their disease
- Pain
- Uncertainty about the future.

Problems with relationships can occur because of the patient's inability to cope and from lack of understanding by others. Sexual relationships can become unsatisfactory because of fatigue, brought about by the cumulative effect of physical disability, disease activity and relationship problems (see Ch. 6).

Patients often try to conceal their handicap which can be stressful and debilitating; stress, anxiety, conflict and responsibility are all contributors to fatigue.

Boredom and monotony result in feelings of dullness and tiredness and this quickly gives rise to day time naps leading to poor sleep patterns.

Environmental factors

The environment in which the patient lives and works can have a profound effect on their fatigue.

Housing. The size and type of the house, location and accessibility of rooms all have a bearing on the situation. For instance, if the bedroom and toilet facilities are upstairs and there is no ground floor toilet, the patient may need to climb the stairs a number of times each day, expending energy and adding to their fatigue. Poor kitchen design and lack of labour saving devices may also contribute.

Uncomfortable seating in the living area and an uncomfortable bed are not conducive to rest, neither is noise, unsatisfactory lighting, or excessive heat or cold. Some patients say that in hot weather they feel more exhausted, and a room that is too hot is fatiguing.

Employment. Many patients find that performing daily living activities is particularly exhausting due to their pattern of morning stiffness (see Ch. 8). Morning stiffness is also a problem when preparing for work; those with arthritis need to allow extra time in order to get ready. To get to work on time frequently involves patients getting out of bed long before they actual start.

The nature of the work undertaken may in itself be very exhausting. Rest periods can be of short duration and the time taken to complete a task may be much longer than previously, leading to an increased work load.

Even when the person arrives home from work, rest may not always be possible. The preparation of meals, other domestic chores and family and social commitments all have to be undertaken.

Lack of knowledge

Lack of knowledge may be a contributory factor that increases a patient's level of fatigue. Patients need to be taught the value of conserving their energy by:

- Resting
- Pacing and prioritising
- Protecting their joints
- Exercise.

Rest is important to restore supplies of energy. Short but frequent rest periods are essential, particularly when the patient is in an active phase of their disease. The value of planning and prioritising activities in order to conserve energy and reduce fatigue are discussed in Chapter 11. Protecting vulnerable joints, by wearing splints, using aids and altering the way in which tasks are undertaken can reduce pain, which leads to reduction in fatigue. Exercise to maintain muscle tone and reduce atrophy needs to be emphasised.

Offering written information to reinforce verbal teaching is essential as it as been shown that patients absorb only small amounts of information at a time (see Ch.15).

Assessment of fatigue

The multifocal dimensions of fatigue makes assessment a difficult process. The ideal person to assess fatigue, either for the outpatient or the patient in hospital, is their named nurse. Assessing the patient's fatigue is an ongoing process as fatigue levels are not constant; they change with the patient's disease activity, treatments and rest. In addition, as patients undergo the process of education and learn how to manage their disease and fatigue, further variation will occur.

Assessment is usually by face to face interview and it is necessary to obtain both subjective (Fig. 9.1) and objective information. The patient should be interviewed in the presence of their spouse, carer or relative if possible.

Observation of the patient's behaviour and mood pattern should be noted and information about their coping mechanisms, laboratory findings, physical problem, dietary assessment and drug history noted. A written assessment form on which to collate the information is useful (Table 9.3).

Table 9.3 Fatigue assessment form

Problem assessed
Disease pattern
Cardiovascular and respiratory problem
Treatments
Symptoms
Laboratory investigations
Sleep and rest pattern
Environmental factors
Work and activity
Coping mechanism and knowledge
Pain
Behaviour and mood
Family
Nutrition
Other relevant information

Management

Recommendations to successfully help patients to manage their own fatigue include:

- Adequate, though not excessive sleep
- Establishment of a work/rest cycle acceptable to the individual
- Elimination of excessive stress, anxiety, or boredom
- Range of movement exercises
- A programme of activity compatible with the individual's capabilities.

Effective use of disease modifying drugs should help to reduce fatigue as the activity of the disease declines and pain, morning stiffness and anaemia lift. Environmental factors should be adjusted to reduce effort required to manage daily activities and to allow for relaxation and adequate rest. The provision of aids aimed at assisting with activities should be considered and information about joint protection and energy preservation should be given. A structured and balanced exercise programme aimed at maintaining function, reducing pain and restoring muscle bulk should be carefully planned with both patient and the physiotherapist.

The approach to management of fatigue is essentially multidisciplinary. Once the assessment is completed the nurse can identify the problems and refer to the appropriate member of the team for suitable intervention (Table 9.4).

Recommended fatigue management interventions for rheumatic diseases

1. Complete the diagnostic fatigue assessments described and initiate cause specific rehabilitation where applicable.

Subjective assessment of fatigue

Please mark an X on the line where it most accurately reflects how you are feeling.

How long do you usually experience fatigue?

Hours _____ Weeks
                        Days

How would you describe the fatigue you usually feel?

Mild _____ Severe
                     Moderate

To what degree do you feel stress usually contributes to the fatigue that you feel?

Not at all _____ A great
                                                                    deal

When I am fatigued I usually feel pain

No pain _____ Severe
                        Moderate   pain

To what degree does sleep usually relieve your fatigue?

No relief _____ Complete
                                                                     relief

Figure 9.1 Subjective assessment of fatigue (adapted from Piper Self reported fatigue scale and based on a 10 cm visual analogue scale).

2. Develop a care plan and set realistic goals with the patient.
3. Assist with medical management including:
   • Treatment of the disease to reduce disease activity
   • Treatment of anaemia if not directly related to the disease process
   • Correction of any chemical imbalance
   • Treatment of locally inflamed joints.
4. Nursing and therapist intervention:
   • Provision of, and advise about convenient appliances
   • Corrective devices to reduce muscle fatigue such as insoles, foot raises, hand splints
   • A safe exercise regime modified regularly according to joint status.
5. Social worker intervention if needed.
6. Education:
   • Patient education is the key to achieving optimal compliance encouraging joint protection and energy conservation.
7. Reduce stress and encourage relaxation.
8. Support Group:
   • Support of peer groups may be helpful particularly if this is backed up by access to professionals.
9. Telephone helpline:
   • Provision of a helpline service makes patients feel less isolated and leads to identification of problems and an early resolution.
10. Sleep management
    • Assess sleep pattern and advise on sleep management.

Box 9.1 Patient Information Leaflet: Coping with your fatigue

For many people with arthritis, fatigue (tiredness) is part of the disease process. There are many reasons for this; the disease itself makes you tired; pain is tiring because it disturbs your sleep and rest; extra effort is required to move stiff painful joints. Drug therapy can also add to fatigue, as can a poor diet and an excess of caffeine or alcohol. Stress and depression may add to your tiredness.

To manage fatigue you need to accept that it is part of the disease process and learn ways to help you to cope.

Hints for dealing with fatigue
• Plan your day.
• Set priorities and do only the things that are most important.
• Do as much for yourself as possible, but take rests. A number of short rests are better than one long one.
• Ask for help from family and friends.
• Rest before you become tired.
• Conserve your energy as much as possible.
• Organise home and work so that tools are handy and plan ahead to minimise activity.
• Try not to sit for more than 20 or 30 minutes before standing or walking about a little.
• If possible sit down for any job that takes more than 10 minutes.
• Try to avoid projects, like cooking a complicated meal, that cannot be stopped at any time should you feel tired.
• Avoid doing jobs which take a long time in one session. It is better to do several short sessions.
• Avoid carrying things by using a wheeled trolley. For example, transport all items for setting the table in one trip.
• An apron with a large pocket is useful for the handyman or housewife, for carrying small objects.
• Store much used items such as plates, cutlery and salt, between eye level and knee level, to reduce the amount of bending and stretching you have to do.

• Do not stay in one position too long and stop frequently when travelling by car.
• When travelling by plane or train, select a seat near the aisle so that you can get up easily and walk around.

Joint protection
• Protect your joints as much as possible.
• Slide objects rather than lift them.
• Use your larger joints where possible. For example carry bags using shoulder or elbow joints not using small joints of the hands.
• Use as many joints as possible to distribute work load. For example, hold a cup in both palms rather than with the thumb and a few fingers.
• Use good posture.
• Take advantage of as many assistive devices as possible. For example use a trolley to carry all the equipment required to prepare a table for a meal.
• A car with power assisted steering is an advantage.

Exercise
• Remember to balance exercise with rest.
• Exercise slowly at first, then gradually increase the amount of exercise you do. Walking and swimming are good forms of exercise.
• Do your range of movement exercises daily.
• Gradually increase the amount of strengthening exercises.

Relaxation
• Practise relaxation techniques.

Diet
• Eat a healthy, well balanced diet.
• Cut down on dairy products, caffeine and alcohol.

Sleep
• Try to improve the quality of your sleep by following the guidelines on how to get a restful night's sleep.

Table 9.4 Treatment of fatigue

Specific	General
Treat specific causes	
Central fatigue	*Central fatigue*
Disease activity	Pain control
Neuropathy	Rationalise medication
Myelopathy	Psychological support
	Improve sleep
	Education about disease management
	Family support
	Correct environment problems
	Adequate well balanced diet
	Weight loss if obese
	Exercise programme
Peripheral fatigue	*Peripheral fatigue*
Keep steroid dosage low	Reverse disuse atrophy with physiotherapy and exercise
Treat localised flare	
Diagnose and treat myositis	

SLEEP

Sleep and rest are essential components of health and lack of either can affect well-being and quality of life. Sleep is also an important element in recovery from illness and sleep deprivation a major impairment to recovery. In addition, sleep disruption makes coping with a chronic illness more difficult. The balance between activity and rest is important in the maintenance of health. However, the effects of rheumatic disease make this balance difficult to achieve, adding to the consequences of the disease. Activity promotes tissue growth and development whilst rest allows restoration and repair, as well as renewal of energies. Assisting patients to balance activity and rest can significantly reduce the effects of the disease and improve their quality of life.

Sleep is a natural process and is a compelling human need. However, for those affected by a rheumatological disease, joint pain and stiffness and physical discomfort significantly reduce the quality or amount of sleep achieved. Disturbed sleep exacerbates the adverse effects of the disease and reduces the quality of life. This, in turn, can feed back negatively to cause increased pain perception, fatigue, anxiety and depression all of which adversely affect sleep. Sleep deprivation can lead to muscle pain and decreased immune response (Moldofsky & Scarisbrick 1976, Palmbald et al 1979). It is important for nurses and patients alike to understand the associations between activity, rest, sleep and fatigue.

Rest and sleep are affected by the physical stresses a person experiences at a given time. The extent of illness will affect the need for sleep and rest. It is likely that the seriousness of the illness will increase the time needed for sleep and rest.

Rest

Rest can be defined as a decrease or change in activity such that physical discomfort and psychological stress are reduced, allowing for renewal of energy. Napping, sleeping, relaxation, changing activity, or simply sitting admiring the view are forms of rest that help renew physical or mental energy. The type of relaxation required and its effect on restoring energy will vary from person to person.

Rest periods are important as they help patients to avoid becoming overtired or overstressed. Rheumatic diseases may cause a deficit in muscle mass, tone, and strength, making muscles less effective. This, combined with mechanical problems resulting from defective joints, requires an overexpenditure of energy. The physiological processes slow down during rest to allow for renewal of energy and rest prevents further exhaustion of already stressed muscles and joints. For this reason, several short rest periods are more beneficial than one long one.

Conditions needed for sleep

Sleep occurs when a person loses conscious awareness of what is happening around them, reducing their ability to respond to environmental stimuli. Most rest occurs during sleep, with human beings spending an average of 7 hours a day or one third of their lives sleeping. Sleep is an active, rhythmic process as can be observed using an encephalogram. The complex physiological processes of sleep and its effects are not fully understood but are thought to be both protective and restorative in nature.

Sleep requires:

- Absence of external stimuli
- Suitable environment
- Daily routine of bedtime
- Relaxation of muscles
- Comfortable bed.

The propensity to fall asleep peaks twice during the day, after lunch and at bedtime. In order to maintain sleep most people need:

- Removal of distracting stimuli such as noise, bright lights, and anxiety
- Suitable ambient temperature
- Ability to relax the body in comfort and safety.

There is an enormous variation in the individual habits adopted by people going to bed with the expectation of sleep. These habits are associated with routines and rituals, especially in childhood, which the individual finds necessary to induce and maintain sleep. Patterns of activity tend to be dictated by work, family and social commitments as well as the individual's particular requirement for sleep. Unfortunately, the complexity and pace of modern life lead to the adoption of behaviour patterns that are antagonistic to the onset and maintenance of sleep. The most obvious examples of factors antagonistic to sleep are a strange environment such as hotels and hospitals, stress and anxiety and the ingestion of central nervous stimulants especially caffeine in the evening (Nicholson & Marks, 1983).

The functions of sleep

Oswald (1984) states that 'there are over 100 research reports showing that the protein synthesis and cell division for the renewal of tissue like the skin, bone marrow, gastric mucosa, bone and brain take place predominantly during that time of day devoted to rest and sleep'. Therefore adequate sleep is essential to those patients who have a chronic illness; sleep will help the healing process and lessen the psychological problems resulting from inadequate sleep.

For many years it has been thought that by permitting the muscles to rest, sleep allows optimal protein synthesis and general recovery to take place. The fact that millions of people go to sleep feeling tired and wake up feeling refreshed supports this theory.

The rate of tissue synthesis is higher during sleep and rest than during activity (Adams & Oswald 1977). During sleep, energy expenditure in the tissue falls and the energy stored within the cells rises to a level sufficient for tissue synthesis to occur. During short wave sleep (see pp. 165–166), the secretion of growth hormone peaks, promoting anabolic activity and stimulating protein, ribonucleic acid and amino acid uptake. Total body oxygen consumption is lower during sleep suggesting lower catabolism (Shapiro et al 1984). A study by Vondra et al (1981) showed changes in enzyme activity and increased lactate acid levels, sampled by muscle biopsy, following 120 hours of sleep deprivation, suggesting increased muscle breakdown. Increased brain protein synthesis occurs during rapid eye movement (REM) sleep supporting the notion that REM sleep is crucial to central nervous system restoration (Drucker-Colin 1979). Another suggested function of REM sleep is the consolidation of learning and memory. Metabolic rate falls by between 5% and 25% during the night, particularly during sleep, thereby conserving energy. This also suggests a link between sleep and major metabolic function. The body temperature and heart rate also fall during the first few hours of sleep.

The physical rest that occurs during sleep helps to conserve energy. The physiological functions of sleep are thought to be multifocal and include genetic, nutritional, and environmental components. Therefore it follows that the purpose of sleep is also multifocal.

Normal sleep

'O sleep, thou rest of all things, sleep mildest of the gods, balm of the soul, who puttest care to flight, soothest our bodies, worn with hard ministries, and preparest them for toil again!' Ovid, *Metamorphoses* XI, 623–625

A good night's sleep and good daytime refreshed wakefulness are interrelated, each depending on the quality of the other. Sleep requirements are subjective and can vary enormously. If the sleeper is satisfied with its duration, continuity and architecture then it may be considered normal, whatever objective recordings might indicate. The average duration is about 7½ hours, but a range of 3–12 hours is considered normal (Johns 1984). Normal habits and needs of individuals bear no resemblance to one another. Some people are early risers whilst others are more active in the evening and tend to go to bed late. Some people habitually take a nap in the afternoon, whilst others do not. It is possible to shorten the normal sleep period by up to 2 hours without any significant effect.

The ability to wake up or arouse from sleep represents an enormously important primary defence mechanism. Stimuli for arousal include light, noise, smell or pain, although the arousal stimuli is perceived at different thresholds by different individuals (Langford et al 1974).

Factors affecting normal sleep

There are many factors affecting normal sleep including:

- Age
- Diet
- Gender
- Ambient temperature.

Sleep patterns are known to change with age. Neonates sleep for 18 hours per day, whilst young adults sleep for about 8 hours and elderly individuals might sleep for 6 hours only. Men are known to have more disturbed nights than women whilst women are known to sleep longer and consume more sleep-inducing drugs (Taylor 1987). Crisp & Stonehill (1971) reported that weight gain was associated with increased sleep duration and weight loss with reduced duration. There is conflicting evidence about the significance of exercise. However, it appears to have a positive effect on sleep promotion, provided that it is not taken late in the evening (Vuori et al 1988). Anxiety and depression frequently interfere with sleep and this is common in patients with musculoskeletal disease, due to uncertainties about the future, work and family tensions. It is easier to relax physically than mentally.

Chronic pain experienced by most patients with musculoskeletal disease represents a major problem affecting sleep. Dyspepsia and pain from gastric ulcers can increase in intensity at night. This is significant for patients taking medication with gastrointestinal side effects who are at greater risk of gastric problems (see Ch. 12). The effects of diet are unclear but spicy foods late at night tend to disturb sleep. A milky night time drink may promote somnolence in some, but does not suit everyone.

Alcohol has an hypnotic effect, increasing stage 2 sleep and reducing REM and short wave sleep early in the night (Jaffe 1980). Later in the night, following the metabolism of the alcohol, rebound effects occur with the increase in REMs, dreams and frequent awakenings. However, alcohol has considerable analgesic properties and may be used by many patients who experience chronic pain, to reduce pain and aid sleep. If it is used frequently and to excess, the overall effect will be to increase insomnia. Drinks containing caffeine should be avoided at night as they act as central nervous stimulants.

The structure of normal sleep

In adults, sleep consists of two different states which have different psychological mechanisms, and behavioural and neurophysiological markers. These two states are commonly known as non-rapid eye movement (NREM) and rapid eye movement (REM) sleep. In addition, NREM can be subdivided into four separate stages.

During a night's sleep, both REM and all four stages of NREM sleep occur many times, usually in cyclic fashion with the NREM sleep periods becoming shorter and the REM sleep periods longer as the night progresses. Most REM sleep occurs during the last third of the night.

Increasing age brings changes to the stage structure and it is usual to experience less 'deep sleep' (stages 3 & 4) and more 'light sleep' (stages 1 & 2) and more arousals in later adulthood.

NREM sleep

NREM sleep is believed to be necessary for tissue restoration and protein synthesis and comprises four stages, as described by Rechtschaffen & Kales (1968). In each stage, cerebral electrical activity progressively slows in frequency and increases in amplitude.

Stage 0 or W (wakefulness). During wakefulness the electroencephalogram (EEG) is characterised by generally low voltage activity at 4–25 Hz.

Stage 1 (drowsing). This is the lightest stage of sleep, being the transition from wakefulness to sleep, in which the subject usually feels drowsy and not fully alert. Day dreams may occur in this stage of sleep. The EEG shows mostly low-voltage, mixed-frequency activity at 2–7 Hz.

Stage 2 (light sleep). This stage of altered consciousness is such that, if awakened most people recognise that they have been asleep. It is in this stage that body movements begin to diminish and dreams involving a story line first appear. Dream recall on waking is less vivid than in REM sleep.

Stage 3 (slow wave sleep). During this stage, body movement continues to diminish and deep sleep occurs. The amplitude of the EEG increases.

Stage 4 (slow wave sleep). There is an high degree of immobility and intense external stimuli are required to arouse the sleeper, who is now in the state of deep sleep. Large increases in the secretion of growth hormone occur at this stage.

Traditionally stages 3 and 4 are considered together and termed short wave sleep (SWS).

Alpha activity is, by definition, a rhythmn of the waking posterior cortex seen with the eyes closed and reducing with the eyes open.

REM sleep

REM sleep is needed for psychological restoration, maintenance of orientation and emotional stability (Chuman 1983). It is characterised by dreaming, muscular relaxation and high levels of physiological arousal. Blood pressure fluctuates, pulse and respiration rates increase and may become irregular and oxygen consumption increases.

During REM sleep, there are rapid darting movements of the eyes under closed lids, occurring in bursts of 3–10 seconds at intervals of 30–40 seconds. These do not always occur, and if absent it is usually during the first period of REM sleep of the night. If subjects are awakened they frequently report that they have been dreaming. Consequently, REM sleep is frequently referred to as dreaming sleep.

Circadian rhythm

Circadian refers to the physiological and behavioural patterns that repeat every 24 hours. Biological rhythms, of which light and dark, wakefulness and sleeping are the most obvious to man, are inherent properties of living (Klietman 1963). Fundamentally, our circadian rhythms dictate when it is time to sleep. Under normal circumstances they are synchronised by external time cues such as the light–dark cycle and by social time cues such as meal times. These synchronising cues are known as Zeitgebers ('time givers'). It appears that there are internal pacemakers or biochemical clocks. Endogenous clocks have been shown to govern the functions of living tissue and are coordinated directly or indirectly by the brain. The sleep/wake cycle coincides with fluctuations in body temperature, heart rate and plasma levels of anabolic and catabolic hormones.

The circadian timing system has two functions:

- To keep us properly timed to the day/night cycle of our environment
- To synchronise various functions of the body.

The human body is programmed to adjust behaviour according to the time of day, with most physiological functions performing to maximum efficiency during the daytime, when there is the greatest need for alertness. Desynchronisation of the circadian rhythm
rature, pulse rate, respiration, arterial
sis and excretion of electrolytes. This
mptoms such as fever, alcohol type
graine, some mental disorders and

Insomnia

Insomnia may be described as a persistent relative lack of sleep, inadequate quality of sleep or both and reflects poor sleep pattern and poor quality sleep for at least three weeks. Subjects may have difficulties with initiation or maintenance of sleep or with early wakening. There should be evidence of poor day time functioning, regardless of the number of hours slept each night, because of the great variability in individuals' sleep requirements. Changes in diet, anxiety sleeplessness phobia, levels of arousal, obsessive thoughts and environmental disturbances all disrupt initiation of sleep.

Interrupted sleep can be random or cyclic. Random awakenings can be caused by pain, sleep apnoea, breathlessness, coughing and nocturia. Waking early in the morning can often occur with depression and daytime fatigue is common in patients with fibromyalgia and active rheumatoid disease.

Effects of lack of sleep

Lack of sleep:

- Reduces motivation and willingness to perform tasks
- Impedes mobilisation and restricts self care
- Reduces efficiency at work
- Decreases attention span
- Affects social and family relationships
- Potentiates the effects of muscle and joint pain and stiffness
- Increases anxiety and depression
- Has the potential to exacerbate the disease
- Impairs memory
- Causes day time sleepiness
- Causes fatigue.

Hospitalisation and sleep

Patients in hospital suffer from disturbed and less effective sleep than in their own environment. Frequent problems suffered by hospitalised patients include sleep latency, interrupted sleep, early awakening and a feeling of not being rested. Factors frequently identified with poor sleep in hospital include:

- Noise
- Anxiety about health
- Separation from family and friends
- Unfamiliar environment

- Monitoring of vital signs
- Administration of medication
- Interruptions
- Discomfort
- Hunger.

Sleep disruption is often intensified by sleep pattern changes, health problems and unfamiliar clinical settings. Hospital routines also prevail over an individual's normal bedtime routine and this often results in disturbed sleep patterns.

Evaluation of a patient's past and present sleep patterns, monitoring of sleep/wake behaviour and implementation of nursing intervention to promote sleep are important when caring for patients in hospital. Sleep assessment should include:

- Observation of the time it takes to fall asleep
- Restlessness during the night
- Number of arousals during each sleep period
- Patient's sense of having a good night's sleep.

The last point is important regardless of other observation.

The number and length of rest periods taken during the day can be recorded, although this depends on the type of rest taken. What constitutes rest depends on the individual and their requirements; it may be sitting quietly gazing at the surroundings or it may be sleeping on the bed. Such variations in rest taken by each individual makes accurate recording difficult. Actual absence of physical activity does not always mean that a patient is resting, and fidgeting or tossing and turning may indicate restlessness.

Unfortunately, in a modern, busy hospital environment such assessments are rarely undertaken.

Nurses should allow hospitalised patients to continue the pre-sleep activities and routines they use at home. Some patients have a night time alcoholic beverage and if they are normally heavy drinkers they may suffer from withdrawal, if they are not allowed an alcoholic drink prior to sleep. Worries regarding the illness, investigations and treatments should be discussed. Realistic measures for sleep onset and maintenance should be set with the patient and evaluated for effectiveness with the appropriate changes made in order to maintain or improve the quality of sleep.

Where possible it is better to deal with causes of insomnia rather than giving medication.

- Temperature should be comfortable
- Lights should be turned out or dimmed
- Patients should be able to get up if they are unable to sleep

- Patients should be encouraged to go to bed only when tired
- Sleep protocols should be implemented, which allow for uninterrupted sleep
- Disturbance during a patient's normal sleep cycle should be forbidden unless essential
- A quiet environment should be maintained with admission units away from areas where patients are attempting to sleep
- Noise from equipment should also be kept to a minimum, since it tends to appear magnified during the hours when a patient is trying to sleep.

Position relates to habit and physical factors such as breathing, temperature and joint pain. Individual position varies greatly and depends on comfort of the joints and muscles but should be conducive to relaxation and lead to sleep. However where possible good body alignment should be considered to prevent undue stress on the muscles ligaments and joints. Encouraging movement when awake may help to reduce stiffness.

Pain has been shown to correlate with sleep disturbances and adequate pain control should be achieved prior to the onset of sleep in order to ensure an adequate night's sleep. When related to musculo-skeletal pain, non-steroidal anti-inflammatory drugs may be more efficacious than opioids, but the two can be used together if necessary.

Important aids to promote rest and sleep include:

- Provision of physical comfort
- Alleviation of psychological stresses
- Structuring of daily activity schedules
- Structuring of a restful environment
- Appropriate choice and time of analgesic administration.

Good personal hygiene aids comfort and thus improves the quality of rest and sleep. Prior to going to bed a warm bath to which essential oils have been added, can be relaxing and help to relieve joint and muscle pain (see Ch. 13). Massage can be comforting and may induce sleep.

Psychological stress can be alleviated by allowing patients the opportunity to discuss fears, anxieties and frustrations. Anxiety about not sleeping and trying too hard to get to sleep can further distress patients and prevent sleep. Quiet relaxing music may help to create a relaxed atmosphere.

Hypnotic drugs such as barbiturates and benzo-diazipines should be carefully controlled and selected since they affect the quality of sleep.

Sleep disturbances in specific rheumatological diseases

Rheumatoid arthritis

In RA, fragmented sleep can be associated with exacerbation of illness, with patients experiencing increased fatigue, morning stiffness, joint and muscle pain and weakness. The increase in pain is consistent with findings that sleep deprivation reduces the pain threshold (Shapiro et al 1993). Alpha-NREM sleep anomaly has been shown to be consistent with increased symptoms with an improvement in rhythm consistent with remission (Moldosky 1986).

The physical and psychological recuperative benefits of sleep are such that the patient with rheumatological conditions should be encouraged to maintain as regular a sleep pattern as the painful nature of the disease will allow. Undisturbed sleep depends on a number of factors. Control of pain and discomfort by use of analgesia, night resting splints, and position are important. An exercise programme, to maintain muscle strength, prevent joint stiffness and improve circulation can also contribute to effective sleep and maintenance of independence.

A study comparing patients with RA whose disease had flared with those whose disease was well controlled, showed reduced sleep times with fragmented and occasionally prolonged awakenings in patients with active disease. In addition, there was a significant relationship between the number of awakenings and pain. The researchers suggested that measures to reduce pain might improve the quality and quantity of sleep in those experiencing RA flares (Crosby 1991). Several studies have shown that a good night's sleep can significantly reduce stiffness in patients with RA (Sharma & Haslock 1979, Vasanthakumar & Haslock 1987, Baumgartner et al 1988). However these studies involved using pain control and it is possible that the improvement in stiffness was caused by the analgesia rather than by the improved quality of sleep.

In patients with RA, the more severe the pain experienced before and during sleep, the more fragmented the sleep. Compared to controls, patients with arthritis have lower indices of sleep quality, less effective sleep, higher levels of activity during sleep and more sleep disturbances (Lavie et al 1992).

Fibromyalgia

About 90% of patients with fibromyalgia describe moderate to severe fatigue with lack of energy, decreased exercise endurance, or the kind of exhaus-

tion felt with the 'flu or with lack of sleep. Often the fatigue is more troubling than the pain and generally, people with fibromyalgia wake feeling tired even after sleeping throughout the night. Sleep studies have shown that people with fibromyalgia have an abnormal sleep pattern, especially an interruption in their deep sleep (Shapiro et al 1993). They may be aware that their sleep has become lighter and that they wake up during the night.

Moldofsky (1986) studied the fibrositis syndrome in a group of patients who had reported severe emotional stress at the time symptoms began. They found increases in muscle tenderness and in subjective symptoms of pain and stiffness. These seemed to be associated with disturbances of sleep and with the development of alpha rhythms in NREM sleep. In normal subjects, sleep disturbances sometimes produced symptoms similar to those in the fibrositis group, including fatigue and musculoskeletal aches and pains. This occurred when sleep disturbance occurred during Stage 4 sleep and the subjects showed a disturbance in alpha rhythm. The symptoms did not occur when sleep disturbances occurred during REM sleep. Studies by have also shown that a wide variety of factors could affect nonarticular rheumatism including psychological stress, physiological disturbances, environmental stimuli and altered central nervous system metabolism (Moldofsky 1986).

Medication to promote sleep may help patients with fibromyalgia. These include amitriptyline, doxepin, cyclobenzaprine and related medications. Although normally used to treat depression, in people with fibromyalgia they are generally used in very low doses and only at bedtime. Thus they are not specifically used as antidepressants or tranquillisers, but may relieve pain and improve sleep.

Even a very gentle exercise programme is thought to improve the quality of sleep. As muscle repair takes place during the 'restorative' phase of sleep, with the production of hormones required to promote repair of muscle, improved sleep is an essential part of the rehabilitation programme for fibromyalgia patients.

Ankylosing spondylitis

The effect of sleep on patients with ankylosing spondylitis was studied by Jamieson et al (1995). Patients with ankylosing spondylitis usually feel worse in the morning, their stiffness and general discomfort easing throughout the day. Good sleep is associated with less nocturnal movement and yet exercise is essential. The study showed that a good night's sleep correlated with increased stiffness, difficulty in awakening, feeling tired and clumsiness in the morning. Pain correlated with subjective measures; difficulty in getting to sleep and a worse quality of sleep; but less well with objective measures of sleep disruption. The study showed that improved sleep integrity, with little nocturnal movement, was related to a decrease in lumbar flexibility. It is suggested that patients with ankylosing spondylitis may benefit from being awakened in the night and that their sleep differs from sleep in healthy people.

Sleep management

Recommendations to improve the quality of sleep include advice about routines that are conducive to sleep onset, maintenance of quality sleep and adequate duration of sleep. The advice given will depend on individualised assessment and care planning with the

patient. Below is a list of information for patients that includes many aspects of advice related to sleep.

Patients with rheumatic disease frequently have poor sleep patterns, due to pain, discomfort and the need for daytime rest. The chronic diseases cause persistent problems that affect sleep on a long-term basis. Consequently, the nurse caring for such patients, requires skills and knowledge to adequately assess sleep patterns and advise on sleep management. A restful night's sleep will significantly reduce disease related fatigue, aid recovery and help patients cope with the effects of their disease.

The traditional management of rheumatoid disease fails to acknowledge the importance of fatigue. As a result, patients may find it difficult to accept that the fatigue they feel is a consequence of the disease process. By helping them to understand that fatigue is an expected part of their disease, health care professionals can improve patients' control and coping mechanisms.

Fatigue is a complex multifactorial and multi-

Box 9.2 Patient Information Leaflet: Advice on how to get a restful night's sleep (adapted from Hauri 1996)

The average person needs 7 to 8 hours sleep to feel refreshed. Many people try to exist on less and are consequently habitually sleep deprived.

If you cannot get sufficient sleep at night try to take 10 to 20 minute catnaps during the day, but not too close to bed time as that can impair your ability to fall asleep at night.

- Make sure your bedroom is favourable to sleep. Keep it free of equipment and smells; for example of cooking, that remind you of daily activity.
- Ensure that the room is at a comfortable temperature.
- The curtains should block out the light.
- The bed should be firm yet comfortable, with covers that are light and suitable to keep your body warm.
- Create a restful pre-sleep atmosphere. Listen to relaxing music, read a suitable book or practise relaxation before you get into bed.
- Avoid strenuous exercise before going to bed. This can speed the body up which tells the brain that it is time to be awake and active. Late afternoon and early evening exercise is best. Avoid strenuous mental activity near bedtime.
- Relaxation and a specific rest/exercise programme may help you to sleep and contribute towards remaining independent.
- Avoid long day time naps and periods of inactivity.
- Aim to go to sleep at the same time each day. This helps to regulate your internal clock to normal sleep/wake rhythms.
- Don't force yourself to sleep or watch the clock if you can't. It's better to get up and read or watch a TV show until you feel naturally sleepy.
- Snacks before bedtime should be light and fluid intake limited. A hot milky drink at bedtime may promote sleep.

- Avoid going to bed hungry or too full. Hunger pains will keep you awake. Over-eating can cause too much acid resulting in heartburn.
- Do not have coffee, tea, cola or a nightcap after dinner. The stimulating effects of caffeine can linger in your body for up to six hours causing a uneven night's sleep. Alcohol may make you sleepy initially, but disturbs sleep later on.
- A warm bath with essential oils taken before bedtime, may relax tired muscles, reduce pain and help to promote sleep.
- Pain should be adequately controlled before going to bed and anti-inflammatory medication may be needed along side analgesia. Other methods of pain control should also be considered such as hot or cold packs, a heat pad or massage.
- Ensure that the joints are in a comfortable position correctly aligned in order not to stress them. Night resting splints may be required to rest joints in a comfortable position.
- Don't get into the habit of relying on sleeping tablets. Many people can use them on a short-term basis without ill effect but used on a regular basis they lose their effectiveness. They also change the structure of sleep and long-term this may be harmful.
- Do not stay in bed if not asleep within approximately 30 minutes according to your own particular habits at bedtime. (Experts recommend only 10 minutes before getting out of bed but this is inappropriate for many people with rheumatological conditions). Get out of bed and sit and relax in another room until you feel sleepy. Repeat as often as required until you fall asleep.

dimensional problem, with numerous causative factors that can be biological, physiological, social and personal in nature. Some of the causes of fatigue are related to everyday life and others to the disease process. Increased understanding of these causes should lead to management aimed at reducing the effects of fatigue.

Since fatigue can result from a variety of causes, acting singularly or in a variety of combinations, it is difficult to give clear cut rules for its control or prevention. The optimum intervention depends on careful, individual assessment by the nursing staff and involvement of the multidisciplinary team. To date, a physiological basis for fatigue has not been identified and the causes remain a multifocal. However, by increasing understanding of the causes and accepting observed behaviour patterns we can start to teach patients and their relatives coping strategies aimed at improving the quality of their life.

> **Action points for practice:**
>
> - Identify the patients in you clinical area who suffer from fatigue. List the possible causes of their fatigue and the relief measures you suggest.
> - In a group session reflect on the effects of lack of sleep on patients with rheumatological conditions. Identify ways you can encourage patients to achieve a good night's sleep in your own clinical area.
> - Conduct a small scale research project into the causes of fragmented sleep in your clinical area. Identify avoidable causes of fragmented sleep.
> - Discuss the components needed to assess and manage fatigue and compile a standard for practice.

REFERENCES

Adams K, Oswald I 1977 Sleep is for tissue restoration. Journal of the Royal College of Physicians, London 11: 376–388

Baumgartner H, Hohmeister R, Blumenberg-Novoselac N 1988 An observer-blind crossover study to compare the efficacies of flurbiprofen, indomethacin and naproxen given orally and rectally in the relief of night pain and morning stiffness due to rheumatoid arthritis. Journal of International Medical Research 16: 189–196

Chuman M A 1983 The neurological basis of sleep. Heart Lung 12: 177–182

Crisp A H, Stonehill E 1971 Aspects of relationships between psychiatric states, sleep, nocturnal motility and nutrition. Journal of Psychosomatic Research 15: 501–509

Crosby L J 1991 Factors which contribute to fatigue associated with rheumatoid arthritis. Journal of Advanced Nursing 16: 974–981

Drucker-Colin R 1979 Protein molecules and the regulation of REM sleep: possible implications for function. In: Drucker-Colin R, Shkurovich M & Sterman M B (ed), The Functions of Sleep. Academic Press, New York, p 99–112

Edwards R H 1981 Human muscle function and fatigue. In: Porter R, Whelon J (eds) Human muscle function, physiological mechanics, Pitman, London

Hashimoto K, Kagi K, Grandjean E 1975 Methodology in human fatigue assessment. Taylor and Francis, London

Hauri Dr 1996 American Sleep Disorders Association. Rochester, Minnesota

Holder-Powell H M, Jones D A 1990 Fatigue and muscular activity: a review. Physiotherapy 11: 672–679 Nov

Jaffe J H 1980 Drug addiction and drug abuse. In: The pharmacological basis of therapeutics. Gilman A G (ed) Macmillan, New York, p494–534

Jamieson A H, Alford C A, Bird H A, Hindmarch I, Wright V 1995 The effect of sleep and nocturnal movement on stiffness, pain, and psychomotor performance in alkylosing spondylitis. Clinical and Experimental Rheumatology 13: 73–78

Johns M W 1984 Normal sleep. In: Priest R G (ed) Sleep: an international monograph. Update Books, ch 1

Klietman N 1963 Sleep and wakefulness, 2nd ed. University of Chicago Press, Chicago

Langford G W, Meddis R, Pearson A J D 1974 Awakening latency from sleep for meaningful and non-meaningful stimuli. Psychophysiology, 11: 1–5

Lavie P, Epstein R, Tzischinsky O, et al 1992 Actigraphic measurements of sleep in rheumatoid arthritis: comparison of patients with low back pain and healthy controls. The Journal of Rheumatology 19(3): 362–365

Moldofsky H, Scarisbrick P 1976 Induction of neurasthenic musculoskeletal pain syndrome in selective sleep deprivation. Psychosomatic Medicine 38: 35–44

Moldofsky H 1986 Sleep and musculoskeletal pain. American Journal of Medicine 81(3A): 85–98

Newham D J, Mills K R, Quigley B, Edwards R H 1983 The strength, contractile properties and radiological density of skeletal muscle before and one year after gastroplasty. Clinical Science 74: 79–83

Nicholson A N, Marks J 1983 Insomnia: a guide for medical practitioners. MTD Press, Boston, p41–44

Oswald I 1984 Good, poor and disordered sleep. In: Priest R G (ed) Sleep: an international monograph. Update Books, ch 2

Palmbald J, Pertrini B, Wasserman J, Akerstedt T 1979 Lymphocyte and granulocyte reaction during sleep deprivation. Psychosomatic Medicine; 41(4): 273–287

Piper B F 1991 Fatigue, current bases for practice. In: Key bases of comfort. Springer, New York, 24: 187–198

Rechtschaffen A, Kales A 1968 A manual of standardised terminology, techniques and scoring systems for sleep stages of human subjects. US Dept of Health, Education and Welfare, Bethesda

Shapiro C M, Goll C C, Cohen G R, Oswald I 1984 Heat production during sleep. Journal of Applied Physiology 56: 671–677

Shapiro C M, Devins G M, Hussain M R G 1993 Sleep problems in patients with medical illness. ABC of sleep disorders. BMJ Publishing Group, London, p 59–62

Sharma B K Haslock I 1979 Night medication in rheumatoid arthritis. The use of Sudilac. Current Medical Research Opinion 10: 592–595

Smith Pigg J, Webb Driscoll P, Caniff R 1985 Rheumatology nursing, a problem orientated approach. Wiley, New York

Tack B B 1990 Self reported fatigue in rheumatoid arthritis. Arthritis Care and Research 3(3): 154–157

Taylor D 1987 Current usage of benzodiazepines in Britain. In: The Benzodiazepines in current practice. Freeman H,

Rue Y (eds) Royal Society of Medicine Services, London, 13–18

Turnbull A 1987 Anaemia in rheumatoid arthritis, does it matter? In: Collected reports on rheumatic disease, Arthritis and Rheumatism Council, Chesterfield

Vasanthakumar V, Haslock I 1987 The effects of differing pharmaceutical preparations of indomethacin on the night pain and morning stiffness due to rheumatoid arthritis. Current Medical Research Opinion 10: 592–595

Vondra, K, Brodan V, Bass A, et al 1981 Effects of sleep deprivation on the activity of selected metabolic enzymes in skeletal muscle. European Journal of Applied Physiology 47: 41–46

Vuori I, Urponen H, Hasan J, Partinen M 1988 Epidemiology of exercise effects on sleep. Acta Physiologica Scandinavica, suppl 574: 3–7

FURTHER READING

Alexander M F, Fawcett J, Runciman P J 1994 Nursing Practice: Hospital and the home: the adult. Churchill Livingstone, Edinburgh

Andrews H, Roy C 1991 The Roy adaptation model: The definitive statement. Appleton, Norwalk

Cooper R 1994 Sleep. Chapman & Hall, London

Skalla K A, Lacasse C 1992 Patient education for fatigue. Oncology Nursing Forum 19(10): 1537–1541

Tack B B 1990 Fatigue in rheumatoid arthritis: condition strategies and consequences. Arthritis Care Research 3(2): 65–70

Tierney A J 1986 Clinical nursing practice. Churchill Livingstone, Edinburgh

Yousaf F, Sedgwick P 1996 Sleep disorders. British Journal of Hospital Medicine 55(6): 353–358

10

Skin and nutrition

Jane Douglas, Jill Byrne

This chapter is intended to promote a holistic and individual approach to skin integrity, discuss the role of a well-balanced diet in the management of the rheumatoid patient, and provide an insight into the relationship between nutrition and the skin. After reading this chapter you should be able to:

- Describe the basic anatomy, physiology and functions of the skin
- Describe factors relevant to the skin of a rheumatology patient
- Identify the causes and prevention of pressure sores and leg ulceration
- Describe the components of a healthy well-balanced diet
- Appreciate the importance of the dietician in the management of the rheumatic patient
- Advise the patient of the effects of both an allergy-free diet and fasting
- Assess the effectiveness of fish oils, evening primrose oil and the supplementation of trace elements in the diet
- Identify the role of education in skin integrity and nutrition.

THE SKIN

There are many common features of rheumatic diseases that effect the integrity of the patient's skin. These include:

- Anaemia
- Poor nutrition
- Immobility

173

- Drug therapy
- Depression.

The contribution that these problems make to the development of pressure sores and leg ulcers needs to be understood by the rheumatology nurse. Possession of an appropriate knowledge of the anatomy and physiology of the skin, and the ability to apply this knowledge to practice is essential if the rheumatology nurse is to attain high quality care (Collier 1994).

The structure of the skin

The skin is one of the largest and most active organs of the body. It is a complex structure weighing approximately 2.5 kg with a surface area of 1.5–2 m^2 in adults. It has two main layers (Fig. 10.1). These are the:

- Epidermis
- Dermis.

The epidermis

The epidermis is the outer layer consisting of tissue known as stratified squamous epithelium. It has several layers of cells (Fig. 10.2) and the surface layer, the stratum corneum, is shed constantly and replaced from the layers below. The complete replacement of the epidermis takes approximately 40 days. The epidermis has no blood vessels or nerve endings and derives its nutrients and oxygen from interstitial fluid from the dermis.

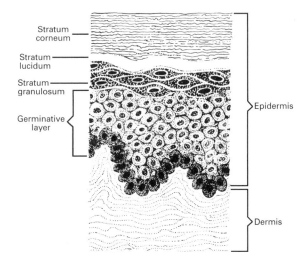

Figure 10.2 The skin showing the main layers of the epidermis (from Wilson & Waugh 1996, p 360, with permission).

One of the properties of the epidermis is that it varies in thickness in different parts of the body, depending upon the need for protection against compression forces. For example, it is thickest on the soles of the feet and the palms of the hands.

The dermis

The dermis is composed of elastic and collagen fibres. It is the thicker of the two layers and is tough and elastic in nature. Superficial fascia or subcutaneous tissue is found beneath the dermis and is attached to underlying organs by, for example, muscle and bone. The tensile strength of skin is provided by the action of collagen fibres binding with water. It is these collagenous fibres that give healing tissues their strength. The blood supply to the skin emanates from the muscles and the vessels and main structures of the dermis are shown in Figure 10.3.

Skin colour

The colour of the skin is determined by three main factors (Collier 1994, Wilson & Waugh 1996). They are:

- A dark pigment known as melanin
- The level of oxygenation of haemoglobin and the amount of circulation in the dermis
- Carotenes in subcutaneous fat and bile pigments in the blood.

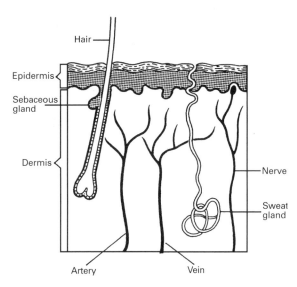

Figure 10.1 Diagram of the skin (from Wilson & Waugh 1996, p 13, with permission).

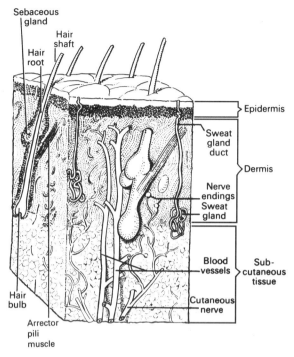

Figure 10.3   The skin showing the main structures of the dermis (from Wilson & Waugh 1996, p 361, with permission).

The functions of the skin

The skin has many functions including:

- Protection
- Formation/synthesis of vitamin D
- Maintenance of body temperature
- Excretion
- Sensation
- Immunity
- Water and energy reserve.

Protection

Skin provides delicate internal organs and structures with a protective barrier. This barrier can protect the body from weak chemicals and most gases, microbes, dehydration, ultraviolet radiation (due to the presence of melanin), and from physical abrasion such as friction and pressure.

Sensory nerve endings in the skin allow the perception of painful or unpleasant stimuli ensuring evasive action against injury through reflex activity.

Formation/synthesis of vitamin D

Ultraviolet light from the sun converts a fatty substance known as 7-dehydrocholesterol, into vitamin D.

Vitamin D assists the utilisation of calcium and phosphorous from the diet which is essential for the formation and maintenance of bone (osseous tissue).

Maintenance of body temperature

Regulation of body temperature is essential to life. The normal body temperature is fairly constant at about 36.8°C and is maintained by a balance of heat produced in the body and heat lost to the environment. Most of the heat loss from the body is via the skin and is regulated by thermoreceptors in the hypothalamus. Heat is lost by:

- Convection
- Conduction
- Evaporation
- Radiation.

The rate of heat loss is controlled through vasoconstriction and vasodilation of the blood vessels supplying blood to the skin.

Excretion

The skin plays a small role in excretion. Urea and sodium chloride are lost in small amounts in sweat and approximately 0.5% of carbon dioxide is excreted via the skin. Aromatic substances such as spices and garlic are also lost via the skin!

Sensation

Sensation plays a role in the normal homeostasis of the body by way of sensory nerve endings found in the dermis. Touch, pressure, temperature and pain are perceived by these nerve endings producing impulses that are transmitted to the cerebral cortex.

Immunity

Cells found in the skin known as keratinocytes, langerhans and granstein promote the normal immune response of the body.

Water and energy reserve

If a haemorrhage occurs the body takes fluid from the dermis to restore blood volume. In the case of starvation, the body calls upon subcutaneous fat to act as an energy reserve (Collier 1994, Hinchliff & Montague 1988, Wilson & Waugh 1996).

The blood supply to the skin

A satisfactory blood supply is essential for healthy

skin and for wound healing. The functions of blood, haemoglobin and oxygen are relevant to the skin and the development of pressure sores and leg ulcers. For instance collagen synthesis can be diminished by hypoxia (Dunne & Robertson 1992).

Functions of blood

Respiration

Oxygen constitutes approximately 21% of atmospheric air. Its presence is required for chemical activities in cells that release energy from nutrient materials and consequently it is essential for the maintenance of human life. The principle role of the respiratory system is to provide an adequate supply of oxygen to the tissues and to remove metabolically produced carbon dioxide. An adult at rest utilises approximately 250 ml of oxygen per minute and produces approximately 200 ml of carbon dioxide per minute. Vigorous exercise can increase these amounts 30-fold.

The lungs transfer oxygen from the air to the blood and carbon dioxide from the blood to the air. The blood transports oxygen from the lungs to the cells and carbon dioxide from the cells back to the lungs for excretion (Fig 10.4). A small proportion of the oxygen and carbon dioxide is transported as aqueous solutions, but the bulk is in the form of chemical compounds of haemoglobin:

- Oxygen combined with haemoglobin to form oxyhaemoglobin
- Carbon dioxide combined with haemoglobin to form carbaminohaemoglobin.

Haemoglobin is a red protein pigment contained in red blood cells. It is synthesised within developing erythrocytes in the red bone marrow during erythropoesis and comprises two main components:

- Haem – an iron containing pigment
- Globin – a protein.

Normal levels of haemoglobin in blood are 13.5–18 g/dl in males and 11.5–16.5 g/dl in females (McGhee 1993).

Oxygen and carbon dioxide are transferred by diffusion between the air and the blood and between the blood and tissue cells. Gases diffuse down the concentration gradient, from areas of high concentration to areas of low concentration. Oxygen is at a higher concentration in the air in the alveoli of the lungs than it is in the blood and so it diffuses from air to blood. Conversely, carbon dioxide is at a higher concentration in the blood than in the air and so it diffuses in the opposite direction, from blood to air (Fig. 10.5). Transfer of gases between the blood and tissue cells is similar. The concentration of oxygen is higher in the blood than in the tissue cells and so oxygen diffuses from the blood to the tissues. The concentration gradient for carbon dioxide is reversed,

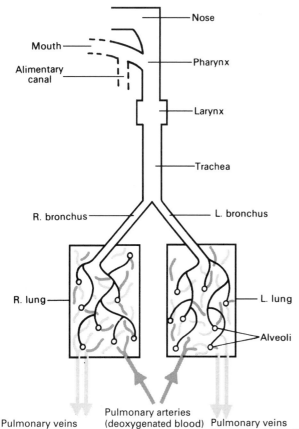

Figure 10.4 Diagram representing the respiratory system (adapted from Wilson & Waugh 1996, p 11, with permission).

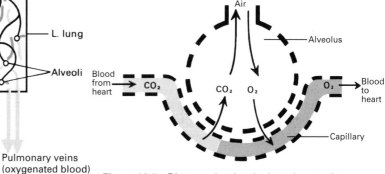

Figure 10.5 Diagram showing the interchange of gases between the air in an alveolus and the blood in a capillary (adapted from Wilson & Waugh 1996, p 11, with permission).

with a higher concentration in the tissue cells than in the blood and consequently, diffusion is from the cells to the blood (Hinchliff & Montague 1988, Wilson & Waugh 1996).

Nutrition

Food taken in at the mouth is broken down into forms that can pass through the walls of the alimentary canal into the blood (Fig. 10.6). These nutrients are absorbed in the small intestine and include monosaccharides, amino acids, fatty acids, glycerol, vitamins, mineral salts and water. They are then transported in plasma to the liver for use in metabolic processes and from there the nutrients are delivered to other tissues.

Excretion

Plasma carries waste products from the tissues and cells to the appropriate organs for excretion. For example urea, uric acid and creatinine are waste products of protein metabolism. Following their preparation in the liver they are transported to the kidneys for excretion.

Regulation of metabolism

Hormones secreted by endocrine glands, and enzymes play a role in the metabolic activities of the body's cells. They are carried in the plasma from the cells of origin to target organs and tissues.

Defence

The body is protected from invasion by microorganisms and their toxins by the phagocytic action of neutrophils and monocytes (white blood cells), and the presence of antibodies and antitoxins.

Prevention of fluid loss

The mechanism of clotting possessed by blood prevents loss of body fluid and blood cells. This homeostasis is due to the function of platelets and a number of clotting and fibrinolytic factors present in plasma.

Protection

Protection is provided by the localised inflammatory response that occurs when tissue is injured.

Maintenance of body temperature

Blood is the medium by which heat is transferred around the body, allowing heat exchange between the tissues and the external environment. Heat loss is controlled by alterations in blood flow to the skin. For example, when the body is too warm the blood vessels near the surface dilate. This increases blood flow and hence heat flow to the surface of the body and so promotes heat loss. Conversely, if the body is too cold or the outside temperature low, the blood vessels constrict, reducing the loss of heat.

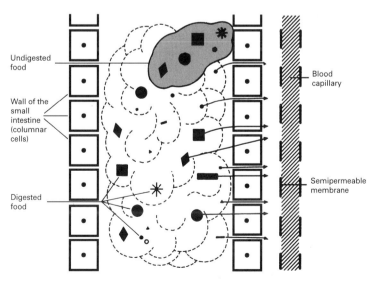

Figure 10.6 Diagram representing the digestion and absorption of food (from Wilson & Waugh 1996, p 11, with permission).

Water, electrolyte and acid base balance

The components of blood and tissue fluid are continually undergoing exchange. Therefore the blood plays a fundamental role in homeostasis and the maintenance of water, electrolyte and acid base balance (Hinchliff & Montague 1988, Wilson & Waugh 1996).

Wound repair

Oxygen is essential for the successful healing of wounds and damaged tissue because of its role in:

- Collagen synthesis
- Growth of new capillaries
- Repair of epithelium.

Wound repair requires a high level of oxygen and any reduction in its availability can result in poor or slow healing. Patients suffering from anaemia, haemorrhage, cardiovascular and and respiratory disorders will have less oxygen and any tissue damage will therefore take longer to repair (Morrison 1992).

CAUSES OF SKIN PROBLEMS IN THE RHEUMATOLOGY PATIENT

There are a number of symptoms of rheumatic diseases that affect the skin integrity of the rheumatology patient. Some are related to the clinical aspects of these diseases, others to the symptoms.

Anaemia

Anaemia is found very frequently in inflammatory arthritides such as rheumatoid arthritis (RA). It takes a number of forms, the most common being:

- Anaemia of chronic disease
- Iron deficiency anaemia
- Megaloblastic anaemia
- Haemolytic anaemia.

These types of anaemia are distinctly different and can sometimes occur together.

Anaemia of chronic disease

Normochromic (red cells normal colour), normocytic anaemia (red cells normal size) is found in patients who have active inflammatory arthritis such as RA. The severity of the anaemia equates to the underlying disease activity. Major factors contributing to this type of anaemia include:

- Under-production of red blood cells from the bone marrow

- Ineffective or reduced concentrations of erythropoietin
- Reduced iron supplies – impaired absorption, transportation and failure to release iron supplies.

Impaired absorption from the patient's diet means that the iron stores are depleted. A higher level of phagocytosis of red blood cells by lymph nodes has also been found.

This type of anaemia will improve only when the underlying disease activity is brought under control (Bird et al 1985).

Iron deficiency anaemia

Patients may also be found to have iron deficiency anaemia. In this instance, the cells are hypochromic (pale coloured) and microcytic (small). This can be due to the disease, for instance oesophagitis which can be present in scleroderma, or it may result from drug induced gastric bleeding or from a diet deficient in iron (Hollingworth 1988, Hart 1984, Kumar & Clark 1990, Matteson et al 1995).

Megaloblastic anaemia

This is a macrocytic anaemia (abnormally large erythrocytes) which is usually due to folate deficiency. Drugs such as methotrexate, a folate antagonist and azathioprine can cause this type of anaemia.

Haemolytic anaemia

This form of anaemia occurs in 10% of patients with systemic lupus erythematosus.

Patients with severe anaemia are at risk of their skin breaking down. Tissue hypoxia occurs due to the reduced level of circulating red blood cells. The resulting lack of oxygen supply to the skin can result in the formation of a decubitus ulcer if preventative action is not taken (Luckman & Sorenson 1980). Dunne and Robertson (1992) suggest that a low level of haemoglobin impairs collagen synthesis if there is also reduced cardiac output, reduced blood volume or protein depletion present.

Poor nutrition

For healthy skin and promotion of healing when skin integrity is broken a healthy diet is essential. If a rheumatoid patient has a pressure sore or leg ulcer to heal, their nutritional requirements will be far greater than that of a healthy individual (Dunne & Robertson 1992). Diet is dealt with in detail later in the chapter.

Steroid therapy

Steroid drug therapy, if used over long periods of time, can cause the skin to bruise easily and tear. This is due to the reduction of collagen and elastin, which leads to the loss of support for blood vessels, leaving them fragile. Oedema can also occur due to the retention of sodium. The combination of oedematous ankles and legs with fragile skin can lead to the development of ulcers if the skin is damaged (Pigg et al 1985).

A raised corticosteroid level delays wound healing and increases susceptibility to infection by suppression of natural immune and inflammatory responses. The delay in wound healing is thought to occur only during the inflammatory and proliferative phases of the response, due to suppression of collagen synthesis and production of fibroblasts (Dunne & Robertson 1992, Hinchliff & Montague 1988, Morrison 1992).

Common problems

Nodular lesions

One of the extra-articular manifestations of RA is the development of nodules. These occur in 20% of patients with seropositive RA, and affect those with severe disease (Hollingworth 1988, Matteson et al 1995).

Nodules are firm, subcutaneous, moveable lesions and are usually painless. They vary in size and have an inner core of necrotised collagen, fibrin and cell debris. They tend to develop over bony prominences such as elbows, ischial and sacral prominences and the occipital scalp, sites that make them very susceptible to mechanical trauma.

Nodules may subside with an improvement in disease activity, but in patients on methotrexate, they may worsen even if disease activity improves.

Gouty tophi

Gouty tophi are solid deposits of sodium urate that appear as irregular, firm nodular swellings. They are yellow/white in colour and appear to shine through the overlying skin. If there is local inflammation the surrounding skin may become erythematous. They typically occur in the digits of the hands and feet, the ear and the olecranon bursa. They can become infected.

Calcinosis

Calcinosis occurs when calcium salts are deposited in the tissues and it is one of the characteristics of systemic sclerosis. These deposits are palpable, intracutaneous and/or subcutaneous and are found located on digits, along the forearm, knees, shins, thighs,

buttocks and elbows. They can ulcerate and a gritty toothpaste like substance drain out (Cohen & Emmerson 1995, Dieppe 1995, Steen 1995). If they ulcerate they can take many weeks to heal.

Pressure sores

Pressure sores are caused by:

- Unrelieved pressure
- Shearing
- Friction.

This is illustrated in Figure 10.7.

Patients with rheumatic disease have an increased risk of developing pressure sores, a risk that can be increased by the presence of other conditions, such as heart disease, respiratory disease or diabetes. Effective prevention can be achieved through individual assessment, and the planning, implementation and evaluation of care. The use of risk assessment tools is also essential for optimum effectiveness (Young 1997).

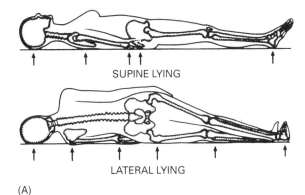

SUPINE LYING

LATERAL LYING

(A)

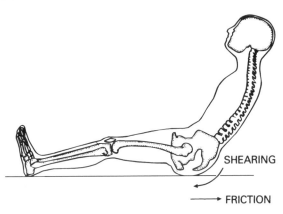

SHEARING

FRICTION

(B)

Figure 10.7 Causes of pressure sores. (A) Unrelieved pressure. (B) Shearing and friction (from Davis 1994 Nursing the orthopaedic patient, p 76, with permission).

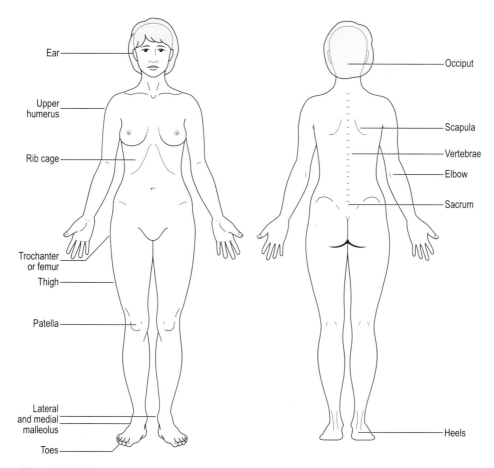

Figure 10.8 Areas at greatest risk of developing pressure sores.

Table 10.1 Factors related to pressure sores.

Causes	Predisposing factors		Preventative measures
	Physical	Common medical conditions	
Unrelieved pressure	Immobility/reduced mobility	Arthritis	Pressure relieving aids
Friction	Altered consciousness	Anaemia	Correct procedures to move
Shearing forces	Sensation loss	Diabetes	patients
	Coexisting debilitating illness	Cardiovascular disease	Promote mobility
	Fragile skin	Respiratory disease	Skin care
	Age	Cerebral vascular accident	Adequate pain relief
	Incontinence	Multiple sclerosis	Healthy diet
	Excessive perspiration	Malignancy	Adequate hydration
	Dehydration	Spinal cord injury	Patient and carer education.
	Malnutrition		
	Pain		
	Depression		

The areas most at risk of pressure sores are shown in Figure10.8 and Table 10.1 summarises their principal causes, predisposing factors and measures for their prevention.

Immobility

One of the largest predisposing factors to the development of a pressure sore is immobility, as unrelieved pressure causes compression of the tissues against bony prominences (Morrison 1992). Immobility is a major problem for patients with rheumatic diseases and can be caused by:

- Pain
- Stiffness
- Joint contracture
- Disorganisation of the joint
- Fatigue
- Depression.

It is important that the multidisciplinary team works towards maximum mobility for each patient. This may require a number of different modalities, for example the use of walking aids or electric chairs, physiotherapy or the prescription of effective analgesia.

The education of the patient, relatives and carers will promote mobility through greater understanding, allowing patients to set their own goals and make their own decisions (Benbow 1996). Knowledge of drug therapy allows the patient to judge the most efficacious time to take their medication, so enhancing mobility (Hill 1990, Hill 1997).

Relieving pressure

Positional changes are the key to pressure relief. The frequency at which this is undertaken will depend on the needs of individual patients, but a minimum of every two hours is recommended (Morrison 1992).

Use of pressure relieving mattresses and seat cushions is often indicated but these should be used as an adjunct to and not instead of positional changes. The range of mattresses and cushions is constantly being improved and articles and up to date information are published regularly in the nursing press (Cowan 1996, Cowan 1997). Care should be taken to assess the research supporting the use of these products and the appropriateness of each to individual patients (Fletcher 1997). Many rheumatology patients find the covers on products make them too hot and others do not like the sensation of the mattresses' changing pressure. Patients often favour mattresses that appear no different to an ordinary mattress and some overlay type mattresses meet these preferences. The appearance of 'normality' can help to promote the patient's self esteem and also acknowledges that they may share their bed with their partner!

Leg ulcers

Leg ulcers can have a great impact on the quality of the patient's life (Hildegard 1995) and immobility plays a part in the development of leg ulcers. For patients with RA, contributing factors are local vasculitis, immobility causing poor venous return, the long term effects on the skin of steroids, poor nutrition, the development of obesity and dependent oedema. However, the lack of understanding of the reasons why patients with RA are susceptible to leg ulcers makes effective treatment very difficult (Cullum & Roe 1995, Morrison 1992, Shipperley 1997).

The causes, contributory factors, factors that delay healing and preventative measures are summarised in Table 10.2.

Table 10.2 Factors related to leg ulcers.

Causes	Contributory factors	Factors delaying healing	Prevention
Arterial disease	Vasculitis	Immobility/reduced mobility	Early recognition of at risk patients
Vascular disease	Poor mobility/immobility	Malnutrition	Planning of appropriate care
(chronic venous hypotension)	Oedema	Psychosocial issues/problems	Promotion of mobility
Diabetes mellitus	Frailty	Leg oedema	Treatment of underlying causes
Rheumatoid arthritis	Previous surgery	Multiple diagnosis (several	Skin care
Malignancy	Smoking	medical problems).	Healthy diet
Trauma			Recognition of and action upon
Metabolic disorders			psychosocial issues/problems
Lymphoedema			Patient and carer education
Blood disorders			Discouragement of smoking.
Infection			

Less common causes in italics

Vasculitis (inflammation of a vessel)

Vasculitis is relevant to skin care because of its manifestation in skin lesions. In connective tissue diseases such as systemic lupus erythematosus and RA, small vessel vasculitis may occur (Kumar & Clark 1990). The initiating factor of a rheumatoid leg ulcer is usually an underlying vasculitis. However its development and chronicity may be progressed by long term use of glucocorticosteroid, arterial and/or venous insufficiency, dependent oedema and trauma (Matteson et al 1995).

Depression

Patients with chronic rheumatic diseases can become depressed from time to time. This is usually when their disease is active and they are in pain and feeling systemically ill. One of the salient symptoms of depression is fatigue and the combination of the fatigue from the two sources can be severely debilitating. Not surprisingly, at these times there is a tendency for the patient to neglect their physical needs and their appearance. To visualise the position many patients find themselves in, take a few moments to consider the following:

- Visualise the things that you do as a matter of routine, such as hobbies, social events, activities of daily living.
- Now imagine that your right arm and leg are in splints, would you still be able to do them?
- Thinking positively, what could you do to maintain your usual quality of life?
- You have worked hard to restore some normality to your life when disaster strikes. Your left arm and leg have to be put in splints.
- You are back to square one; now what will you do?

Your imagined situation is analogous to that faced by many people with RA, who have to cope with their disease through flare after flare. However, your postulated condition was relatively benign. You had only to cope with loss of function and independence. Many patients have to cope with a multitude of additional problems including, deformity of joints, altered body image, chronic pain and stiffness, fatigue and frustration (Arthur 1994).

Under these circumstances it is hardly surprising that patients frequently respond to rheumatic disease with feelings of depression and despondency (Bird et al 1985, Pigg et al 1985, Shipley & Newman 1993). However, this can only add to their problems if it manifests itself as sleeplessness, loss of appetite and lack of motivation. If the depression is chemical in nature or becomes a major episode, medical intervention must be sought (Pigg et al 1985). It is frequently assumed that anxiety and depression relate to the level of disease activity. However, socioeconomic factors rather than physical factors appear to be more relevant (Gordon & Hastings 1995).

Nurses should watch for signs of this potential reaction, and act before it becomes a problem. The first indication may be the patient withdrawing or becoming 'snappy'. You can use your own counselling skills or call upon the expertise of a colleague. Often patients will talk to someone they have come to know very well and feel comfortable with. This may be the qualified nurse, ward domestic, health care assistant or home help. Patients must be given support and encouragement but most importantly, time and a listening ear. Patient education can help dispel fears and anxieties and can maintain or improve health and promote self management (Bird et al 1985, Hill 1995, Lorig 1996). Involvement in patient support groups such as Arthritis Care can be a great benefit.

EDUCATION

Patients who do not adhere to the pattern of care prescribed by their health professionals often become labelled as non compliant. However, this non compliance may stem from lack of understanding and ignorance of their condition and situation. Education can increase a patient's knowledge and provide them with the resources upon which to make judgements and decisions regarding their disease. Encouraging patients to actively contribute to their own care planning can be seen as a genuine move towards empowerment (Ertl 1993, Hill 1990, House 1996, Ruane-Morris et al 1995).

Skin integrity should form one part of a holistic care programme, and this should be reflected in the content of any patient education programme. The subject of patient education is dealt with in depth in Chapter 15 and so only those factors relevant to skin integrity are included here.

What to teach is always a concern. However, a starting point for an individual programme can be to establish what the patient already knows and what they would like to learn. With regard to the skin, the emphasis should be on prevention and early recognition of signs of a leg ulcer or pressure sore developing and should include the following:

- The use of soaps and the avoidance of highly perfumed varieties
- The need to carefully rinse all traces of soap from the skin
- Use of moisturisers, taking care to avoid sensitivity

reactions. Use of emulsifying creams can be recommended

- Occasional use of favourite toiletries is in order, to promote self esteem and improve impressions of body. We all must have experienced the benefits of a self indulgent bath!
- Skin must be thoroughly dried by gentle patting rather than rubbing to prevent damaging friable blood vessels
- Keep finger and toenails short to prevent accidental scratches and tears (may require referral to a chiropodist)
- How leg ulcers develop
- How pressure sores develop
- Recognition of early signs of a leg ulcer or pressure sore developing
- Pressure relief
- Use of pressure-relieving equipment
- Elevation of legs
- Nutrition (may require referral to a dietician)
- Why the patient is at risk
- Effects of medication if applicable
- What to do if they detect a problem (provision of contact names, addresses and telephone numbers can be useful as well as supportive).

When providing patient education, it should be remembered that it is not just useful to the patient. It is also important to include relatives and carers in any education programme (Benbow 1996, Ertl 1992).

DIET AND ARTHRITIS

Throughout history we have been aware of the relationship between what we eat and our health. Teachings about the various elements in the diet have been documented as far back as 2000 years. However, over the past century, the science of nutrition has heightened this interest and diet is now a composite part of the management of health and ill health.

Over the years, there have been many advances in drug therapy in the management of arthritis, but some nurses and physicians have also postulated the effect of dietary manipulation and a well balanced diet as a safer therapeutic option than toxic drug therapy. To many traditionally trained health professionals, diet as a component of the management of arthritis, has been perceived as an alternative or fringe medicine and has been dismissed accordingly (Darlington 1985). However, patients often have queries about diet such as 'does it cause arthritis?' or 'what should I eat?' It is understandable that patients seek alternatives when consideration is given to the long term nature of the disease, the relative ineffectiveness and side effects of many drugs. Patients strive to find a therapy guaranteed to be effective, safe, user friendly and free from side effects.

It is interesting that patients' questions are usually addressed to the nursing staff, as many feel that their queries are too trivial for the doctor! It is therefore vital that nurses are sufficiently informed about diet and its effects to address these questions and they should encourage discussion about the patient's diet.

If patients feel unable to talk to health professionals, they may take it upon themselves to manipulate their diet and some patients have used diet as a replacement for their drug regime, which can be detrimental to their health.

THE DIETICIAN

The dietician can offer current, evidence-based advice to patients and health professionals and is a vital member of any multidisciplinary team. Wherever possible, the dietician should be involved in regular ward meetings and case conferences, but unfortunately where resources are limited, the dietician may only be available on an appointment basis.

Although diet and nutrition is an area primarily assessed by the nurse, in some locations nurses may not be able to refer patients directly to the dietetic department. Unfortunately, some units insist that a physician makes the referral! This issue should be addressed on an individual basis within the realms of professional practice. The individual making the referral must ensure that the request is explicit. Inappropriate or inexplicit referrals can result in misunderstandings and a reluctance to ask for further help.

Dietetic training provides the dietician with the skills needed to maintain overall dietary adequacy whilst introducing and varying the diet to meet the individual's needs. There are a variety of situations where the dietician's help is invaluable to the rheumatic patient, for instance:

- Weight reduction for the obese patient
- Dietary supplementation for the malnourished patient
- Dietary manipulation during systemic ill health in acute disease
- Advice regarding liquid diet for those patients with swallowing and chewing difficulties.

A WELL-BALANCED DIET

A healthy well-balanced diet will help the patient with arthritis to maintain optimum health. The skin is sensitive to changes in nutritional status, consequently the malnourished patient is susceptible to pressure sores, and vitamin A is known to be required to maintain the integrity of skin. A well-nourished body will recover more easily from the frequent flares of disease and episodes of ill health that rheumatic patients endure.

How can a well-balanced diet be defined?

Individuals perceive 'good eating' in different ways. Opinions are influenced strongly by:

- Childhood experiences
- Money available to spend on diet
- Socioeconomic group.

Dieticians tend to define a healthy diet as one that incorporates all the essential nutrients such as amino acids, vitamins, carbohydrates, fibre and those fatty acids essential to cell function which maintain an optimum body weight. Most foods contain some of these nutrients, but most are deficient in one way or another and so a variety of foods must be eaten to ensure that the diet is well balanced. All the essential nutrients can be found in animal products such as meat, fish, cheese, eggs and milk in combination with vegetables and fruit.

Dietary protein and amino acids

The protein requirements of the body vary with each individual, depending on the metabolic rate and the health status. Pregnant and breast feeding mothers need an increase in intake for growth in foetal and maternal tissue. Similarly, the rheumatic patient who has increased tissue damage and so greater repair requirements needs an adequate protein intake. Protein is constantly being broken down into amino acids and re-synthesised. Some amino acids are lost early on in the process but many are re-utilised to ensure adequate serum and tissue protein levels. This process is under hormonal and metabolic control, allowing the body to adjust to the health status of the tissues. For example in an acute inflammatory episode there is an increase in the utilisation of amino acids. Consequently the dietary source needs to be adequately maintained to meet the increased demand from the tissues. The body can cope with a temporary reduction in protein, but if it persists, a deficiency will result in detrimental effects on tissue healing and general health status.

In general, animal proteins such as fish, meat and dairy products are more readily digestible than vegetable proteins. However, a high fibre diet can increase protein digestibility by as much as 10%.

Protein supplementation

In cases of hypoproteinaemia, protein supplementation may be indicated. If the patient is able to eat a normal diet, the regular consumption of foods rich in protein such as milk, eggs, meat, fish, vegetables and fruit may suffice. However, if the patient is systemically unwell and has anorexia, the addition of skimmed milk powders to drinks may be a better method. The dietician will be able to offer further advice about protein supplementation from the wide range of supplementary feeds available.

Patients with liver or renal dysfunction may experience impaired synthesis and/or excretion of protein and in these cases, manipulation of dietary protein must be managed with great care.

Dietary fats

Dietary fats comprise:

1. Triglycerides
2. Phospholipids
3. Cholesterol.

Triglycerides are the largest group and comprise about 95% of body fat. They consist of one molecule of glycerol combined with three fatty acid molecules. There is only one form of glycerol, but many fatty acids and the nature and nutritional value of the fat is determined by the particular fatty acids it contains. Fats are insoluble in water and weight for weight yield more energy on combustion than carbohydrates. Consequently they are a very convenient form in which energy yielding molecules, the fatty acids, can be stored.

Phospholipids are important in the composition of some cell structures. They have a structure similar to that of the triglycerides, but in phospholipids, one of the three fatty acids is replaced by phosphoric acid.

Cholesterol is structurally different to typical fats but has many similar properties, including insolubility in water and solubility in organic solvents.

Fatty acids

The structure of stearic acid, a typical fatty acid is shown in Figure 10.9A. It consists of a chain of carbon atoms to which hydrogen is attached (a hydrocarbon chain) and ends in the form of an acid carboxyl group. In this particular example, each carbon atom has two hydrogen atoms bonded to it, with the result that there is a hydrogen atom at every possible site on the hydrocarbon chain. Fatty acids that have this feature are termed *saturated* fatty acids. Another common fatty acid, oleic acid, has a different structure as shown in

A

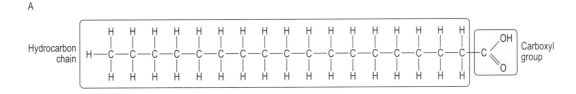

B

Figure 10.9   Molecular structure of fatty acids. (A) Saturated fatty acid – stearic acid. (B) Unsaturated fatty acid – oleic acid.

Figure 10.9B. Here, there is a double bond between two of the carbon atoms in the middle of the chain. Because of this, these two carbon atoms have only one site available for a hydrogen atom, and so the chain does not contain the maximum possible number of hydrogen atoms. Fatty acids having this feature are termed *unsaturated* fatty acids.

There are 21 fatty acids found in the diet. Amongst the most common are:

• Palmitic
• Stearic
• Oleic
• Linoleic
• Linolenic
• Arachidonic.

Essential fatty acids

The body is able to synthesise most fatty acids. However, linoleic, linolenic and arachidonic acids, all unsaturated fatty acids essential to tissue function, must be provided in the diet. These are referred to as the essential fatty acids. They are precursors of prostaglandins, the chemicals involved in the inflammatory process, substances that promote platelet aggregation and anticoagulants.

Dietary effects of saturated and unsaturated fats

Saturated fatty acids are known precursors of cardiovascular disease. It is thought that a reduction in their intake could reduce heart disease.

Obesity, lack of exercise, systemic illness and smoking are predisposing factors to heart disease. This places the rheumatic patient at potential risk because:

• Their ability to exercise is reduced
• Their systemic health is impaired
• A large percentage of patients smoke.

To reduce the risk, patients should be provided with the following advice about the fat content of their diet.

1. Substitute saturated fats with polyunsaturated fats.

Polyunsaturated fats do not contain cholesterol and are a safer option for dietary fat consumption as they reduce low density lipoprotein concentrations, the group of cholesterols that are associated with heart disease. Polyunsaturated fats are contained in some margarines and vegetable oils.

2. Reduce excessive fat intake.

A high intake of fat can precipitate weight gain and obesity that is particularly detriment to patients with joint dysfunction. Obesity hinders mobility, lowers moral and self esteem and greatly increases the load carried by weight bearing joints.

Carbohydrates

Carbohydrates are taken in the diet in the form of sugars and starches. Starches are carbohydrates derived from plants and sugars can be described as their soluble form. Carbohydrates are classified according to their chemical complexity:

• Monosaccharides – single units or molecules: glucose, fructose, galactose

- Disaccharides – two monosaccharide molecules: sucrose, maltose, and lactose
- Polysaccharides – large numbers of monosaccharide molecules: starches, glycogen, cellulose and dextrins.

The main functions of carbohydrates are to:

- Provide a rapid source of energy and heat
- Store energy
- Spare protein.

Foods which supply carbohydrate, include sugar, jams, bread, pasta, cereals fruit and vegetables. No matter from which dietary source the carbohydrate is derived, it is converted to and absorbed into the blood in the form of glucose. All bodily tissues, especially the brain need carbohydrate as a vital fuel for their function. To meet these demands the body attempts to maintain a steady level of glucose in the blood stream at all times.

Under normal circumstances the blood glucose rises after eating:

- If there is a surplus of glucose it is stored in the liver or muscles as glycogen
- If the level of carbohydrate exceeds that required to maintain blood glucose level and glycogen levels in the tissues, it is converted to fat for storage.

Once exercise is initiated these glycogen stores are released back into the blood stream to maintain a steady level.

The normal blood glucose level is between 2.5 and 5.3 mmol / litre and maintenance at these levels is vital for normal bodily function. Homeostasis is maintained by insulin and glucagon acting in a complementary manner.

- Blood glucose levels are increased by glucagon
- Blood glucose levels are reduced by insulin.

If insulin function is abnormal the blood glucose level remains excessively high. If the level falls excessively, a feeling of hunger prevails, associated with a sense of agitation and depression, symptoms that frequently present in the patient with arthritis. If the diet is tuned to maintain a steady glucose level, the symptoms associated with these peaks and troughs may be avoided. More complex carbohydrates such as those found in potatoes, pasta and rice are digested at a slower rate and can help to maintain the levels of blood glucose. If they are eaten in their most natural form, for example potatoes with their skins, brown rice, wholemeal pasta, they are more likely to appease the appetite as they remain in the stomach longer and maintain a more stable blood sugar level.

Dietary fibre

Dietary fibre is a complex mixture of carbohydrates that consists of plant cell walls. It is indigestible and therefore offers little value to nutrition. Its functions are to:

- Provide bulk
- Stimulate peristalsis
- Attract water that softens and bulks the faeces
- Prevent constipation
- Prevent gastrointestinal disorders such as diverticular disease.

The recommended intake of fibre is 18 –20 grams per day but in developed countries where a more refined diet is eaten, the average intake is 11–12 grams per day. This is made up of vegetables and cereals in almost equal parts. If fibre intake is increased then health will benefit.

Benefits of increased fibre

Satiation of appetite. The first beneficial effect is the feeling of fullness. For the overweight person extra fibre will help to satisfy the appetite and can help tremendously in weight reduction. Fibre is a very natural slimming aid and also has the advantage of being relatively cheap.

Relief of constipation. The second benefit is to those patients who suffer from constipation. The increased bulk and water retention can help to regulate bowel habit. Analgesia usually forms part of the drug therapy regime of patients with rheumatic conditions and analgesics, particularly those containing codeine, can cause severe constipation.

Many rheumatic diseases cause pain, stiffness and debility which leads to immobility and lack of exercise. This can cause stasis of the bowel. Extra fibre will stimulate peristaltic action.

Lower blood cholesterol. High fibre diets have the advantage of lowering blood cholesterol and are thought to reduce the incidence of cancer of the large intestine.

Vitamins

Vitamins are defined as any organic compound required by the body in small amounts for metabolism and health. They assist in the:

- Formation of hormones
- Blood cells
- Nervous system chemicals
- Genetic material

- Skin integrity
- Muscle regeneration
- Recovery from acute episodes of inflammation.

Generally they act as catalysts, combining with proteins to produce metabolically active enzymes that in turn produce hundreds of important chemical reactions throughout the body. Without vitamins many of these reactions would slow down or cease.

There are 13 well-defined vitamins that are classed according to their solubility in fat or water.

The fat-soluble vitamins A, D, E and K are generally consumed along with fat-containing foods. Because they are stored in body fat they do not need to be consumed every day. In contrast, the eight water-soluble B vitamins and vitamin C cannot be stored and must be replenished frequently, preferably daily. The only vitamin that can be produced by the body is vitamin D. All others must be derived from the diet.

Vitamin supplementation

Vitamin supplementation has often been claimed to be a 'cure for all' and large sums of money are spent on vitamin supplements. In reality, the body eliminates most of these supplemented vitamins quite rapidly. Dieticians suggest that a well-balanced diet will provide all 13 vitamins in adequate amounts.

Many patients with rheumatic diseases request advice regarding vitamin supplementation. When answering these questions it should not be assumed that they are able to provide themselves with a well-balanced diet. Many patients eat what is easiest for them to manage or what their relatives or carers prepare. When assessing a patient's intake of vitamins it is useful to ask them to outline their daily diet. One way of doing this is to ask them to describe the meals they had the previous day and how they were prepared. If a broader picture is needed, request them to keep a diary of everything eaten during a week. This will enable specific vitamin deficiencies to be highlighted. If further specialised advice is need, consult the dietician.

Obesity in the rheumatoid patient

Weight will remain stable if the dietary intake balances the energy expended by the body. However the patient with arthritis may have difficulty achieving this balance. Weight gain and subsequent obesity is a very common problem in disabled patients, particularly those with osteoarthritis. Many find it extremely difficult to exercise actively even when their disease is well controlled. Factors influencing the extent to which patients can exercise include:

- Joint pain
- Stiffness
- Muscle weakness
- Muscle wasting.

Obviously the degree of joint pain and the level of disease activity varies between patients, but very few are able to sustain a programme of exercise that is vigorous or regular enough to burn off excess calories.

The boredom and frustration of immobility compound the problem of weight gain and the temptation to indulge in comfort eating is understandable. Patients who are housebound also find themselves alone for long periods and derive solace from eating.

Chronic disability can degrade and demoralise a person and poor body image results in personal neglect. Medications such as steroids can induce weight gain and clothes do not look or feel good to wear. This sometimes results in non compliance with the drug therapy involved.

The patient with weight problems needs to be treated with compassion and understanding. Nurses can be a source of great support and comfort, especially those who are 'pleasantly plump' themselves! Advice must be practical and sensible and there is a plethora of information available from the figure conscious media.

Literature should be made available regarding:

- Sensible diets
- Local slimming clubs
- Exercise facilities that cater specifically for the disabled or less able patient.

Exercise must be modified to meet individual needs and many sports centres are recognising this and offering specialised sessions. Some local rheumatology units hold sessions for patients at their local pools, but it should be noted that swimming pools need to be about 10°F (6°C) warmer than usual to provide an environment more conducive with hydrotherapy. There are many local initiatives. For instance one was started by a rheumatology occupational therapist and physiotherapist who gave their time voluntarily to initiate an exercise programme that the patients could perform. Another unit began a slimming group for the patients with the physiotherapist providing a gentle exercise programme to music. These innovations are time consuming and expensive, but considering the long term side effects of excess weight on the damaged joint these interventions must be worthwhile.

For the patient with osteoarthritis (OA) of the weight bearing joints, weight reduction can be a very successful therapeutic option. Walking can result in the knee experiencing an impulse loading of up to eight times body weight. Therefore joint pain and discomfort are very likely to be reduced if obese patients reduce their weight.

The underweight or malnourished patient

Acute and chronic inflammatory disease can result in an increased metabolic rate where energy expended exceeds dietary intake. The patient may eat normally but still loose weight. This in association with tiredness and malaise leads the patient to wonder whether they have an additional, more serious illness such as cancer or AIDS. Although weight loss is associated with inflammatory rheumatic disease, it is important to think holistically and rule out other, non-related pathology.

There are several points to consider:

• Has the patient actually lost weight?

They often feel unwell, don't want to eat and so feel thinner, but this doesn't always mean they have lost weight. A reduction in mobility can reduce muscle bulk making the legs and arms look particularly emaciated and thin.

The best method of verifying weight loss is to monitor the weight over a period of weeks. Use the same scales each time as the variation from one set to another can be dramatic. Weight documentation should be shared with the patient to reassure them if the weight is steady, and discuss diet or further investigations if it is not.

If the weight loss is confirmed, consider whether this is solely a result of disease or due to a concurrent disease. Medical and nursing management will vary according to the history but it is vital that nurses obtain a concise history from these patients. Questioning should include:

• How much weight have you lost and over what time period?
• Has the weight loss been in parallel with your disease activity?
• Do you have an adequate appetite?
• Is your diet well balanced?
• If your diet and appetite are poor can you think of a reason why?

Practical difficulties may form part of the problem. For instance:

• The patient may not drink to avoid walking to the toilet
• Food preparation may pose such great difficulties that it is easier not to eat
• The patient may be too fatigued to bother to cook
• Manual dexterity may inhibit food preparation.

Some patients have severe problems with manual dexterity and so one of the first considerations is whether the patient can use their hands efficiently enough to cut up or prepare food. If not, referral to the occupational therapist for adapted cutlery and kitchen equipment (see Figs 11.6 and 11.7) can often retrieve much of their independence (Douglas 1980). Some patients may then have difficulty lifting the food to their mouths due to stiffness, weakness or contractures.

Rheumatic diseases are energy depleting and fatigue may increase the demand for, but reduce the will to prepare a meal. Pain may also contribute to difficulties with nutrition; opening packets and jars, stirring or lifting pans can prove impossible for some patients. Medical review of medication and assistance from the occupational therapist and physiotherapist can be of great benefit (Arthur 1994, Crosby 1991, Ryan 1995).

If weight loss is due to other medical problems an assessment of the general health of the patient should not rely on the skills of the medical practitioner alone. Nurses can use their questioning skills to provide a background to the problem. Many doctors confirm that the patient is often happier and more confident answering questions posed by a nurse. If communication between the nurses and doctors is good then true multidisciplinary assessment of the patient can be undertaken.

Gastrointestinal problems

Disorders of the gastrointestinal tract can often result in weight loss and anorexia. Problems can be identified by asking patients:

• Do you have mouth ulcers or a sore mouth?
• Do you have a dry mouth?
• Is the process of chewing painful because of jaw pain?
• Do you have difficulty swallowing?
• Do you experience indigestion, heartburn or vomiting?
• Have you ever seen blood in the vomit?
• Have you any history of hiatus hernia, gastric ulceration?
• Is constipation and/or diarrhoea evident?
• Have you ever noticed blood in your stools? If yes

do you have haemorrhoids? They can be the source of bleeding rather than a site higher up in the tract.

Many of these problems can be addressed and treated by the nurse. For instance advice regarding mandibular pain, mouth care and mouth sprays for a dry mouth caused by Sjögren's syndrome. Advice about constipation and swallowing difficulties due to scleroderma can also be given. If the nurse can provide a concise patient history, this will aid the doctor to plan medical management and save the patient time.

COMMON QUESTIONS REGARDING DIET

There are a number of questions that reoccur regarding diet and the rheumatic patient. The most frequently asked are discussed in this section.

Can fasting influence the disease activity in RA?

The suggestion that the gut may be involved in the immune mediated process of RA suggests the possibility that elimination of antigenic material in the gut could result in a reduction of inflammatory symptoms. It is therefore relevant to discuss the role of the gut in the inflammatory process of RA.

Involvement of the gut in disease activity

It is possible that the gut may be involved in the inflammatory process of RA. In normal health the intestinal mucosa forms a selective barrier which keeps material within the intestinal lumen completely separate to the internal body fluids. The mucosal gut wall contains enterocytes and these along with the overlaying mucous layer, the glycolax, ensure that this separating function is maintained (Jenkins et al 1987). The mucosa selectively absorbs necessary nutrients once enzymatic digestion has broken them down into dipeptides, triglycerides, fatty acids and disaccharides (Seeley et al 1992).

In addition to nutrients, small structured molecules such as ions, vitamins, and certain drugs can pass through the gut wall relatively freely. Some diseases or infections can render the barrier ineffective, allowing antigenic (foreign to the immune system) material within the dietary contents or within bacterial colonisation to penetrate the gut walls (Buchanan et al 1991). The literature suggests that this intestinal presentation of 'non-self' material can trigger an autoimmune response and a number of rheumatic diseases such as RA, ankylosing spondylitis and reactive arthritis are known to be related to the passage of antigens across the barrier (Darlington & Ramsey 1993).

The role of fasting

Fasting can be defined as 'the voluntary refraining from food for a limited period of time' (Palmblad et al 1991). It has been advocated as treatment for depression, hypertension, obesity and arthritic conditions.

Fasting causes a sudden and dramatic fall in exogenous energy that would normally be supplied by the diet. After a relatively short time the shortage of energy must be compensated to supply metabolic needs and this is achieved by release of endogenous energy from the liver glycogen, muscle protein and fat tissue (Landsberg & Young 1976). When these compensatory changes occur, metabolic hormones are readjusted and it may be at this point that the inflammatory process of RA is influenced.

The literature confirms that fasting reduces disease activity in RA when measured using subjective and objective criteria. However, the benefit is short lived and deterioration is noted within several days of reintroduction of food (Skoldstam et al 1983, Sundvist et al 1982).

The immediacy of remission is a great attraction to the patient despite the antisocial nature of fasting. Patients often embark on such dietary regimes without the support of their physician or specialist nurse. This is of great concern as the patient may be at risk of malnutrition and dehydration if the fast is undertaken in an uncontrolled manner. Equally important, the patient may attempt to use fasting not as an adjunct to but as a replacement for drug regimes. If the patient is taking steroids this could be life threatening. Overall, there is no clinical evidence to support the promotion of fasting as an adjunct therapy in the management of RA.

What is the effect of an allergy-free or elemental diet on a patient with RA, and can an allergic factor be clinically identified?

The immunological presentation of certain antigenic substances in the gut may be a precursor to an inflammatory process in RA. If foods likely to be antigenic are removed from the diet, improvement in disease activity may be expected. An elemental diet is a hypoallergenic protein-free diet that contains:

- Amino acids
- Glucose
- Trace elements
- Vitamins.

It provides food in its simplest form; protein as amino acids, carbohydrates as glucose and fat as medium-chain triglycerides (Kavanagh et al 1995).

Research shows that the introduction of an elemental diet has dramatic immediate benefits to the RA patient. Unfortunately, as with fasting, the effects are short lived and disappear rapidly after the reintroduction of food. Reintroduction of specific foods appears to produce a variety of individual responses. Some respond significantly to one food, whilst others respond to a lesser degree. It is concluded that allergy to diet is not a major causative factor contributing to the aetiology of RA (Kavanagh et al 1995, Van de Laar & Van Der Korst 1992, Panush 1990, Beri et al 1988, Felder et al 1987, Darlington et al 1986).

Many patients report symptoms associated with certain food substances such as dairy products, but the literature does not offer any evidence that these substances should be avoided in the wider rheumatoid population.

Does supplementation with omega three fatty acids such as fish oils and evening primrose oil influence disease activity in RA?

This is one of the commonest diet related questions asked by patients. Essential fatty acids are derived from the diet and are divided into two groups:

- Linoleic acid – omega six fatty acids
- Alpha-linolenic acid – omega three fatty acids.

Omega six acids are found in abundance in corn, safflower, soy and other vegetable oils.

Omega three acids are found in fatty fishes such as tuna, sardines, salmon and in certain plants such as the evening primrose.

Essential fatty acids provide energy and are an integral part of cell membranes. They are also the precursors of prostaglandins, thromboxanes and, collectively termed eisoanoids. This group of chemicals is involved in the development and regulation of immunological and inflammatory processes (Sperling 1991).

When cells involved in immune reactions are stimulated, the body's existing store of essential fatty acids are mobilised from the phospholipid pools for synthesis of prostaglandins. The type of prostaglandins produced is dependant on the type of essential fatty acids present (Meade & Mertin 1978). If the essential fatty acid store is rich in omega three fatty acids of the five series, for example PGE3, then prostaglandins that demonstrate beneficial anti-inflammatory properties will be produced. However, if the diet contains a majority of essential fatty acids from the omega six group, far more active prostaglandins will be activated that promote the inflammatory process.

The production of beneficial and antagonistic prostaglandins from the dietary intake of certain essential fatty acids begs the question as to whether manipulation of their intake could benefit the RA patient.

The most well known sources of essential fatty acids are fish oils. Many claims, the majority anecdotal, have been made as to the efficacy of increasing the dietary intake of fish oils and fish oil supplements. They have been of interest but caused confusion to the patient (Cerrato 1992).

There is considerable interest in taking omega three fatty acids and many patients already subscribe to them as an adjunct therapy (Darlington & Ramsey 1993). They are persuaded of their efficacy because of the tremendous amount of anecdotal evidence published by the media. The research appears to support the anecdotal claims that the supplementation of omega three fatty acids results in a subjective improvement in symptoms in a percentage of patients (Cleland et al 1988, Darlington 1988). However, there is no statistical evidence to demonstrate correlation with biochemical indices despite obvious clinical improvement demonstrated by some patients (Brzeski et al 1991, Cleland et al 1988). Further research is being undertaken in the form of a multicentre study involving 300–400 patients with RA being treated at high doses (Darlington 1994).

Fish and evening primrose oils have been shown to provide a safe and efficacious adjunct therapy in the management of RA and many patients believe in their efficacy. Given that the aim of medicine is to provide both physical and psychological support, patient should not be discouraged to take these medications. Nevertheless, the patient will need to be kept fully informed about the research findings regarding these therapies, and any new information should be shared.

Evening primrose oil is prescribed for psoriasis as gamolenic acid, but it is not available on prescription for the person with RA. Evening primrose oil is expensive and the quality of the preparation varies; patients need to be informed of this.

Is there a correlation between trace elements and RA and does supplementation of these elements reduce disease activity?

Trace elements are essential to basic function in animals (Kumar & Clark 1994). These elements include:

- Iron
- Copper
- Iodine
- Fluorine
- Selenium
- Calcium
- Phosphorus.

Normal physiology and metabolism depend upon blood and tissue concentrations of trace elements and supplementation is frequently used in diseases where the body is unable to absorb the required amount (Kennedy et al 1975).

The possible link between trace elements and RA is of considerable interest and in particular the functions of selenium, zinc and copper suggest that they could be of therapeutic value. However, whilst much work has been carried out on the effects of trace elements in other disease processes there is little information regarding selective supplementation to modulate the immune response in rheumatic disease. Some evidence has been offered in the past to support correction of some immunological abnormalities in rheumatic disease.

Corman (1974) reviewed three trace elements:

- Selenium
- Zinc
- Copper.

Selenium

Selenium forms a component of the cellular defence mechanism, protecting membrane lipids, proteins and nucleic acids from the damaging oxidant effects of inflammation. In active RA, selenium serum levels are lowered but rise when disease activity is suppressed by drugs (Tarp et al 1985).

Although selenium is widely advertised as a cure-all for arthritis, very little work has been carried out on its use in RA.

Zinc

Diets deficient in zinc affect several aspects of the immune system:

- T-cell activity
- Circulating immunoglobulin concentrations
- Cytokine activity.

Zinc is also associated with collagen formation (Ferendez-Madrid et al 1971) and promising results have been obtained on its effects on collagen and the immune system. This raises the possibility that zinc has a role in a connective tissue disorder such as RA. However, little if any improvement has been found in this disease if zinc is supplemented (Simkin 1976, Honkanen & Lamberg 1991).

In common with selenium, serum levels of zinc are lowered in active RA, but to a lesser extent when disease activity is suppressed by drugs (Balogh et al 1980, Tarp et al 1985).

Copper

Copper is essential for the functioning of many enzymes, but it can be toxic in high concentrations or when dissociated from its carrier protein. In RA, serum levels of copper are elevated but no correlation has been found with disease activity, and levels depend on the patient's drug regime. Insufficient rigorous research relating to copper and RA has been undertaken and to allow recommendations to be made for clinical practice (Bajpayee 1975, Honkanen & Lamberg 1991, Scudder et al 1978).

The available research on the role of trace elements in rheumatic disease is scanty and any link remains unproven. Overall, there is no demonstrable improvement in RA when the level of these trace elements in the serum is manipulated (Tarp et al 1985).

RECOMMENDATIONS FOR CLINICAL PRACTICE

1. Fasting should not be routinely employed as an adjunct therapy in the management of RA.

2. Allergy to food substances should not be considered as a major causative agent in the aetiology of RA.

3. No specific foods should be routinely restricted from the patient's diet to reduce allergic response, as no specific agent can be identified as provoking an allergic reaction in a wide population of RA patients.

4. The subjective clinical improvement found with omega three fatty acids should be relayed to the patient with RA. They should also be informed of the lack of biochemical evidence. Patients should then be allowed to make their own decision.

5. Manipulation of the dietary intake of copper, selenium and zinc is not recommended for the management of RA.

6. Patients should be offered support, advice and guidance about their diet, taking into account their own beliefs. This will allow them to make informed, efficacious and safe decisions.

Action points for practice:

1. Write a case study on a rheumatology patient with a leg ulcer or pressure sore discussing potential and actual causes and any preventative measures that can be taken.

2. Reflect upon your risk assessment methods and tools. Do they truly take into consideration the multiple problems of rheumatology patients? If they do not, then change them!

3. Develop two education programmes specifically relating to skin integrity. One should be suitable for your students and colleagues, another for your patients and carers.

4. Produce an information package for your patients relating to the nutritional aspects of their care.

5. Undertake a literature search on the effects of diet on arthritis and critique the findings.

6. Choose a patient and complete a case study relating the influence of diet to their disease.

REFERENCES

Arthur V 1994 Nursing care of patients with rheumatoid arthritis. British Journal of Nursing 3(7): 325–331

Balgoh Z, Ahmed F, El-Ghobarey A F et al 1980 Plasma zinc and its relationship to clinical symptoms and drug treatment in rheumatoid arthritis. Annals of the Rheumatic Diseases 39: 329–332

Bajpayee D P 1975 Significance of copper and caeruloplasmin concentrations in rheumatoid arthritis. Annals of the Rheumatic Diseases 34: 162

Benbow M 1996 Pressure sore guidelines: patient/carer involvement and education. British Journal of Nursing 5(3): 182–187

Beri D, Malaviya A N, Shandily A, Singh R R 1988 Effects of dietary restrictions on disease activity in rheumatoid arthritis. Annals of the Rheumatic Diseases 47: 69–72

Bird H A, Le Gallez P, Hill J 1985 Combined care of the rheumatic patient. Springer Verlag, Berlin

Brzeski M, Madhok R, Capell H A 1991 Evening primrose oil in patients with rheumatoid arthritis and side effects of non-steroidal anti-inflammatory drugs. British Journal of Rheumatology 30: 370–372

Buchanan H M, Preston S J, Brookes P M, Watson-Buchanan W 1991 Is diet important in rheumatoid arthritis? British Journal of Rheumatology 30: 125–134

Cerrato P L 1992 Fish oils: food fad or therapeutic tool. Research Nurse 75–77

Cleland L G, French J K, Betts W H, Murphy G A, Elliott M J 1988 Clinical and biochemical effects of dietary fish oil supplements in rheumatoid arthritis. Journal of Rheumatology 15: 10

Cohen M G, Emmerson B T 1995 Gout. In: Klippel J H, Dieppe P A (eds) Practical Rheumatology. Mosby, London, ch 25, pp 255–262

Collier M 1994 Anatomy of the skin and the healing process. Educational leaflets No.1 and 2 (revised) Vol 2 (1). Wound Care Society, Huntingdon

Corman L C 1974 Effects of specific nutrients on the immune response. Journal of Infectious Diseases 129: 597–600

Cowan T 1996 Pressure relieving aids for community use. Professional Nurse 12(2): 131–138

Cowan T 1997 Pressure support systems for hospital use. Professional Nurse 12(7): 511–520

Crosby L J 1991 Factors which contribute to fatigue associated with rheumatoid arthritis. Journal of Advanced Nursing 16: 974–981

Cullum N, Roe B H 1995 Leg ulcers nursing management. A research based guide. Scutari, Harrow

Darlington L G 1985 Does food intolerance have any role in the aetiology and management of rheumatic disease? Annals of the Rheumatic Diseases 801–804

Darlington L G 1994 Dietary therapy for rheumatoid arthritis. Clinical and Experimental Rheumatology 12: 235–239

Darlington L G 1988 Do diets rich in polyunsaturated fatty acids affect disease activity in rheumatoid arthritis? Annals of the Rheumatic Diseases 47: 169–172

Darlington LG, Ramsey N W 1993 Review of dietary therapy for rheumatoid arthritis. British Journal of Rheumatology 32: 507–514

Darlington L G, Ramsey N W, Mansfield J R 1986 Placebo controlled blind study of dietary manipulation therapy in rheumatoid arthritis. The Lancet (1) 8475: 236–238

Dieppe H 1995 Clinical features and diagnostic problems in osteoarthritis. In: Klippel J H, Dieppe P A (eds) Practical rheumatology. Mosby, London, ch 12, pp 141–155

Douglas J 1980 Occupational therapy, rehabilitation and resettlement. In: Panayi G S (ed) Essential rheumatology for nurses and therapists. Baillière Tindall, London, ch 15, p 160–183

Dunne C, Robertson J 1992 Wound healing in rheumatoid arthritis. Wound Management 2(4): 13–14

Ertl P 1993 The multiple benefits of accurate assessment. Professional Nurse 9(2): 139–144

Ertl P 1992 Look beyond the ulcer itself. Professional Nurse 7(4): 258–262

Felder M, De Blecourt A C E, Wuthrick B 1987 Food allergy in patients with rheumatoid arthritis. Clinical Rheumatology 6(2): 181–184

Ferendez-Madrid F, Prasad A S, Oberleas D 1971 Allergy and rheumatoid arthritis. Journal of Laboratory Clinical Medicine 78: 853

Fletcher J 1997 Pressure relieving equipment: criteria and selection. British Journal of Nursing 6:6 (suppl) Focus on pressure sore management

Gordon D A, Hastings D E 1995 Clinical features of rheumatoid arthritis: early, progressive and late disease. In: Klippel J H, Dieppe P A (eds) Practical Rheumatology. Mosby, London, ch 15, pp 169–182

Hart F D 1984 Practical problems in rheumatology. Methuen, Australia

Hildegard C 1995 The impact of leg ulcers on patients' quality of life. Professional Nurse 10(9): 571–574

Hill J 1997 A practical guide to patient education and information giving. Ballière's Clinical Rheumatology 11(1): 109–127

Hill J 1995 Patient education in rheumatic diseases. Nursing Standard 9: 25–28.

Hill J 1990 Patient education: what to teach patients with rheumatic disease. Journal of the Royal Society of Health 110(6): 204–207

Hinchliff S M, Montague S E 1988 Physiology for nursing practice. Baillière Tindall, London

Hollingworth P 1988 Rheumatology. Heinemann, London

Honkanen L, Lamberg A 1991 Plasma zinc and copper in RA – influence of dietary factors on disease activity. American Journal of Clinical Nutrition 54: 1082–1086

House N 1996 Patient compliance with leg ulcer treatment. Professional Nurse 12(1): 33–36

Jenkins R T, Rooney P J, Jones D B, Blenenstock J, Goodache R L 1987 Increased intestinal permeability in patients with rheumatoid disease. British Journal of Rheumatology 26: 103–107

Kavanagh R, Norkman E, Nash P, Smith B, Hazleman J, Hunter J O 1995 The effects of elemental diet and subsequent foods reintroduction on rheumatoid arthritis. British Journal of Rheumatology 34: 270–273

Kennedy A S, Fell G S, Rooney P J, Stevens W H, Carson-Dick W, Watson-Buchanan W 1975 Zinc: its relationship to osteoporosis in rheumatoid arthritis. Scandinavian Journal of Rheumatology 4: 243–245

Kumar P, Clark M L, 1994 Clinical Medicine, Baillière Tindall, London

Kumar P J, Clark M L 1990 Clinical medicine, 2nd edn. Baillière Tindall, London

Landsberg C S, Young J B 1976 Fasting, feeding and regulation of sympathetic nervous system. New England Journal of Medicine 298: 1295

Lorig K 1996 Patient education: a practical approach, 2nd edn. Sage, Thousand Oaks

Luckmann J Sorenson K C 1980 Medical-surgical nursing, 2nd edn. W.B. Saunders, Philadelphia

McGhee M 1993 A Guide to laboratory investigations, 2nd edn. Radcliffe Medical Press, Oxford

Matteson E L, Cohen M D, Conn D L 1995 Clinical features of rheumatoid arthritis: systemic involvement. In: Klippel J H, Dieppe P A (ed) Practical Rheumatology. Mosby, London, ch 16, pp 183–190

Meade C J, Mertin J 1978 Fatty acids and immunity.

Advanced Lipid Research 16: 127–165

Morrison M J 1992 A colour guide to the nursing management of wounds. Wolfe Publishing, London

Palmblad J, Hafstrom I, Ringertz B 1991 Anti-rheumatic effects 17(2): 351–361

Panush R S 1990 Food induced 'allergic' arthritis: clinical and serological studies. Journal of Rheumatology 17: 3: 351–361

Pigg J S, Driscoll P W, Caniff R 1985. Rheumatology nursing: a problem oriented approach. John Wiley, New York

Ruane-Morris M, Thompson G, Lawton S 1995 Supporting patients with healed leg ulcers. Professional Nurse 10(12): 765–770

Ryan S 1995 Nutrition and the rheumatoid patient. British Journal of Nursing 4(3): 132–136

Scudder A, Al-Timini A L, McMurray W, White A G, Zoo B, Dormendy I 1978 Serum copper and related variables in rheumatoid arthritis. Annals of the Rheumatic Diseases 37: 67–70

Seeley R R, Stephens T D, Tate P L 1992 Anatomy and physiology, Mosby Year Book, USA, p 807

Shipley M, Newman S P 1993 Psychological aspects of rheumatic diseases. 7(2): 215–219

Shipperley T 1997 The importance of assessing patients with leg ulceration. British Journal of Nursing 6(2): 71–80

Simkin P A 1976 Oral zinc sulphate in rheumatoid arthritis. The Lancet 1: 539–542

Skoldsam L, Jorfelt L, Lindell B, Martensson J 1983 Specific plasma protein as indices of inflammation during a modified fast in patients with rheumatoid arthritis. Scandinavian Journal of Rheumatology 12: 161–165

Sperling R I 1991 Dietary omega three fatty acids: effects of lipid mediators of inflammation of rheumatoid arthritis. Rheumatic Diseases Clinics of North America 17: 2

Steen V D 1995 Systemic sclerosis. In: Klippel J H, Dieppe P A (ed) Practical Rheumatology. Mosby, London, ch 34, p 343–350

Sundvist T, Lindstrom F, Magnusson K E, Skoldstam L, Stjernstrom I, Tagesson C 1982 Influence of fasting on intestinal permeability and disease activity in patients with rheumatoid arthritis. Scandinavian Journal of Rheumatology 1: 33–35

Tarp U, Overad K, Jansen C, Thorling E B 1985 Low selenium levels in severe rheumatoid arthritis. Scandinavian Journal of Rheumatology 14: 97–101

Van De Laar M A F, Van Der Korst J K 1992 Food intolerance in rheumatoid arthritis. A double blind, controlled trial of the clinical effects of elimination of milk allergens and azo dyes. Annals of the Rheumatic Diseases 51: 298–302

Wilson J W, Waugh A 1996 Anatomy and physiology in health and illness, 8th edn. Churchill Livingstone, New York

Young T 1997 Pressure sores: incidence, risk assessment and prevention. In: Focus on pressure sore management (suppl). British Journal of Nursing 6: 6

FURTHER READING

Bender D A 1992 Nutritional biochemistry of the vitamins. Cambridge University Press, Cambridge

Community Nutrition Group of the British Dietetic Association 1986 Diet and arthritis. Nutrition Group Information Sheet. British Dietetic Association, London

Edmunds J, Hughes G 1985 Lecture notes on rheumatology. Blackwell Scientific Publications, London, p 45

Ewles L, Simnett I 1985 Promoting health a practical guide to health education. John Wiley, Chichester

Thomas B 1994 Manual of dietetic practice. Blackwell Scientific Publications, London

11

The team approach to mobility and self care

Joan Stamp

The aim of this chapter is to describe how the nurse and other members of the multidisciplinary team can help and encourage patients to care for themselves and retain or achieve optimum mobility. After reading this chapter you should be able to:

- **Describe the pivotal role of the nurse in the team approach to patient-centred care**
- **Outline the role of the other professionals' in the team and their contribution to the package of care**
- **Discuss the importance of assessment of the patient and their environment in relation to self-management and coping strategies**
- **Discuss self-management techniques for patients with rheumatic diseases including care of the feet and skin, joint protection, exercise and energy conservation**
- **Identify the contribution of the nurse in encouraging the patient to access resources such as Arthritis Care and other support agencies.**

THE CENTRAL ROLE OF THE NURSE

The Royal College of Nursing Rheumatology Nursing Forum Philosophy in the 'Standards of Care' (1989) states 'the patient should participate fully in their healthcare in order to achieve their own optimum level of good health'. It also suggests that the primary goal of care must be to teach the patient sound principles of healthcare and disease management, tailored to living with their illness. The rheumatology nurse plays a central role in helping the patient and their carers achieve these objectives. By virtue of being a constant presence, especially in the inpatient setting, the nurse is best placed to be the key player building up a rapport with the patients and carers. By working within the team the nurse is ideally placed to act as facilitator, communicator and patients' advocate and to ensure the highest possible standard of seamless care is delivered by enlisting the skills of the other professionals (Fig. 11.1). The very nature of nursing encompasses the needs of the patient. This begins when the diagnosis is made, and continues with the care and support of the patient through the disease, until end stage care is needed.

To fulfil their role in rheumatology nursing, a clear understanding of the disease, its progression and its consequences, is essential. This should be combined with a comprehensive knowledge of the elements of care which their fellow professionals can contribute to the management package required if the patient is to achieve 'their own optimum level of good health'.

The nurse will need good interpersonal skills in communication and negotiation. An educational approach is fundamental to meeting the needs of the patient, their carers and fellow professionals. To function effectively as facilitators and coordinators, nurses must first gain an understanding of the skills of all the other professionals in the team. This will allow maximum utilisation of each professional's skills to the benefit of the patient.

For the team to function effectively each member should be professionally robust enough to share expertise and information. Failure to do this will hinder the effective management of the patient by causing duplication of effort or disjointed interventions that are not in the patient's best interests. It is the seamlessness of the service from the team that is important in the package of care planned with the patient. This care should be re-evaluated constantly to enable it to respond to the changing needs of the patient in a timely fashion.

Newly diagnosed patients and their carers should receive information and education on all aspects of the disease and its management from each member of the team (see Ch. 15). Each professional will repeat certain elements of good management, especially topics such as:

• Joint protection
• Energy conservation
• Rest
• Exercise.

There is no harm in repeating this important information that will equip the patient and their carers to be in better control of their illness. This knowledge will help to remove some of the anxieties which arise when coming to terms with a chronic disease which is erratic in its progress and can only be controlled not cured (Hill 1997a).

During the patient's life a number of different professionals will be called upon to participate in their care. They will make any alterations to the patient's home and management and then withdraw until they are needed again. The medical and nursing staff will keep the patient under review and refer them back when their help is needed again.

THE ROLE OF THE MEDICAL STAFF

The general practitioner is usually the first member of the team to be involved with the patient. This often happens when the patient's symptoms do not subside with drugs that they can buy over the counter. The general practitioner may treat diseases such as osteoarthritis (OA) with analgesics, advice on weight control and by teaching the importance of exercise. They may also feel competent to treat patients with conditions such as tennis elbow and frozen shoulder with intra-articular injections and exercise. They may feel less well equipped to diagnose and implement treatment for patients whom they suspect have a more complex disease such as rheumatoid arthritis (RA), or in whom they are unable to reach a diagnosis from the symptoms the patient presents. In this case they are likely to suggest to the patient that a hospital specialist opinion should be sought and refer them to the local rheumatology department. It is important that such patients should not have to wait for months for a

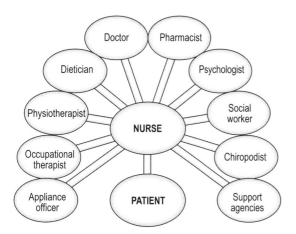

Figure 11.1 The role of the nurse within the multidisciplinary team.

hospital appointment. If they do have RA, ankylosing spondylitis, systemic lupus erythematosus or one of the other complicated rheumatic diseases, it is important that a diagnosis is reached and appropriate treatment started with the minimum of delay. This is because the window of opportunity for introducing disease-modifying drugs is within months rather than years. A deterioration of the patient's health, with the associated reduction in mobility, can lead to loss of employment or the ability to care for their home, family and perhaps themselves. Once a patient has lost their job, they may experience difficulty in getting another one even when they are physically able after their disease has been brought under control.

THE ROLE OF THE RHEUMATOLOGIST

When the patient first visits the hospital a medical history and full medical examination is undertaken. Particular emphasis will be placed on the locomotor system. Once completed, investigations may be undertaken to aid diagnosis. When all the information is to hand an explanation of the diagnosis will be given to the patient.

The next stage is to discuss appropriate treatment. This is often centred on drug therapy, and it is at this point that the nurse has an important role to play (Arthur 1995a). Once the initial information about the type of drug treatment offered has been given by the doctor, the nurse should then spend some time educating the patient and answering any further questions.

The nursing consultation should include:

- An explanation of the benefits of the drugs
- Possible side effects
- Drug interactions
- Methods of taking the drug
- Any other information the patient requests at that time.

If a second-line drug is being considered, the patient will need to know if regular blood tests and other safety monitoring, such as urine testing is required (Hill 1997b, Ryan 1997). This information will enable the patient to make an informed decision on whether or not to accept the advice and embark on the suggested therapy.

Written information on the drug and its effects and side effects are invaluable to the patient (see Ch. 15). This should be given in addition to a verbal explanation, not as an alternative to it. It can be confusing and unhelpful for the patient if they are merely handed a leaflet and told to go away and read it. They will almost certainly take notice of all the adverse effects and concentrate less on the virtues of the drug. However, leaflets and information sheets do have a place as re-enforcer and source of reference for the patient if they have problems with their drugs at any point in the future.

Although a few patients need minimal treatment in the early stages of their disease, others will need the investment of many resources to gain an improvement. They may need a combination of:

- Drug therapy
- Physiotherapy
- Occupational therapy
- Chiropody.

These modalities will need to be combined with education to gain maximum effect and mobility. This is sometimes achieved by increasing the dose of drugs or by adding an extra drug. It may be necessary to change the medication regime completely if it is not controlling or maintaining the disease effectively. If the patient has unacceptable side effects, or the drug is not effective, the rheumatologist will discontinue it.

If the patient's disease is generally under control but one particular joint is swollen and painful, an aspiration of the excess synovial fluid may be necessary to relieve their symptoms. The addition of an intra-articular corticosteroid to damp down the inflammation of the joint may also be carried out.

Yttrium synovectomy can be helpful if the patient has persistent synovitis in just one or two joints. In this procedure radioactive yttrium is injected into the joint space destroying the synovium which is producing excessive synovial fluid. The synovectomy reduces the painful swelling which lessens the stress upon the supporting joint structures that can lead to joint instability. A supra-scapular nerve block can sometimes give relief from a painful shoulder that has failed to respond to intra-articular injections.

The doctor is probably the team member with whom the nurse will need to liaise most frequently concerning the day to day management of patients. However, the patient should be able to rely on easy access to the nursing staff for problem solving and ongoing support.

THE SPECIALIST NURSE

Suitably trained and experienced nurses in all specialities are increasingly developing skills in areas that have previously been in the domain of the medical staff. Rheumatology is no exception to the extension or expansion of the nurses role (Hill 1997c). In many centres suitably experienced rheumatology nurses manage the second line drug safety monitoring. In other centres the junior doctor may carry out this task. The two most important points to keep in mind when deciding who does what in a rheumatology department are:

- What is in the patients best interests?
- What resources are available?

The nurse is there not to compete with the doctor, but to act as a professional in her own right, enabling her to compliment the skills of the rheumatologist (Hill et al 1994, Hill 1992). Authors have encouraged nurses to broaden their role in the rheumatic diseases as they can have a positive effect on the patient's outcome (Cohen 1994). For example, specialist nurses can help patients increase their self care skills and so enhance their ability to cope (Newbold 1996).

The UKCC has recognised the need for advice and guidance for nurses who are developing their role, and who carry out tasks that were not included in their normal training for registration. They have recently issued several documents that suggest that the onus is on each individual nurse to recognise their own level of competence. Nurses should decline any duties or responsibilities that they feel unable to perform in a safe and skilled manner (see further reading).

The Royal College of Nursing Rheumatology Nursing Forum has also identified the need for guidance and has recently issued a document outlining the nurses' responsibilities when they administer intra-articular injections (Appendix 3.1).

THE ROLE OF THE PHYSIOTHERAPIST

Physiotherapists are essential members of the multi-disciplinary team and one of their most important contributions is functional assessment. This applies whether patients are attending as outpatients or have been admitted to a ward for rehabilitation as part of the package of care. Clarke et al (1987), give an outline of the initial physiotherapy assessment of patients with RA and spinal disease. They suggest that both a subjective and objective approach to assessment is fundamental to designing a plan of treatment. The initial assessment takes place before embarking on a plan of treatment and is repeated throughout the course of the therapy. The final assessment will be made when the physiotherapist believes that the patient has achieved maximum benefit from their intervention. At this point a discharge report should be sent to the referring practitioner indicating any unresolved problems.

Initial assessment

At the initial assessment a patient history will be taken that includes information about the duration of their disease, its progress and the presenting problem. It is important to discover:

- The amount of pain the patient is experiencing
- The amount of disability present
- Whether the pain and disability has been as bad as this before
- What helped to resolve the problem in the past.

A patient may have attended for physiotherapy treatment in the past and found a particular form of therapy helpful. Conversely, they may have found that they reacted badly to some element of treatment and have no wish to be subjected to it again. In order to set realistic goals for treatments the patient's expectations about the intervention should be sought. This will enable the therapists to use their time and energies most effectively.

A thorough physical assessment need not be time consuming but it is important for the physiotherapist to have a clear picture of the presenting problems. A note is made of the extent of any swelling in or around the joints and any level of disability caused by the disease process. An accurate measurement of factors such as range of movement and muscle power should be made and noted. Only when the therapist has all this information can they then start to plan the course of treatment.

It is important that patients are made aware that physiotherapy is not merely 'something that is done to you to help make you better'. It is a form of self-care that requires their commitment and involvement. This is especially important if it is intended that the patient continues time-consuming therapy at home, such as an exercise regime, hot or cold packs, or wax hand baths.

Treatments

The therapist will decide which modality is an appropriate treatment for the presenting complaint and embark upon the chosen therapy only after discussion with the patient. The therapy may include:

- Hydrotherapy
- Ultrasound
- Traction
- Heat or cold
- Exercises
- Acupuncure
- Transcutaneous electrical nerve stimulation.

Hydrotherapy has a significant role to play in the mobilisation and rehabilitation of patients attending rheumatology departments. The non weight-bearing nature of the therapy encourages the patients to put irritable joints through a wider range of movement than may otherwise be possible. It also has the advantage of exercising many joints simultaneously. Once the patient's condition allows, active hydro-rehabilitation can be undertaken on all weight-bearing joints plus non weight-bearing joints such as the shoulders, elbows and hands. If it is indicated, further mobilisation can be carried out immediately after hydrotherapy whilst the joints remain warm and supple.

Ultrasound is used for reducing soft tissue swelling and pain. It can ease the joint symptoms prior to other therapies being used to mobilise the affected joint.

Traction is sometimes indicated for relief of pain in back and neck. This treatment may be continuous or intermittent.

Heat or cold in the form of wax baths and ice packs are commonly used in conjunction with other forms of treatment. The application of heat or cold reduces pain and stiffness which enables the patient to regain their function.

Acupuncture is sometimes used for pain relief (see Ch. 13).

Transcutaneous electrical nerve stimulation (TENS) machines are often used to control pain. They can be particularly helpful in the treatment of crush fractures in osteoporosis and on patients with OA at just one or two sites. Thought should be given to whether the patient can manage to site the electrode pads and manipulate the controls of the machine without help. If not, this form of therapy may be impractical.

Walking aids

Walking sticks assist balance and provide moderate support for the lower limbs. They provide pain relief by decreasing the amount of body weight transferred through the lower limb. The provision of walking aids such as walking sticks often falls within the remit of the physiotherapist. To ensure that the aid is at the correct height, it must be properly measured. This is usually done by placing the handle of the stick on the floor at the side of the patient, who is standing in an upright position wearing their walking shoes. The lower end of the stick should be at wrist level. When the stick is reversed and held in the hand, the elbow should be flexed at 30°.

The choice of stick is particularly important for those with multiple joint involvement. A conventional stick (Fig. 11.2A) may be suitable for a patient with OA of

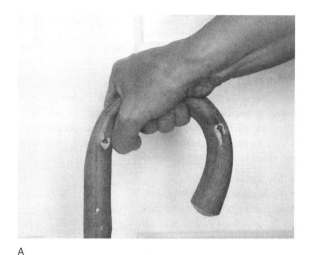

A

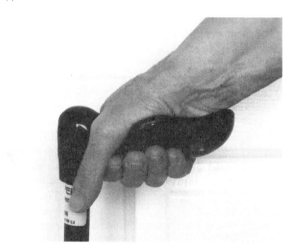

B

Figure 11.2 Walking sticks. (A) A conventional walking stick, (B) a Fisher stick.

the hip or knee, as they probably have little or no hand involvement. However, a patient with RA may develop a disfigured, painful hand, and a made to measure Fisher stick with a moulded handle (Fig. 11.2B) may be necessary. Instruction on the use of the stick is important. It is surprising how many patients attend the outpatients clinic using a stick belonging to a friend or relative which they are holding in the wrong hand. A walking stick should normally be used on the opposite side to the affected joint.

Whichever treatment is used, it is important that patients do not have to wait an inordinate length of time for their therapy, as their condition can deteriorate rapidly. Lack of treatment may lead to loss of mobility, increasing dependency and prolongation of the length of treatments needed.

Exercise

Exercise is likely to reduce the risk of disability and there is increasing evidence to support its efficacy (Gecht et al 1996, Minor 1996). It is likely that patients with systemic rheumatic disease will develop inflamed, painful joints, leading to:

• Muscle loss
• Reduction in muscle power
• Reduced range of movement.

To counter this, the early adoption of an exercise programme would appear to be logical but there is little research to show the optimum time for intervention. The use of simple pieces of apparatus such as soft balls and plasticine type material can be used to increase hand function. A pulley system can be an integral part of a shoulder exercise regime to encourage the patient to achieve maximum mobility.

The physiotherapist plays an important role in the education of the patient. Patients with ankylosing spondylitis, OA and RA can contribute significantly to their own mobility and management by including a home exercise plan in their daily routine. It is important that the patient understands that regular exercise is their contribution to an investment in their future.

Although beneficial, the patient may find exercise to be tiring, painful, boring and time consuming, which make adhering to such programmes difficult, but patients most likely to exercise are those who:

• Believe in the positive benefits of exercise
• Feel confident about their ability to exercise.

Patients need to be encouraged and motivated; simply knowing how to exercise will not necessarily lead to an increase in its practice. This means that it is essential to involve the patient in their care and so when planning their exercise regime, the physiotherapist and the patient will work together. In addition to the patient requiring a programme that can be incorporated into their lifestyle, some diseases require specific regimes.

Exercise and ankylosing spondylitis

Ankylosing spondylitis needs particular attention in the area of the spine as disease outcome can be influenced by diligent daily exercise. Many patients benefit from initial one to one instructions from the physiotherapist and then go on to join their local National Ankylosing Spondylitis group (NASS). These groups meet regularly under the supervision of a physiotherapist and the treatment usually consist of:

• Hydrotherapy
• Gym exercises
• Advice on posture.

The latter is particularly important as the maintenance of good posture whilst standing, sitting and lying down, can lead to less severe functional problems as fusion occurs.

Physiotherapy and scleroderma

The fibrosis of scleroderma causes contraction of the fingers (see Ch. 2, page 51), causing drastically impaired functional ability. The use of wax hand baths and intense physiotherapy may be necessary at an early stage of the disease to maintain hand function, or at a later stage to retrieve it.

Wax therapy

The patient plunges their hands into a bath of warmed wax that coats the skin. The hands are then wrapped in towels and the hands are rested for approximately 10–15 minutes. The cool wax is then peeled off, and whilst the hands are still warm, the patient is encouraged to perform straightening and strengthening exercises.

Serial splinting

Serial splinting is sometimes used to regain function caused by contracture of the skin and other structures. The occupational therapist makes a specialised splint to hold the fingers in the best position that can be achieved, and gradually straightens the fingers by adjusting the position of the splint. Meanwhile, the physiotherapist will encourage the patient to mobilise the hand with exercises.

Multidisciplinary working

The physiotherapist works closely with the occupational therapist to help overcome any functional difficulties that the patient encounters. It is thought that appropriate working or resting splints supplied at an early stage of the disease can maintain the patient's function and independence for longer. They also can help relieve pain and delay deformity.

THE ROLE OF THE OCCUPATIONAL THERAPIST

Whether they are working in hospital or in the community the occupational therapist has close links with other agencies such as:

- Social workers and the social service departments
- Disability centres
- Vocation advisors and retraining officers.

The training received by occupational therapists prepares them to recognise the physical and psychological consequences of disease, regardless of which area of the speciality they are working in. Their role is to help the patient to:

- Maintain independence
- Maximise their abilities
- Minimise limitations imposed by disabilities
- Advise on a safe environment
- Adapt the environment to the patient's needs

Regular reassessment is necessary to ensure that the needs of the patient continue to be met, and so some departments offer open access to patients once they have had an initial assessment by the occupational therapist.

Safe environment

It is important for the occupational therapist to assess both the patient and their environment. An occupational therapist assessment will include the patient's function and coping skills in areas of personal care, their home, workplace and leisure actives. They will also assess the patient's emotional needs.

Education

Ideally the occupational therapist should be involved in the education of the newly diagnosed patient, as patients or carers can inadvertently compound the problems presented by rheumatic disease. For instance, placing a pillow under painful knees to alleviate pain can rapidly lead to a flexion deformity. This can effectively immobilise the patient, and it is very difficult to regain a range of movement once it is lost.

The occupational therapist will also teach:

- Joint protection
- Provide aids and adaptations to assist in joint protection
- Relaxation techniques
- Energy conservation.

Joint protection

The claims that joint protection can prevent deformity have been moderated over the years. Many occupational therapists now believe that 'reducing the risk of deformity' is a more acceptable definition. In a paper by Hammond (1994) the objectives of joint protection are defined as:

1. Pain relief
2. Reduction of internal and external stresses on joints
3. The possibility of decreasing inflammation.

Many occupational therapists have established patient education programmes that focus on joint protection, and research into the effect of these programmes has been undertaken (Hammond 1994, Nordenskiöld 1994). In the former study joint protection was taught in two sessions, lasting a total of 3.25 hours. This programme brought about changes in attitude but not behaviour. The author concluded that the programme was probably too short and the content needed refining. In contrast the latter study, a 13 hour course extending over 3 weeks, resulted in greater use of assistive devices, which brought about a significant reduction in pain.

Splint making and fitting

The appropriate use of working splints may save the patient much pain and frustration and help to delay some of the deformities that interfere with function and daily activities. They can be ready-made splints with a metal insert that can be bent to the most supportive position (Fig. 11.3). They can also be made of canvas or neoprene rubber.

Night resting splints keep the hand in a good position whilst at rest and the patient should benefit by having less pain (Fig. 11.4). They may also help delay deformities of the hand and wrist. These splints are usually made to measure using a material that can be moulded into the required shape when heated. They are often held in place using Velcro. If resting splints are needed for both hands it may be impractical for the patient to wear them simultaneously, as they would be unable to adjust bedcovers or even turn over or get out of bed. The patient is best advised to use one splint each night and alternate the procedure. Splints can be made for many other joints, such as the lower limbs and the neck.

Reducing stress on the joints

Simple advice such as using a trolley in the supermarket instead of a basket, or alterations to housework

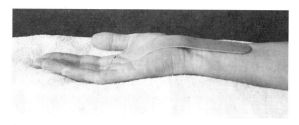

A

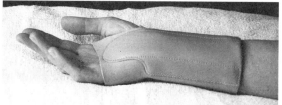

B

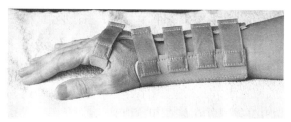

C

Figure 11.3 Working wrist splint. (A) Metal insert bent to the optimal position. (B) Underside of the splint. (C) Velcro fastenings.

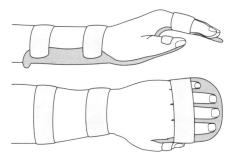

Figure 11.4 Night sleeping splint.

procedures may help the patient maintain their independence. As with other areas of disease management, the patients needs to be encouraged to assume a realistic amount of responsibility for their own care. This requires education and instruction on what they can do to avoid unnecessary joint stress. They need advice on what activities will cause undue stress to their joints, such as lifting heavy items. Any forced twisting

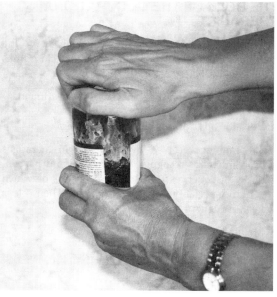

A

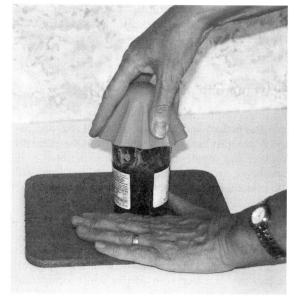

B

Figure 11.5 Correct method of opening a jar. (A) Wrong way causing joint stress. (B) Correct way minimising stress.

movements of the wrist such as turning stiff taps, wringing out cloths and undoing tight lids will hasten damage to vulnerable joints. These harmful movements can be avoided. For instance, jars should be placed on a non-slip pad and opened with the flat of the hand (Fig. 11.5).

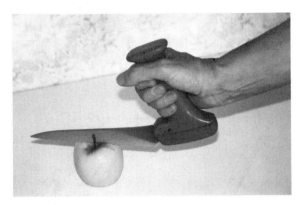

Figure 11.6   Adapted kitchen knife.

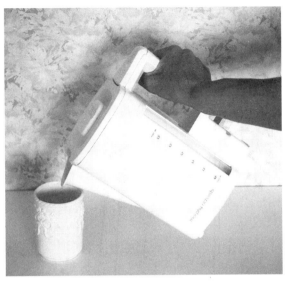

A

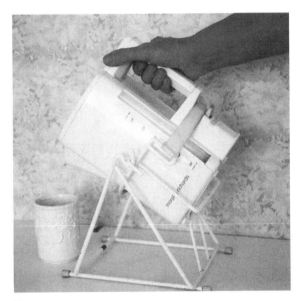

B

Figure 11.7   Kettle tipper. (A) Poor joint protection technique. (B) Reduced stress on the small joints and wrist.

Aid to daily living assessment (ADL)

An aid to daily living assessment may highlight the need for further adaptation to cutlery and crockery. The provision of kitchen utensils (Fig. 11.6) and tap turners may mean that the patient can continue to cook meals. Other adapted items include, electric tin openers, microwave ovens, kettle and teapot tippers (Fig. 11.7), and wire baskets for use in pans. These can help the patient remain independent for many years. If the patient has functional problems in the kitchen and in carrying out domestic chores, it is likely that they will also have problems with personal hygiene and may need a home assessment by the occupational therapist.

Home assessment visits

Seeing the patient in clinic or in the hospital environment is never quite as revealing as seeing them function in their own home. A home assessment visit may highlight needs in the living area such as seat raisers. The bathroom may need adaptation to the bath or shower, well placed grab rails and perhaps a raised toilet seat (Fig. 11.8). Toothpaste tubes and stiff taps all conspire to make a frustrating start to each day if the patient is unable to manage them because of early morning stiffness and painful hands and wrists.

It is understandable that the illness can cause depression and dismay to patients and carers. When providing adaptations, the occupational therapist should be sensitive to the feelings of the patient and to the family who share the home. Some patients may resist adaptations, seeing them as an ever-visible sign of the disability caused by the illness. Some carers will see adaptations as a signal that the patient is becoming increasingly dependent upon them.

THE ROLE OF THE CHIROPODIST OR PODIATRIST

Podiatrists are experts who understand the structure and dynamics of the foot and their skill goes far beyond cutting nails and treating calluses and corns. In order to avoid unnecessary stresses on the vulnerable joints of the foot, their advice should be sought at an

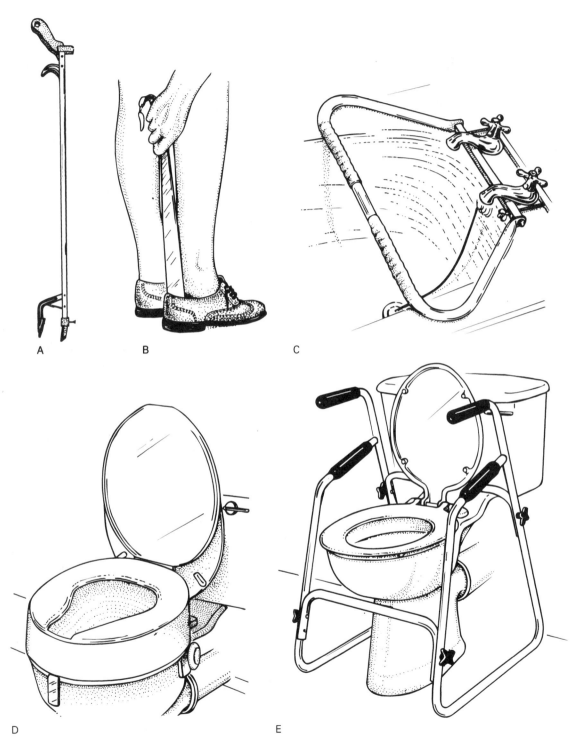

A   B   C

D   E

Figure 11.8 Aids to independence.

early stage in the patient's disease. Unless patients fully understand the service the podiatrist offers, they might decline an appointment and thereby be deprived of essential advice. For example, simply being taught about foot care and the choice of footwear may stop patients inadvertently contributing damage to their feet. Well fitting supportive footwear may accommodate the patient's foot problems for quite some time and may delay the need for insoles, surgical shoes and ultimately foot surgery.

When giving advice on skin care and care of nails, the patient's ability to reach their feet and grip the handles of scissors or nail clippers needs to be taken into account. Some patients will depend on others to perform their pedicure for them.

An annual review of the patient's podiatry needs, whether they are looking after their own feet or attending a podiatrist serves to identify the need for insoles or prostheses. Extra depth shoes are necessary to accommodate these inserts. Ready made, extra depth shoes are available commercially and if indicated are cheaper than made-to-measure surgical shoes. However, ill-fitting shoes cause damage to the skin and other tissues and so made-to-measure footwear will be needed if the patient's feet become very deformed.

Some podiatrists have undertaken post registration training in the surgical treatment of diseases affecting the foot. After a period of supervised training they are qualified to perform some surgical procedures. Gait analysis is a measurement of walking patterns that can be carried out by the physiotherapist or podiatrist. This analysis can be used to plan any alteration to footwear intended to correct deviation, which in turn would stress other weight-bearing joints.

In liaison with the physiotherapist and orthotist, the podiatrist can supply or recommend items such as:

• Callipers to support an unstable ankle
• A built-up shoe to correct uneven leg length
• A remedial sole to tilt the foot into a better alignment for weight-bearing.

All these measures can help to maintain the patient's mobility.

THE ROLE OF THE APPLIANCE FITTER/ORTHOTIST

A range of useful prostheses can be prescribed to help with specific disabilities caused by rheumatic diseases.

A knee brace may be the treatment of choice for a patient with an unstable knee who is unsuitable for corrective surgery (Fig. 11.9). Callipers can support an

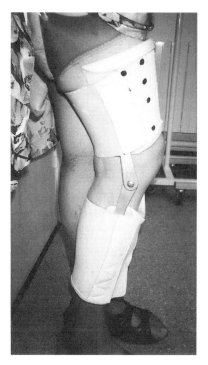

Figure 11.9   Knee brace.

unstable ankle joint and so help the patient to return to reasonable mobility. Insoles, extra depth or made-to-measure shoes can be manufactured to accommodate foot deformities that occur if arthritis progresses.

A corset is occasionally prescribed for patients with osteoporotic crush fracture of the spine, whilst pain control and bone bulking agents are being implemented.

THE ROLE OF THE PSYCHOLOGIST

A chronic disabling disease will undoubtedly have emotional as well as physical effects (Bird et al 1985). The erratic nature of rheumatic diseases and the pain and disability they can cause can place an intolerable burden upon the patient and their carers. Not all patients need the individual expertise of the clinical psychologist, some will choose to share anxieties, worries and problems with a professional within the team with whom they feel rapport. This may be all that is needed to resolve the problem. However, some patients will need the support of the psychologist in coming to terms with their illness and its consequences. The psychological aspects of the disease are discussed more fully in Chapter 5 of this book.

As well as helping patients, the psychologist may

also act as a resource to members of the staff who are helping patients and their carers through difficult times.

The psychologist is a valuable member of the health education team contributing to group education programmes and perhaps running sessions or study days for patients and their carers on general topics such as pain management, self image and coping strategies.

THE ROLE OF THE DIETICIAN

A healthy well-balanced diet contributes to overall good health but people with rheumatic diseases face particular problems (Ryan 1995).

Obesity

Inactivity, caused by illness, immobility and energy depletion, can lead to obesity in some patients with rheumatic disease. The excess weight poses an extra burden on the already damaged joints, leading to further immobility and pain. The dietician is able to help by planning a nutritious weight reducing diet for these patients, and reassessing their progress until their target is reached.

Emaciation

The systemic effects of RA can cause patients significant weight loss to the extent that they become emaciated and unwell. In these circumstances, the dietician's advice on weight gain should be sought. The addition of supplements to a nutritious diet may help to reverse unacceptable weight loss. The role of nutrition is discussed more fully in Chapter 10 of this book.

THE ROLE OF THE SOCIAL WORKER

Ideally the rheumatology ward should have a designated social worker on a sessional basis which enables them to build up a rapport with the patient and their family. Using the duty officer from a pool of social workers means that there is no continuity in the service and the patient may have a brief acquaintance with many different social workers and an affinity with none. This fragmentation causes difficulty for the social worker who has to start from the beginning of the patient's social case history each time they are involved. No matter how meticulous the record keeping, it is unlikely that all information concerning the patient can be written in a case report.

The social worker is a resource to both inpatients and outpatients, giving advice on any financial allowances or pensions that the patient may be entitled to. Working with the occupational therapist, a social worker experienced in the problems encountered by the patient with a rheumatic disease can ensure that the home environment is adapted to suit their changing needs. This will help to maintain the patient's mobility, self care abilities and consequently their independence.

It should be borne in mind that the lack of timely social worker input can delay the patient's discharge from hospital and cause unnecessary pressure on specialist beds. Discharge planning should start on admission to the ward, and so when undertaking an initial assessment, the nurse should identify problems which will need to be resolved before the patient can return home.

THE ROLE OF THE PHARMACIST

In the ward setting the pharmacist will explain any changes to drug therapy to the patient. Pharmacists supplement the information given by the doctors when they prescribe the drugs and nurses when they dispense the medication.

Most hospitals provide written information about medication that is usually prepared by the nursing staff, pharmacist, or a partnership of both. It is immaterial who writes the information leaflets as long as the information is accurate and understandable (Arthur 1995b). Ideally the writing of the leaflet should involve input from the patients, medical and nursing staff as well as the pharmacist.

Written information should always be discussed with the patient, allowing them time to ask questions and clarify any points that they are unsure about. Written information should not be seen as a substitute for verbal explanations, it is an adjunct that will help patients comply with the drug regime and manage their own medication effectively.

Self medication

The introduction of a self-medication programme onto a rheumatology ward is an excellent way to ensure that patients understand their drug therapy, and such schemes have been evaluated on rheumatology wards (Thornett et al 1994). To confiscate the patient's medication because they are in hospital is contrary to the philosophy that patients are taught skills to encourage them to contribute fully to their own disease management. If there is any doubt about compliance, a well run self-medication programme can highlight misunderstandings which may lead to poor compliance, and the patient can be taught to make best use of the drugs prescribed. The topic of drugs used in rheumatic disease is covered more fully in Chapter 12.

PRIMARY CARE TEAM

As with any chronic disease requiring life long treatment, patients with rheumatic disease will rely upon the primary care team. However, liaison with the hospital team is vital if seamless care is to be provided in the location that is best for the patient. Whilst the doctors, nurses, therapists and other members of the community team will not have the depth of specialist experience found in a hospital rheumatology department, they make an important contribution to patient centred care.

Monitoring the safety of drug therapy is often more convenient for the patient if it is carried out in their own general practitioner's surgery. Guidelines and protocols are written by the staff in the specialist centre in conjunction with the primary care team. When patients visit the general practitioner's surgery for monitoring, it is usually the practice nurse who reports any problems that indicate deterioration in the patient's condition. If her district nurse colleague goes to the patient's home to take a blood sample or change a dressing, she will be the one to signal that there is a problem.

Because care is being shared it is important that the primary care team know that they can rely on the support and co-operation of the hospital team when advice and practical help for the patient are needed. Chapter 16 of this book discusses the role of the primary care team in providing shared care with the specialist hospital team.

STAFF ON NON-RHEUMATOLOGICAL WARDS

People with rheumatic conditions are not exempt from other health problems and a proportion of patients will be admitted to orthopaedic, surgical and medical wards at some time. Unless it is absolutely necessary, it is important that such events do not result in alterations to the treatments that are keeping the arthritis under control. Once good control is lost it can be some time before it is regained. Staff on other wards may be unfamiliar with the drugs used to control arthritis and may discontinue therapies such as the second line drugs, not because it is necessary, but because they are unsure about using them. There may also be a problem

in making sure medicine rounds are flexible enough to allow drugs such as non-steroidal anti-inflammatory drugs to be taken with food. Good pain control should not be sacrificed to fit in with the next medicine round and analgesics should be available when they are needed.

The nurses on the specialist rheumatology ward should share information and expertise with their colleagues elsewhere and the expertise of a clinical nurse specialist is an invaluable resource to non-specialist staff (Ryan 1996). More and more specialist rheumatology nurses are visiting their patients who are in other wards and acting as a resource to their fellow professionals throughout hospital specialities. This is a great advantage to the rheumatology patient.

THE TELEPHONE HELPLINE

Many rheumatology departments are using the telephone as a means of communication between the specialist unit and patients, carers and professionals who are sharing the care of the patient. This allows problems to be resolved quickly and encourages minimum disruption to the patient's treatment.

This applies particularly when the patient presents at the surgery to see the general practitioner or practice nurse and a drug side effect is reported. Often the drug is stopped unnecessarily, but sometimes it is continued when it would be wiser to withhold the drug. If the doctor or nurse at the surgery knows that advice is just a phone call away they will confer with the staff in the rheumatology department before making a decision.

THE DISABILITY LIVING CENTRE

Hospitals or social services provide disability living centres, which are an excellent resource to patients and their carers. A visit to such a centre allows the patient to view an extensive range of aids, adaptations and appliances. Patients with functional problems can try items from adapted cutlery through to electric easy chairs and stair lifts. Patients often feel reassured that many of the mobility problems that they felt were insurmountable can be overcome with suitable adaptation.

The disability living centre also keeps a directory of addresses of useful agencies and suppliers.

LOCAL SUPPORT GROUPS

The nurse should familiarise herself with the role of the support agencies in the locality and how these groups function. This will enable them to give accurate information to patients about meetings locally. Arthritis Care, ankylosing spondylitis, lupus and psoriatic arthritis support groups often thrive locally and fill a social gap for patients out in the community.

CONCLUSION

One aim of this chapter is to demonstrate the importance of the team approach to the effective management of patients with rheumatic diseases. Having briefly described the role of the team members and the central role of the nurse in that team, this chapter has touched generally on many topics which have had an entire chapter specifically devoted to them. Perhaps it has given an indication of the breadth of experience needed by the rheumatology nurse if they are to use their communications skills to facilitate best possible package of care for their patient. By understanding and utilising the skills of the team in a timely fashion they can contribute significantly to helping the patient maintain their 'optimum good health'.

Action points for practice:

- Discuss ways in which you could improve communication with other health professionals within the multidisciplinary team.
- Describe how patient education can influence the patient's ability to manage their rheumatic disease effectively.
- Produce a drug information leaflet for patients starting on a second line agent.
- A 50-year-old man has severe OA in both knees. Discuss the mobility problems he is liable to face and describe the care he will require from the multidisciplinary team.
- Assess the problems facing the following newly diagnosed patients and identify the team members who would be involved in planning their care:
  - A 4-year-old girl with juvenile chronic arthritis.
  - An 18-year-old policemen with ankylosing spondylitis.
  - A 24-year-old woman with RA who is 6 months pregnant.

REFERENCES

Arthur V 1995a Drug therapies for patients with rheumatoid arthritis. British Journal of Nursing 4(11): 616–621
Arthur V 1995b Written patient information: a review of the literature. Journal of Advanced Nursing 21: 1081–1086
Bird H, LeGallez P, Hill J 1985 Combined care of the rheumatic patient. Springer Verlag, Berlin
Clarke A, Allard L, Braybrooks B, 1987 Rehabilitation in Rheumatology The team approach. Martin Dinitz, London
Cohen 1994 Joint efforts. Nursing Times 90(2): 18
Getcht R, Connell K J, Sinacore J M, Prohaska T R 1996 A survey of exercise beliefs and exercise habits among people with arthritis. Arthritis Care and Research 9: 82–88
Hammond A 1994 Joint protection behaviour in patients with rheumatoid arthritis following an education program. Arthritis Care and Research 7: 5–9
Hill J 1997a A practical guide to patient education and information giving. Baillière's Clinical Rheumatology 11(1): 109–127
Hill J 1997b Management of arthritis. Community Nurse 3(6): 20–22
Hill J 1997c The expanding role of the nurse in rheumatology. British Journal of Rheumatology 36(4): 410–412

Hill J 1992 A nurse practitioner rheumatology clinic. Nursing Standard 7(11): 35–37
Hill J, Bird H A, Harmer R, Wright V, Lawton C 1994 An evaluation of the effectiveness, safety and acceptability of a nurse practitioner in a rheumatology outpatient clinic. British Journal of Rheumatology 33: 283–288
Minor M A 1996 Arthritis and exercise: the times they are a changing. Arthritis Care and Research 9: 79–81
Newbold D 1996 Coping with rheumatoid arthritis. How can specialist nurses influence it and promote better outcomes? Journal of Clinical Nursing 5: 373–380
Nordenskiöld U 1994 Evaluation of assistive devices after a course in joint protection. International Journal of Technology Assessment in Health Care 10: 293–304
Ryan S 1997 Nurse led drug monitoring in the rheumatology clinic. Nursing Standard 11(24): 45–47
Ryan S 1996 Defining the role of the specialist nurse. Nursing Standard 10: 27–29
Ryan S 1995 Nutrition and the rheumatoid patient. British Journal of Nursing 4(3): 132–136
Thornett S, Heasman S, Bentley D 1994 Evaluation of self administration on a rheumatology ward. Journal of Clinical Nursing 3(2):pages

---

FURTHER READING

Carson D, Montgomery J, Montgomery E, 1993 Nursing and the Law 1993 Macmillan Publishing
United Kingdom Central Council for nursing, midwifery and health visiting:

Exercising Accountability (1989)
Scope of Professional Practice (1992)
Code of Professional Practice (1992)
Standards for Administration of Medicine (1992)

Therapeutic interventions

SECTION CONTENTS

The multifaceted nature of rheumatic disease requires a combination of therapies. In addition to conventional treatments such as drug therapy and surgery, this section includes complementary therapeutic interventions such as aromatherapy and acupuncture. Continuing the theme of empowering and working with the patient, the section is underpinned by a chapter on patient education and is completed by the inclusion of a chapter on seamless care.

12

Medication in rheumatic diesase

Jill Byrne

The aim of this chapter is to provide a clearer understanding of the drug therapies available to treat the rheumatic patient. The history, modes of mechanisms and indications for use will be discussed, and the provision of safe monitoring and education of the patient is also considered. After reading this chapter you should be able to:

- Describe the current concepts of drug management of rheumatic disease and the need for early intervention
- Discuss the actions and indications of first and second line therapies
- Outline the indications for steroid therapy and the potential adverse reactions
- Prepare or obtain drug information literature to provide the patient with an individual education package
- Appreciate the need for vigilant drug monitoring and the importance of providing the patient with the most convenient option for drug monitoring
- Describe how patient education can enable the patient to make informed decisions about therapeutic options.

Drug therapy plays an important role in the management of rheumatic diseases and yet nurses receive a minimal training in pharmacology. To provide a comprehensive service to their patients, nurses need an in depth understanding of the mechanisms and actions of drugs on rheumatic diseases and knowledge of the available therapeutic options. Although the pharmacist is sometimes involved, the nurse provides the majority of drug education to patients. If the teaching is to be effective, it is essential to include the:

- Potential benefits
- Potential adverse reactions
- How to cope with any side effects
- Routine monitoring.

Although information is produced for patients, there is a dearth of literature specifically produced for nurses regarding the pharmacokinetics and pharmacodynamics of rheumatology drugs. Information is needed at a more detailed level than patient literature but a little more simply than the medical and pharmacology texts offer. This chapter is intended to bridge this gap.

THE HISTORY OF DRUG THERAPY

Since the late 1960s the therapeutic options available for the management of inflammatory joint disease have been transformed. Greater understanding of the involvement of the immune system and the pathology of these diseases has led to a tremendous development in drug management.

Initially, the use of analgesia, non-steroidal drugs and physical modalities were the only treatments available. Scientific development has now provided new therapeutic agents with sophisticated drug delivery systems based on a clearer understanding of some of the aspects of the inflammatory process. The discovery of the inflammatory cascade with its prostaglandin and cyclooxygenase (COX) systems has provided the insight to develop 'designer' drugs which have the capability of producing their own individual immuno-suppressive effects. The specificity of these drugs is improving and products that combine preparations such as misoprostol should help to avoid adverse reactions such as gastrointestinal bleeding and peptic ulceration.

Analgesia and non-steroidal anti-inflammatory agents (NSAIDs) are referred to as first-line agents and are usually the first groups of drugs used to suppress symptoms. However, the use of first-line agents alone does not significantly influence the natural progression of erosive development that eventually leads to destructive joint changes in some diseases. Long-term outcomes do not appear to be influenced in a beneficial way if undue reliance is placed upon first line therapies alone.

The primary rationale of drug therapy is to restrict or prevent destructive change in musculoskeletal tissues and to combat the systemic ill health that is frequently associated with inflammatory joint disease,

particularly rheumatoid arthritis. Inflammatory triggers and immunological mechanisms play an important part in joint destruction and cartilage degradation in rheumatoid arthritis (RA). Therefore drugs that have an influence on the immune response have recently gained considerable attention. Such agents have been shown to modify the natural progression of these diseases and are referred to as disease modifying anti-rheumatic drugs (DMARDs), second line agents, or slow acting anti-rheumatic drugs (SAARDs).

There is now a clear recognition that early intervention, preferably in the predamaged state of these disorders, is likely to lead to improved treatment outcomes. As a result of these developments there is emerging a consensus and a hierarchy of treatment options. Until the late 1980s it was deemed best practice to offer therapy in a pyramidical format, starting with first line therapies such as analgesics and non-steroidal anti-inflammatory drugs. In addition, physical modalities such as physiotherapy, joint splinting and rest would be prescribed. If these actions proved ineffective as time progressed, second-line agents such as sulphasalazine or plaquenil would be considered. If these were not effective, progression to more potent and toxic agents, such as penicillamine or intramuscular gold would be made.

The disadvantage of this model of care is the gross joint destruction that occurs in the intervening period before an effective disease-modifying agent was introduced. Current practice is to suppress early inflammatory disease with more aggressive agents as the first port of call (Emery 1994). The disadvantage to this early aggressive therapy is that the patient is exposed to drug toxicity that is associated with the more potent immunosuppressants. The concept of risk versus benefits is still a contentious issue in the management of rheumatic diseases. As yet there are no therapies that are effective in all patients or any that are risk free. Development in genetic studies may improve the selection of treatment regimes suited to individual patients.

At present there is great diversity in prescribing practice. Different drugs are preferred by individual rheumatologists, monitoring protocols vary and overall management strategies differ dramatically. Hopefully, all agree with one fundamental philosophy, therapeutic interventions must be shown to be as effective as possible and offered at an early stage of the disease.

FIRST-LINE THERAPY

Analgesia

'Arthritis may not kill you but it sure as hell makes you wish you were dead!'

This profound quote from an anonymous patient cited in Smith Pigg et al (1985) portrays the despondency and despair that a chronic long-term illness can have. Health professionals may have the ability to sympathise with patients but few have ever experienced such pain that they can offer true empathy. Can we truly understand how it feels to crawl into bed at night in pain and wake up the next morning still in pain and with such a degree of stiffness that walking to the bathroom is agony? If pain remains severe and uncontrolled the day ahead becomes a potential nightmare. It is impossible to even think ahead, let alone function independently.

Severe, unrelenting pain can result in profound psychological deterioration that can alter the patient's perception of self, loved ones and what life may hold for them. If this were to continue unchecked, the patient's future would indeed be grim. It is important that the issue of pain is addressed at an early stage in the disease process and the nurse must gain the patient's trust, reassuring them that everything possible will be done to help them to control their pain.

The patient with inflammatory arthritis is further disadvantaged because of the very nature of the pain. Pain associated with tissue damage results in its amplification. It is thought that this results from inflammatory mediators such as histamine, prostaglandins and serotonin producing peripheral sensitisation (see Ch. 8).

General management of pain with analgesia

Nearly every rheumatic patient relies on a form of analgesia at some point in time, and therefore they are the commonest group of drugs used in the treatment of rheumatic diseases. Nurses are involved in advising the patient about their analgesics and so a sound understanding is required of the:

- Types of analgesics available
- Which are best to take in different situations
- Potential adverse reactions.

In the rheumatic diseases, analgesics are seldom used in isolation. When a combination of drugs is used consideration needs be given as to whether the interaction may enhance or diminish the effects of either drug. For instance, non-steroidal anti-inflammatory drugs potentiate the effects of warfarin leading to an increased risk of bleeding. Drug interactions need to be understood, particularly in those most susceptible such as the elderly and those with impaired renal or liver function.

Analgesics can be divided into two groups:

1. Non-opioid analgesics
2. Opioid analgesics

Non-opioid analgesics

Drugs such as paracetamol and low dose aspirin are non-opioid analgesics. Higher doses of aspirin (3.6 g daily) have an anti-inflammatory effect and would be classed as a non-steroidal drug. Single dose non-steroidal anti-inflammatory drugs are used as analgesia and therefore also fall within this category. All these drugs are suitable for treating mild to moderate pain.

Paracetamol. Paracetamol is thought by many patients to be too simple an analgesic to relieve their pain. This may be because it can be purchased over the counter and is considered by patients to be a safe and possibly less effective home remedy. In fact, paracetamol can be very effective. When pain has not responded to what patients consider to be 'stronger' analgesia and they switch back to paracetamol, they have found it to be remarkably effective. Paracetamol is indicated for mild to moderate pain and also has an anti-pyrexial property due to its action on the hypothalamus. This property can be very beneficial when patients experience a raised body temperature in acute flares of RA and gout. Paracetamol is also very effective in the short-term management of osteoarthritis (OA) demonstrating similar levels of pain relief to ibuprofen (Bradley 1991). The advantage of giving paracetamol rather than a non-steroidal anti-inflammatory drug is that it does not appear to cause gastric side effects.

Adverse reactions

Side effects are usually mild but occasionally haematological reactions occur. They include:

- Thrombocytopenia
- Pancytopenia
- Neutropenia
- Agranulocytosis.

Pancreatitis and skin reactions also occur occasionally. A few patients have shown to be hypersensitive to paracetamol and this is characterised by urticaria, dyspnoea and hypotension (Stricker 1985). Patients with impaired renal and hepatic function should only be prescribed paracetamol with caution as it can cause further deterioration to these systems.

There is also a danger that as paracetamol is considered a very simple analgesic, patients may exceed the recommended dose of 4 g per day for adults. Over-dosing with paracetamol can cause devastating liver damage within 24 hours of ingestion. If it is not treated within 12 hours with antidotes such as acetylcysteine and methionine that can limit the damage, severe poisoning can result in coma and death.

Compound analgesics

If effective pain relief cannot be achieved with non-opioid preparations it will probably be necessary to progress to stronger analgesia. Compound analgesia combines drugs such as aspirin or paracetamol with a low or full dose of an opioid agent, which is often codeine phosphate.

- Low dose = 8 mg per compound tablet with 500 mg paracetamol (8/500) e.g. co-codamol 8/500
- High dose = 30 mg per compound tablet with 500 mg paracetamol (30/500) e.g. co-codamol 30/500, Kapake, Tylex, Solpadol

Other compound analgesia combine paracetamol with other opioid compounds:

- Co-proxamol = dextropropoxyphene hydrochloride 32.5 mg/paracetamol 325 mg
- Fortagesic = pentazocine 15 mg/paracetamol 500 mg
- Lobac = chlormezanone 100 mg/paracetamol 450 mg.

The introduction of opioid compounds must be approached with careful consideration, as the side effect profile is considerably greater with this group of drugs. Codeine is often the choice of opioid for compound analgesia because its adverse reactions seem to be best tolerated. Adverse reactions include:

- Nausea
- Vomiting
- Drowsiness
- Dizziness
- Severe constipation
- Potential dependency if the dose is high and given long term.

Although compound analgesics contain relatively low doses of opioid, it should be noted that a percentage of patients are particularly sensitive to any dose of opioid. Dizziness, nausea, vomiting and constipation are the most common complaints. The latter is potentiated by the lack of exercise and mobility in the patients with arthritis. If constipation occurs, it is advisable for patients to take a laxative such as lactulose. Alcohol potentiates central nervous symptoms and therefore should be avoided when taking such drugs.

Opioids

If combined analgesia does not prove successful the use of stronger opioids should be considered. However, adverse reactions are far more common and are of a more serious nature. It has been suggested that side effects and dependency occur in the majority of patients (Justins 1996).

The use of opioids for the management of rheumatic disease is a controversial area and causes much concern for many practitioners. When consideration is given to the long-term nature of a disease such as RA, it is clear that analgesia may be needed for many years. The tendency towards dependency on these drugs points towards their avoidance as a long-term solution to chronic non-malignant pain.

However, opioids can be used effectively and safely for short periods in very acute episodes of pain. These include drugs such as:

- Buprenorphine
- Dihydrocodeine
- Tramadol.

Buprenorphine (Temgesic) and dihydrocodeine are used fairly commonly for moderate to severe pain but still demonstrate significant side effects; nausea, vomiting and dizziness. Tramadol has been reported to have less typical opioid effects and seems to be well tolerated.

Morphine remains the most valuable opioid and it is the standard that other opioids are measured against. However, its use should only be considered in the terminally ill patient when the objective is to provide a pain free period until death.

Non-steroidal anti-inflammatory drugs

Non-steroidal anti-inflammatory drugs are widely used in the management of rheumatic diseases. They are usually taken on a regular basis in combination with analgesics, and where indicated, with second line agents. There are over 20 non-steroidal preparations available. They are not described individually in this section, as this would be too time consuming, but they are all documented in the British National Formulary.

History of non-steroidal anti-inflammatory drugs

Anti-inflammatory treatment has been used since the sixth century in the form of willow and poplar bark. Similarly, extracts of autumn primrose, containing colchicine were also used for gout but the chemical formulation of colchicine was not identified until 1820.

Colchicine is still recommended for the management of acute phases of gout. In 1900 salicylic acid and aspirin were identified (Rodnan & Benedek 1970) but the term non-steroidal was not used until it was applied to phenylbutazone in 1949. The anti-inflammatory properties of indomethacin were first identified in rats in 1965 and many non-steroidal anti-inflammatory drugs have since been shown to be efficacious by this method.

Since the late 1960s research has resulted in a vast array of non-steroidal anti-inflammatory drugs and they can now be administered by several different routes:

- Oral
- Intramuscular
- Rectal
- Transdermal.

The effects of non-steroidal anti-inflammatory drugs

Anti-inflammatory drugs have the potential to reduce the signs and symptoms of inflammation by their anti-inflammatory, analgesic and anti-pyrexial properties. In single doses, non-steroidal anti-inflammatory drugs have an analgesic effect similar to paracetamol, but in regular full strength doses they have both a longer lasting analgesic and anti-inflammatory effect. In some instances, pain, heat, stiffness and swelling of the joints and most connective tissue, begin to reduce within hours of absorption. The full benefits can be noticed within several days (British National Formulary 1994). This improvement in symptoms and the subsequent easing of movement allows patients to improve their functional capacity. Consequently, many patients wonder why there is a need to introduce disease-modifying drugs to control their disease.

Unfortunately there is no evidence that non-steroidal anti-inflammatory drugs effect the course of the disease. They offer no protection to tissue from inflammatory injury, and so damage to the joints continues despite the obvious reduction in clinical symptoms. It has even been suggested that they may actually accelerate the rate of cartilage destruction in patients with OA (Rashed 1989). In addition symptom relief is lost very rapidly following cessation of non-steroidal anti-inflammatory drugs. Sound patient education is essential, as this will help patients to appreciate the need for symptom relief and the additional immunosuppressive effects of the disease modifying drugs.

Pharmaceutical companies claim considerable differences in the mode of action of individual non-steroidal anti-inflammatory drugs but in practice, approximately 60% of patients will respond to any anti-inflammatory. Of the remaining 40%, some find certain preparations more beneficial than others, and so it is often necessary to try several different drugs before a suitable anti-inflammatory is identified. From a medical viewpoint the most important differences between non-steroidal anti-inflammatory drugs is the incidence of side effects. In these circumstances the prescriber must balance efficacy against potential side effects.

The use of non-steroidal anti-inflammatory drugs

Non-steroidal anti-inflammatory drugs are widely used in the management of many rheumatological conditions. They may be employed in the following ways:

- As additional therapy for patients taking disease modifying drugs and who still experience inflammatory symptoms.
- As a single medication in mild RA, OA or gout.
- Patients whose disease is well controlled may take them during a flare, or occasionally on an ad hoc basis.
- In combination with analgesics. Many patients are unaware of the potential benefit of combining these two groups of drugs and so suffer unnecessarily.

When commencing an non-steroidal anti-inflammatory drug, the dose should be gradually increased to the necessary maximum over 1 to 2 weeks and if response is inadequate after a 4-week period an alternative non-steroidal anti-inflammatory drug should be tried. The ever increasing number of non-steroidal anti-inflammatory drugs with their various release mechanisms should allow the practitioner to select the best drug for the patient. Many patients take preparations that must be taken twice or three times daily and find them effective. Other preparations can be taken in a single daily dose and this is ideal for the patient whose daily routine makes more frequent tablet taking an inconvenience. For those patients with pain that disturbs them through the night, it maybe beneficial to use a slow release preparation so that the serum level of the drug is maintained over a longer period.

The most familiar non-steroidal anti-inflammatory drug is aspirin. Aspirin is associated with a number of side effects even when taken at doses below 3.0 g daily. They include:

- Nausea
- Dyspepsia
- Gastrointestinal bleeding.

Unfortunately, at the anti-inflammatory dose of 3.6 g daily, the side effect profile is much higher and includes the additional problem of salicylate intoxication. This is characterised by:

• Dizziness
• Tinnitus
• Deafness.

As these side effects are dose-related, it is difficult to use aspirin effectively. It is therefore used infrequently in the management of the patient with arthritis who needs a safer option for long term use. The non-steroidal anti-inflammatory drugs include ibuprofen, acemetacin, azapropazone, diclofenac sodium, etodolac, indomethacin, ketoprofen and mefenamic acid to name but a few. Amongst the 20 available there are numerous preparations leading to a vast amount of choice or confusion for the prescriber!

Mode of action

The principle of non-steroidal anti-inflammatory drugs is to inhibit the production of a group of fatty acids called prostaglandins, which play a large role in the inflammatory response, resulting in pain, joint stiffness and swelling. The synthesis of prostaglandins is complex. They are derived from arachidonic acid and rely on its presence for their formation. Arachidonic acid is found in the cell membrane of all cells and is released into the cell cytoplasm by the action of phospholipase A2. It can then be converted into prostaglandins by the action of two enzymes:

• Cyclooxygenase
• Lipoxygenase.

Non-steroidal anti-inflammatory drugs prevent the action of cyclooxygenase and hence reduce the production of prostaglandins. For those patients experiencing pain, stiffness and swelling, the reduction in prostaglandins would seem to be an ideal treatment. However in reality it is not quite as straightforward as it would first appear. Not all prostaglandins are detrimental to the body's tissues. They have many functions, some of which are very beneficial including:

• Prevention of platelet aggregation
• Stimulation of smooth muscle action
• Regulation of renal blood flow
• Inhibition of gastric acid production.

The latter is particularly important. The inhibition of gastric acid protects the lining of the gastrointestinal tract and so prostaglandins are referred to as being 'cytoprotective' (Whittle 1977).

It is therefore clear to see that if all prostaglandins are inhibited, symptoms normally controlled by the beneficial prostaglandins may present and it would be ideal if non-steroidal anti-inflammatory drugs could be selective in the type of prostaglandins they suppress. Much research has been performed and the pharmaceutical industry has spent large sums of money attempting to refine and produce a selective non-steroidal anti-inflammatory drug. A drug called meloxicam is being used more often which claims to selectively inhibit the inflammatory prostaglandins leaving the beneficial ones relatively undisturbed. The mode of action of this drug lies in the fact that there are two recognised forms of cyclooxygenase referred to as COX 1 and COX 2.

Broadly speaking:

COX 1 is responsible for the production of those prostaglandins that are protective of the tissue i.e. protect gastric mucosa.

COX 2 are involved in the production of specific prostaglandins that are actively involved in the inflammatory process.

It is the inhibition in the action of COX 1 and the subsequent reduction in beneficial prostaglandins that are specifically responsible for gastric symptoms.Some drug companies claim that their non-steroidal anti-inflammatory drugs have a balanced inhibition of the two types of prostaglandins, whereas meloxicam is said to inhibit COX 2 slightly more than COX 1 and is therefore referred to as a 'selective COX 2 inhibitor'. This process is demonstrated diagrammatically (Fig. 12.1). A drug with this profile, should it fulfil its expectations, could revolutionise the use of non-steroidal anti-inflammatory drugs in the treatment of rheumatic disease.

Adverse effects of non-steroidal anti-inflammatory drugs

Side effects to non-steroidal anti-inflammatory drugs are common and for ease of reference these reactions may best be categorised into the following groups:

• Gastrointestinal
• Hepatic
• Renal
• Hypersensitivity
• Haematological
• Central nervous system.

Gastrointestinal. This is by far the commonest type of side effect to non-steroidal anti-inflammatory drug therapy. Taking non-steroidal drugs with or directly following food helps to overcome this side effect.

Prostaglandins have been shown to suppress gastric acid secretion, which offers a degree of protection to

Roles of COX 1 and COX 2 isoenzymes

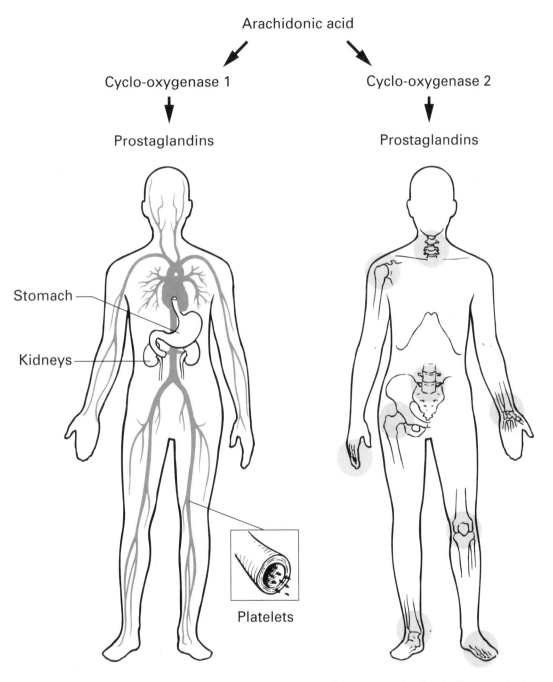

Tissue distribution sensitive to
NSAID mediated COX 1 inhibition

Rheumatological disease-induced
distribution of COX 2

Figure 12.1   Roles of COX 1 and COX 2 isoenzymes (adapted with kind permission from Boehringer Ingelheim).

the gastric mucosal barrier. When non-steroidal anti-inflammatory drugs are taken this protective effect is reduced and in some patients it makes little difference clinically and no gastric symptoms are observed. However some patients notice dramatic effects, demonstrating varying degrees of gastritis ranging from mild inflammation to life threatening erosive ulceration. These patients may never be able to tolerate any non-steroidal anti-inflammatory drug therapy.

It should be noted that the incidence of more severe damage is noted in the elderly. Approximately one peptic ulcer complication occurs for every 10 000 non-steroidal anti-inflammatory drug prescriptions in patients of 60 years and over in the United Kingdom (Langman et al 1994).

The symptoms commonly experienced with gastrointestinal reactions are:

- Heartburn
- Indigestion
- Nausea
- Vomiting
- Bloated sensation
- Anorexia.

Bowel disturbance with the inflammation resulting in diarrhoea can also occur. The presence of blood in the stools or blood stained vomit are symptoms of underlying problems. Less commonly stomatitis, perforation of the colonic diverticular and pancreatitis has been reported (O'Brien & Bagby 1985). Because of the high risk of non-steroidal anti-inflammatory drug induced gastrointestinal problems, patients should be considered at risk if they have a history of:

- Oesophagitis
- Hiatus hernia
- Gastritis or gastric ulceration
- Duodenitis or duodenal ulceration.

Any patient with a history of peptic ulceration should only be given non-steroidal anti-inflammatory drugs after all other therapeutic options have been considered. However when acute joint inflammation is present one must assess the benefits against the potential disadvantages.

Research has shown that certain non-steroidal anti-inflammatory drugs are more likely to induce gastric problems. Azapropazone and ketoprofen appear to carry higher risks than ibuprofen, which has been found to show a lower incidence ratio of gastric bleeding (Langman et al 1994). However, in clinical practice, many patients can remain on a non-steroidal anti-inflammatory drug deemed likely to induce side effects without experiencing problems. When they change to a safer option, they can develop side effects from these safer drugs. Whether this is due to individual chemistry or the fact that the patient has become tolerant of the drug over several years is uncertain and open to dispute. Gastrointestinal side effects from non-steroidal anti-inflammatory drugs are unpredictable and potentially life threatening in a few patients, but armed with research based evidence safer decisions can be made for those patients at greater risk.

Hepatic effects. There is little research evidence available relating to the effect of non-steroidal anti-inflammatory drugs on the liver, but hepatic side effects are uncommon. In clinical practice, even when liver function tests are elevated the patient tends to remain asymptomatic and once the drug is withdrawn or the dose reduced the elevations usually subside.

Renal effects. Non-steroidal anti-inflammatory drugs decrease renal blood flow. This can result in fluid retention which may subsequently cause hypertension (Harris 1992). This is more prevalent in patients who are already taking antihypertensive therapies than those who are not (Johnson 1994). The elderly population may need closer blood pressure screening as the chances of their needing blood pressure control using antihypertensive drugs is increased if they are taking non-steroidal anti-inflammatory drugs. Elderly patients are also prone to renal failure because of the reduction in blood flow (O'Callaghan 1994).

If the patient is taking diuretics or has a concurrent illness such as cirrhosis or congestive heart failure, there is an increased risk of renal toxicity. Acute nephritis can also result from hypersensitivity to non-steroidal anti-inflammatory drugs and if this does occur, the patient may present with fever, arthralgia, skin rashes and acute renal failure. Less commonly, non-steroidal anti-inflammatory drugs may induce renal capillary necrosis, nephritis and nephrotic syndrome (Griffiths & Emery 1996).

Hypersensitivity. One of the beneficial actions of prostaglandins is that of dilatation of the airways. If non-steroidal anti-inflammatory drugs artificially influence the prostaglandin balance, bronchoconstriction can occur and an acute asthma attack can prevail. This only tends to affect the patient who has a tendency to asthma. It has been surmised that when COX 1 and 2 are inhibited, arachidonic acid is more actively involved in producing lipoxygenase products such as leukotriens that can precipitate bronchospasm (Szczeklik 1993). It appears that if patients have demonstrated this reaction to one non-steroidal anti-inflammatory drug then they are likely to be sensitive to all, and therefore all non-steroidal anti-inflammatory drugs should be avoided in this type of patient.

Haematological. The principal action of non-steroidal anti-inflammatory drugs is to inhibit cyclooxygenase and hence limit prostaglandin formation. Because of the widespread inhibition of these enzymes, platelet cyclooxygenase is also impaired which reduces the effectiveness of platelet aggregation. This reduced effect should be considered with patients who may be at risk of bleeding from the stomach or those who are scheduled for surgery. It is not the norm but some doctors insist that patients take no non-steroidal anti-inflammatory drugs for several days prior to surgery to allow full excretion from the body. Other rare haematological adverse effects of non-steroidal anti-inflammatory drugs include:

- Anaemia
- Thrombocytopenia
- Neutropenia
- Eosinophilia
- Agranulocytosis.

Central nervous system. Headaches, dizziness, anxiety, drowsiness, tinnitus and deafness are all symptoms that have been attributed to non-steroidal anti-inflammatory drug therapy (Hoppman 1991). Rare effects include memory loss, forgetfulness, confusion and paranoid tendencies.

There is no doubt that non-steroidal anti-inflammatory drugs can be extremely effective drugs but that they are clearly not without potential adverse effects. Elderly patients are more at risk of developing reactions especially those who have other illnesses and are taking several medications. The most frequently documented side effects are those associated with gastric damage. There is evidence to show that those patients who have a proven history of gastric irritation or ulceration are most at risk of developing further problems and should be screened with great caution. Non-steroidal anti-inflammatory drug associated ulcers are more common in females. Those who smoke are especially at risk. This is of particular relevance when one considers that RA predominantly affects women and that many patients smoke. Because of the potential for gastric problems, many general practitioners and hospital doctors decide to treat their patients with an anti-ulcer drug therapy as soon as they commence non-steroidal anti-inflammatory drugs. This concept of prophylactic treatment is extremely expensive and the debate of cost versus safety continues.

Drug interactions

Non-steroidal anti-inflammatory drugs can interact with numerous other drugs. A detailed list can be found in the relevant section of the British National Formulary.

Corticosteroids

Corticosteroids have been used in the management of inflammatory diseases since the 1920s when they were heralded as the ultimate answer to controlling the inflammatory process. Unfortunately their success was thwarted because of the side effect profile that long term, high dose steroids can cause. There is some controversy about their use. Some rheumatologists are very averse to using any steroids whilst others use them as a method of inducing remission.

How do steroids work?

Steroids are produced by the adrenal cortex and can be grouped into three categories:

- Glucocorticoids
- Mineral corticoids
- Sex hormones – mainly androgen.

The glucocorticoid group include cortisone, hydrocortisone or cortisol and they have an action on glucose formation and glycogen storage in the body (Martindale 1996). They also exert an influence over protein, calcium and lipid metabolism. In inflammatory disease, glucocorticoids are particularly important because of their anti-inflammatory properties. They are known to have an effect on tissue repair, the heart, kidneys and central nervous system.

Mineral corticoids have more specific effects and act predominantly upon electrolyte and water metabolism.

Many synthetic analogues (chemical copies) have now been produced that can mimic the action of naturally produced steroids. The principle of supplementing the body's normal steroid compliment is to increase the beneficial effects, for example the anti-inflammatory action, without increasing the adverse effects like fluid and electrolyte retention.

Routes of administration

In the rheumatic diseases synthetic steroids are administered via the following routes:

- Oral
- Intramuscular
- Intravenous
- Intra-articular.

Oral corticosteroids

Oral administration has become less popular because of the side effects of long term systemic steroids (Table 12.1). They tend to be reserved as a last resort for those patients in whom disease modifying agents have proven to be ineffective.

Their use is seen more often in the elderly population when the benefits outweigh the adverse reactions and quality of life can be balanced against longevity. There are also a number of aggressive connective tissue diseases such as polymyalgia rheumatica and temporal arteritis in which corticosteroids are recognised as being the safest and most effective first-line therapy.

Corticosteroids are not thought to suppress the underlying disease in RA, and are therefore usually given in combination with a disease modifying drug. For instance, an azathioprine / corticosteroid combination appears to be particularly effective.

Dosage. Adverse reactions are more prevalent at doses above 7.5 mg daily and so for long term use, 7.5 mg per day or below is used. The best dose is the lowest dose at which symptoms are controlled. For instance if a patient is not controlled on prednisolone 5 mg per day, increasing the dose to 7.5 mg on alternate days may suffice. In cases of acute flare, a rheumatologist may sometimes prescribe a short course of higher dose therapy. Enteric coated products produce far less gastrointestinal symptoms.

Table 12.1 Adverse reactions associated with synthetic corticosteroid therapy

Reduction in inflammatory symptoms	The immunosuppressive effects of steroids down-regulate the inflammatory process. Also masks other signs of inflammation and infection until it has progressed to an advanced stage. • Renders the patient susceptible to infection including TB, fungal and viral infections.
Oedema and hypertension	Electrolyte balance is influenced by corticosteroids: • Results in water and sodium retention. • Excess secretion of potassium leads to cardiac failure in susceptible patients.
Nausea, vomiting, indigestion, gastritis	Long term treatment with steroids can result in peptic ulceration. • Research indicates this only occurs in 2% of patients taking steroid therapy (Spiro 1983). • Because of the low incidence rate prophylaxis is not routinely recommended.
Hyperglycaemia/polyuria/polydipsia	Corticosteroids have an effect on glycogen metabolism. • Abnormal synthesis and release of glycogen into blood results in hyperglycaemia, polyuria and polydipsia. • Diabetics may require more insulin. • Non diabetics can develop hyperglycaemia requiring sugar free diet/insulin. • If dose is high and long term glycogen stores become so low muscle weakness can result.
Osteoporosis	Calcium metabolism is influenced by corticosteroids. • Increase in the metabolic rate mobilises too much calcium from the bone. • Bones become thin and brittle and susceptible to fracture. • Occurs in 50% of patients on long term steroids. • Bone loss more rapid in early stage of the disease, most noticeable in spine, hip, distal radius, pelvis and ribs. 7.5 mg prednisolone and over causes significant loss in most patients (Lukert & Raisz 1990).
Hyperlipidaemia	Steroids control lipid and cholesterol production. • Over production can result in hyperlipidaemia and hypercholesterolaemia. • If untreated arthromatous plaques can lead to ischaemic heart disease (Durlington 1990).
Depression and mental disturbance	High dose steroids are linked with mental disorders especially psychosis, euphoria and depression. Patients taking intravenous steroids have demonstrated depression, restlessness and sleeplessness (Mitchell & Collins 1984). These side effects have been observed to continue after withdrawal of the steroid therapy (Wolkowitz & Rapaport 1989).

Intramuscular corticosteroids

There is an increasing use of the intramuscular route for a rapid induction of remission of acute flares of RA. It is particularly useful when admission to hospital is not an option.

It is becoming commonplace for patients to have a short course of intramuscular Depomedrone 120 mg over a period of a week. It may be given three times or on alternate days or even daily. Some rheumatologists use it on a weekly basis for several weeks. These regimes can have a dramatic anti-inflammatory effect but during the acute stage of the disease their use must be supported with advice on:

• Rest
• Planning and pacing
• Joint protection
• Exercise.

Intravenous corticosteroids

Intravenous steroids can also be used to induce a rapid remission of rheumatoid disease in those patients with acute exacerbation. However, there are no nationally agreed protocols and so there is a wide diversity in practice regarding dosage and time scales. One example is solumedrone 1 g given intravenously over a 4 to 6 hour period. This may be given two or three times on alternate days depending on the level of disease activity. Although intravenous steroids can be administered to outpatients, some units are fortunate enough to be able to admit patients to dedicated rheumatology units for induction of remission and it is in these units that intravenous steroids are commonly used.

Intra-articular corticosteroids

The introduction of corticosteroids into the synovial joint reduces synovial inflammation. This in turn helps to resolve effusion that results in pain relief and an increase in functional capacity of the joint. The indications for intra-articular injection are:

• Relief of pain resulting from inflammatory arthritis localised to one or a few joints
• Relief of discomfort from soft tissue pain
• To aid mobilisation
• To improve function and rehabilitation.

Rheumatoid synovitis is sometimes suppressed for months with such treatment.

Corticosteroids can also be helpful in treating a number of other problems such as:

• Bursitits
• Nodules
• Tendonitis.

Inflammation, which is localised specifically at the site of muscle insertion, responds well to corticosteroid injections (Doherty 1992). Resting the joint from strenuous exercise for 48 hours following an intra-articular injection enhances benefits and patients should be informed of this.

Contraindications. There is no evidence that intra-articular steroids spare cartilage degradation and so frequent use is not recommended, especially in weight bearing joints. It is suggested that intervals between injections should not be normally less than 3 months (Williams & Gumpel 1980). Intra-articular steroids should not be given when the patient has a:

• Local infection
• Intra-articular fracture
• Taking anticoagulant therapy
• Has a bleeding disorder.

Historically, doctors have always administered intra-articular injections, but more recently an increasing number of nurses, physiotherapists and occupational therapists are performing this procedure. The expansion in role of nurses and other health professionals can provide a more holistic care package to the patient. However, it is important that they receive the correct training and feel competent to perform such tasks as intra-articular injections in a skilled and safe manner. In the UK the Royal College of Nursing Rheumatology Nursing Forum has produced useful guidelines for nurses undertaking this procedure (Appendix 3.1).

Side effects

Despite the potentially life saving benefits of corticosteroids, this group of drugs has a very high adverse effect profile. Side effects to most systems of the body have been documented and this is expected when we consider that our own steroid production influences virtually every mechanism essential to life. Table 12.1 provides a list of the commoner side effects with brief descriptions of how corticosteroid therapy produces these symptoms.

When steroids have been given long term or in high doses, symptoms similar to Cushing's syndrome can occur. Cushing's syndrome refers to the clinical state of increased free glucocorticoid that normally occurs following the therapeutic administration of synthetic steroids.

Cushingoid symptoms are listed below:

- Weight gain
- Change in appearance
- Amenorrhoea / oligomenorrhoea
- Poor libido
- Thin skin
- Easy bruising
- Increase in body and facial hair
- Acne.

Supervision of steroid therapy

Patients taking oral steroids must carry a Steroid Information Card, which is often provided by the pharmacist or prescribing doctor. Patients should be requested to carry the card on their person so that it is available at all times. The steroid card carries written instructions for the patient (Fig. 12.2) and documents the dose and duration of therapy.

Patients must be fully aware of the side effects of therapy and that they must never stop taking their tablets suddenly. The danger is that when synthetic steroids are taken, the adrenal cortex produces less or even ceases to produce its own steroid. If therapy is stopped suddenly, the cortex may not activate quickly enough to start to produce sufficient endogenous steroid. If sufficient levels are not maintained this is referred to as adrenal crisis and is potentially fatal.

Doses of steroid need to be increased in times of serious illness, infection, stress or accident. For this reason all doctors, anaesthetists and dentists should be informed that the patient is taking steroid therapy.

I am a patient on

STEROID

TREATMENT

Which must not be stopped abruptly

and in the case of intercurrent illness may have to be increased.

Full details are available from the hospital or general practitioners shown overleaf

---

INSTRUCTIONS

1. **DO NOT STOP** taking the steroid drug except on medical advice. Always have a supply in reserve.

2. In case of feverish illness, accident, operation (emergency or otherwise), diarrhoea or vomiting the steroid treatment **MUST** be continued. Your doctor may wish you to have a **LARGER DOSE** or an **INJECTION** at such times.

3. If the tablets cause indigestion consult your doctor **AT ONCE**.

4. Always carry this card while receiving steroid treatment and show it to any doctor, dentist, nurse or midwife or anyone else who is giving you treatment.

5. After your treatment has finished you must still tell any doctor, dentist, nurse or midwife or anyone else who is giving you treatment that you have had steroid treatment.

Figure 12.2 Steroid card.

SECOND-LINE THERAPY – DISEASE MODIFYING ANTI-RHEUMATIC DRUGS

This section addresses a group of drugs that are thought to influence and modify the natural progression of some rheumatic diseases. They exert individual effects, many relating to specific components of the autoimmune process, particularly the inflammatory cascade. Unlike first-line medication they have been proven, to varying degrees, to influence both the long and short-term outcomes of the disease. Disease modifying anti-rheumatic drugs are often referred to as second-line drugs, indicating the progression from symptom relief to disease suppression.

These drugs are not listed in any order of priority or popularity, as different rheumatic conditions respond more favourably to specific drugs and each patient is also different. Some drugs are more potent than others and as a general rule those agents that have a greater influence on the immune system have a higher adverse reaction profile. The number of potential side effects is vast and for ease of reference the adverse reactions are compiled together with recommended monitoring guidelines (Table 12.2).

Sulphasalazine

Sulphasalazine was first developed in Stockholm, Sweden in the late 1930s from a combination of salicylate and a sulphonamide (Wolfe 1990). At that time it was thought that the aetiology of RA was closely related to a bacterial infection. It was surmised that the anti-inflammatory effects of salicylate and the anti-bacterial effects of sulphonamide, the components of sulphasalazine, would be an ideal drug with which to suppress RA. Early trials of sulphasalazine suggested that it was ineffective as a treatment in RA but very effective in Crohn's disease. It was not until the late 1970s that interest in sulphasalazine resurfaced and it is now accepted as a proven second-line drug. Current research has demonstrated that sulphasalazine inhibits the production and release of certain cytokines (Symmons et al 1988).

Indications.

- Treatment of RA which has failed to respond to non-steroidal anti-inflammatory drugs.
- Sulphasalazine is also an effective treatment of ankylosing spondylitis and HLA-B27 associated diseases (Ferraz et al 1990).
- There have also been suggestions that it can have a protective effect on cartilage degradation and for this reason it is being prescribed by some rheumatologists in the treatment of OA.

- Induction of remission of ulcerative colitis and the treatment of active Crohn's disease.

Administration. For the treatment of rheumatic disease sulphasalazine is prescribed in the enteric-coated oral form, salazopyrin EN tablets. Sulphasalazine is available as an uncoated tablet, but this is inappropriate for rheumatic patients as it causes them gastric side effects.

The maximum recommended dose is 3 g per day. Many patients experience an increase in side effects if they start on too high a dose and therefore a gradual introduction may avoid symptoms. Patients are usually advised to start with 1×500 mg tablet each day for the first week, and increase the dose by 500 mg per day each week to the maximum prescribed.

Taking them with or after food decreases the possibility of gastric side effects. The most common adverse effect is nausea. This can occur in up to 30% of patients and ranges from mild to very severe. If patients experience nausea, they are advised to reduce their dose until the nausea ceases and then very gradually, try to increase it. The disease modifying action of this drug can take up to 12 weeks and as it has no analgesic properties the patient should be advised to remain on their non-steroidal anti-inflammatory drug and to take simple analgesia if necessary.

Special precautions. Sulphasalazine should not be given to patients with allergy/sensitivity to sulphonamides or salicylates. Patients with renal or hepatic disease should be treated with caution. Sulphasalazine can reduce the uptake of digoxin and folate.

Penicillamine

Penicillamine was originally introduced as a treatment for Wilson's disease in which copper accumulates in the brain. Penicillamine aids the elimination of copper ions from the body, hence its effect in Wilson's disease. It was observed that those patients who also had RA experienced an improvement in their symptoms. Research into the efficacy of penicillamine in RA was first documented in a multi-centre trial conducted in the United Kingdom (Multi-Centre Trial Group 1973). It is a component of the penicillin molecule and can be produced from penicillin or made entirely synthetically (Joyce 1989). The mechanism of action is unknown; it is thought to be neither anti-inflammatory nor immunosuppressive but it has been shown by American workers to selectively inhibit T-helper cell activity (Lipsky & Ziff 1980).

It is particularly beneficial in the management of RA when extra-articular manifestations such as vasculitis,

Table 12.2 Essential monitoring and adverse reactions to disease modifying anti-rheumatic drugs

Drug	Monitoring	Adverse reactions
Sulphasalazine	Typical pretreatment assessment: FBC, LFTs (inc. AST or ALT) Typical monitoring: FBC two weekly and LFT's (inc. AST or ALT) 4 weekly for the first 12 weeks. FBC and LFTs (inc. ALT or AST) 12 weekly thereafter. If during the first year of treatment blood results have been stable, 6 monthly tests will suffice subsequently.	*Haematological* – potentially fatal leucopenia, aplastic anaemia and thrombocytopenia. *Renal* – crystalluria, haematuria, proteinuria and nephrotic syndrome. *Hypersensitivity* – skin eruptions, exfoliative dermatitis, pruritus, photosensitivity, anaphylaxis, arthralgia, polyarteritis nodosa, fibrosing alveolitis. *Gastrointestinal* – nausea, vomiting, stomatitis, pancreatitis, hepatitis. *CNS* – vertigo, tinnitus, peripheral neuropathy ataxia, convulsion, insomnia, depression, hallucination. *Fertility* – reports of oligospermia (all reversible). Consider sperm donation prior to treatment.
D–Penicillamine	Typical pretreatment assessment: FBC, urinalysis, U&E's Typical monitoring: weekly urinalysis and two weekly FBC until on a stable dose and thereafter monthly.	*Haematological* – thrombocytopenia, leucopenia, agranulocytosis, aplastic and haemolytic anaemia. *Gastrointestinal* – anorexia, nausea, vomiting, oral ulceration and stomatitis taste impairment. *Skin* – occur early in treatment, often allergic in nature. Pruritus, urticaria. Affects skin collagen and elasticity in long term use. *Renal* – proteinuria is frequent, may progress to glomerulonephritis or nephrotic syndrome. *Other toxicity* – Goodpasture's syndrome, myasthenia gravis, polymyositis, pancreatitis.
Hydroxychloroquine	Typical pretreatment assessment: U&Es, FBC and creatinine. Typical monitoring: No blood monitoring required. Yearly ophthalmic review suggested.	*Gastrointestinal* – nausea, vomiting CVS – ECG changes *Ophthalmic* – visual disturbances including diplopia and blurring vision often with headaches. Rarely due to irreversible retinal damage, corneal opacities. *Skin* – depigmentation of skin and hair. *Haematological* – very rare. Thrombocytopenia, agranulocytosis and aplastic anaemia.
Auranofin – oral gold	Typical pretreatment assessment: FBC, urinalysis, U&Es, LFTs Typical monitoring: monthly FBC and urinalysis. Patient should be asked about the presence of rash or oral ulceration each visit.	As for IM gold but adverse reactions far less common *Gastrointestinal effects* – profuse diarrhoea common occurrence.
Sodium aurothiomalate – IM gold	Typical pretreatment assessment: FBC, urinalysis, U&Es, LFTs Typical monitoring: FBC and urinalysis at the time of each injection. The results of the FBC need not be available before the injection is given but must be available before the next injection, it is permissible to work one FBC in arrears. Patient should be asked about the presence of rash or oral ulceration before each injection.	*Skin* – accounts for 60–80% of all adverse gold reactions. Rash, dermatitis and stomatitis. *Renal* – proteinuria, microscopic haematuria, nephrotic syndrome. *Blood* – eosinophilia, leucopenia, agranulocytosis, thrombocytopenia, anaemia, pancytopenia. *Pulmonary* – cough, shortness of breath, pleuritic chest pain and pulmonary crackles. *Gastrointestinal effects* – uncommon – may include diarrhoea, nausea, vomiting.
Methotrexate	Typical pretreatment assessment: FBC, U&Es, LFTs (inc. AST or ALT). Chest x-ray. Typical monitoring: FBC weekly until 6 weeks after last dose increase and provided it is stable monthly thereafter. LFTs (inc. AST or ALT) 2–4 monthly. U&Es 6–12 monthly (more frequent if there is any reason to suspect deteriorating renal function)	*Haematological* – these may occur suddenly, leucopenia, thrombocytopenia, megaloblastic anaemia, pancytopenia. *Pulmonary* – non-productive cough, dyspnoea, pulmonary fibrosis. *Gastrointestinal* – anorexia, nausea, vomiting, diarrhoea, weight loss, mouth ulcers. *Other toxicity* – alopecia, urticaria, cutaneous vasculitis, transient oligospermia, liver toxicity, potential for foetal abnormality due to teratogenic effects.

Table 12.2 (cont'd)

Drug	Monitoring	Adverse reactions
Azathioprine	Typical pretreatment assessment: FBC, U&Es, LFTs Typical monitoring: FBC weekly for first 8 weeks, then monthly once stable. LFTs monthly throughout. After each dose increase return to weekly FBC for 4 weeks.	*Hypersensitivity reactions* – malaise, dizziness, vomiting, fever, rigors, jaundice, arrhythmias and hypertension. *Haematological* – bone marrow suppression resulting in potential pancytopenia. *Gastrointestinal* – nausea and vomiting, rarely pancreatitis. *Other toxicity* – hair loss, susceptibility to infections, rarely pneumonitis.
Cyclosporin	Typical pretreatment assessment: FBC, U&Es, creatinine on 2 separate occasions, LFTs, serum magnesium, serum uric acid, fasting lipids, urinary proteins and 3 separate blood pressure (BP) recordings. Typical monitoring: two weekly BP, U&Es and creatinine to be maintained until maximum dosage is reached. Once stable reduce monitoring to monthly.	*Renal* – commonest is tubular and vascular dysfunction which if reversible. Structural change in proximal tubule also reversible. Changes in afferent arteriole structure are less common but irreversible. *Other toxicity* – excessive growth of body hair, tremor, hypertension, hepatic dysfunction, fatigue, GIT disturbance. Less common symptoms include headaches, rashes, mild anaemia, hyperkalaemia, gout, weight increase and confusion.
Cyclophosphamide	Typical pretreatment assessment: FBC, LFTs, U&Es, creatinine. Typical monitoring: oral = weekly FBC for 6 weeks then monthly once stable. Weekly urinalysis for blood to be maintained throughout. Intravenous = FBC day 7, 10 and 14 after first dose then prior to each dose.	*Haematological* – bone marrow suppression = leucopenia, thrombocytopenia and anaemia. *Gastrointestinal* – nausea and vomiting. *Renal* – haemorrhagic cystitis. *Other toxicity* – alopecia, hyperpigmentation of skin especially palms, soles and nails, hepatotoxicity, disturbance of carbohydrate metabolism, gonadal suppression.

Felty's syndrome, amyloidosis and rheumatic lung disease are present.

It does not appear to show any beneficial response in seronegative arthropathies.

Indications.

- Severe active RA
- Wilson's disease.

Administration. Penicillamine (penicillamine, distamine, pendramine) is taken orally at 125 mg daily increasing at two/four weekly intervals to a maintenance dose of 500–750 mg daily. Occasionally, doses are increased to 1000 mg per day. Penicillamine is usually taken at least one hour before food as it is a metal chelator and mops up essential metals, including iron. If the patient takes oral iron, it should be taken 2 hours before or 2 hours following penicillamine. The presence of antacids hinders the absorption of the penicillamine and if they are needed they should be taken at a different time of day. Improvement takes up to 12 weeks. If penicillamine does not induce remission within a 12 month period, then it should be withdrawn.

Hydroxychloroquine

Hydroxychloroquine is one of the family of antimalarial drugs that comes from the bark of the Peruvian cinchona tree. Pelletier & Caventau first identified the active ingredients, quinine and cinchonine in 1820 (Rynes 1993). Its action is not truly known, but it is thought to be related to the inhibition of cellular enzyme release and interference with intracellular function. The theory is that lysosomal membranes inhibit the release of lysosomal enzymes that may be involved in the inflammatory process. It may also inhibit interleukin-1, which is involved in cartilage degradation. As antimalarials are particularly effective in the management of discoid lupus, they may also have a photo-protective quality that helps the skin lesions.

Indications. In the rheumatic diseases hydroxychloroquine is used to treat:

- Systemic and discoid lupus erythematosus
- Active RA.

Administration. 400 mg hydroxychloroquine sulphate tablets (plaquenil) are given initially in divided doses daily. Maintenance doses range between 200–400 mg daily.

Special precautions. Ocular toxicity is the main concern with antimalarial drugs. They have high affinity to the retina, and if retinal damage is not detected early, their effects cause blindness. In the past, vigilant ophthalmic monitoring has been carried out but due to the relatively low incidence rate, patients are often advised to have 6-monthly eye examinations by their own optician.

Ocular toxicity is dose related, and dosage is limited to 6.5 mg/kg/day for safety. However, hydroxy-chloroquine is thought to be a very safe drug and it requires minimal monitoring otherwise.

Hydroxychloroquine should be avoided in patients with severe renal and hepatic disease and should not be given to those with psoriatic arthritis.

Myasthenia gravis may be exaggerated.

Gold compounds

Gold therapy has been used in the management of diseases for many years; it was used for the treatment of tuberculosis by Koch in 1890. In 1929 a French rheumatologist called Forestier pioneered the use of intramuscular gold for the treatment of RA, working on the assumption that both tuberculosis and RA were infectious in their aetiology (Kean et al 1985). Gold compounds act on inflammatory cells such as monocytes, lymphocytes and their mediators, thereby producing immunosuppressive effects (Scharf & Christophidis 1995).

There are two compounds of gold:

- Sodium aurothiomalate
- Auranofin.

The former is administered by intramuscular injection, whilst auranofin is an oral preparation. Although both are gold preparations, they are not interchangeable as they have very different profiles of efficacy and safety (Miller 1996).

Indication

- Active RA.

Sodium aurothiomalate

Administration. Intramuscular gold induces clinical improvement in about 70% of patients. Unfortunately, 30% experience adverse effects. In the 1980s many patients had their intramuscular gold therapy terminated because of adverse reactions, but recently compliance and tolerance have seemed to improve. It

has been postulated that this may be due to improved physician experience, which allows patients to continue treatment despite minor adverse reactions.

The injectable form, sodium aurothiomalate (myocrisin) is given by deep intramuscular injection into the buttock and the area massaged gently. Because of the potential for hypersensitivity reactions, a test dose is always given (5–10 mg) and if no reaction is reported, weekly injections of 50 mg are continued. Gold has a cumulative effect and benefit is not usual until 300–500 mg have been given (6–8 weeks of treatment). However it may take 3 to 6 months for improvement to occur. When improvement is apparent, the frequency of treatment can be reduced to 50 mg per month. Treatment can continue indefinitely subject to efficacy and tolerance. Guidelines for the administration of intramuscular gold are shown in Appendix 3.2.

Oral gold

Auranofin (Ridaura) is given by mouth. The initial dose is 6 mg that can be divided into two doses. If benefits are not noted an increase to 9 mg daily can be made. This can be given in three divided doses. If no benefit is observed after 3 months, the treatment should be discontinued. Its most troublesome side effect is diarrhoea.

Special precautions. Ideally gold compounds should be avoided in patients with renal and hepatic disorders, history of blood disorders, severe dermatitis and pulmonary fibrosis.

Methotrexate

Methotrexate was first employed as a disease modifying drug in the late 1950s and has evolved as one of the most commonly used therapies over the past 35 years. Low-dose methotrexate was approved in the United States of America in 1988 as a therapy for active RA. Originally it was only used in severe cases of refractory arthritis, but is now used by many rheumatologists as the drug of first choice in the early stages of the disease.

Historically methotrexate was used for childhood leukaemia but its utilisation in the rheumatic diseases has now expanded and it is currently being used for the treatment of psoriatic arthritis and Reiter's syndrome. It is still widely used as a chemotherapy agent, especially for acute lymphoblastic leukaemia and in the treatment of meningococcal meningitis.

Methotrexate is an anti-metabolite. This term describes a substance that competes with or replaces a particular metabolite (a product of metabolism). In this case the metabolite is folate which is essential for the production of blood cells. Therefore methotrexate is also classified as an antifolate agent. Folates are essential for the formation of blood cells and hence methotrexate has the ability to slow down blood cell production. The advantages in leukaemia are clear to see, but it is less obvious how methotrexate influences disease activity in rheumatic diseases. Antifolate agents not only slow down blood cell production, but are potent inhibitors of connective tissue cell division.

Methotrexate inhibits folate action and folates are required for deoxyribonucleic acid (DNA) synthesis. The drug exerts its most powerful influence in cells that are actively undergoing deoxyribonucleic acid synthesis, particularly those cells in the S phase of the cell cycle. Those cells most susceptible are rapidly dividing cells in the epidermis (hence its benefit for psoriasis), and the gastrointestinal tract. This action accounts for side effects such as mouth ulcers, nausea and vomiting.

Indications

- Severe active RA
- Severe uncontrolled psoriasis
- Malignant disease.

Administration. For the management of rheumatic diseases, methotrexate is given as a weekly dose by either the intramuscular or oral route, the latter being used more often.

Oral methotrexate

This can be given as one dose or spread over a 24 hour period. It should not be given more frequently because of a greater risk of liver toxicity. The initial dose is commonly 7.5–10 mg weekly. If the patient cannot tolerate this dose, 5 mg can be given and gradually increased. If there is no response over the next 4–8 weeks the dose can be increased if no adverse reactions have occurred. The optimum dose varies, but most rheumatologists use doses ranging from 7.5–25 mg per week.

Patients with psoriatic arthritis usually require doses in the higher range of 25–30 mg per week to benefit their joint and skin symptoms.

Intramuscular methotrexate

In some patients intramuscular methotrexate appears to be better tolerated than oral administration. Most patients are started on oral methotrexate because of its ease of use and switched to the intramuscular route if they experience unacceptable side effects. As methotrexate is a cytotoxic drug, the nurse must be aware of the local policy regarding handling, administration and disposal of cytotoxic agents. The Royal College of Nursing Rheumatology Nursing Forum has produced guidelines for the administration of intramuscular methotrexate (Appendix 3.3).

Folate supplementation

Because of methotrexate's action on folates, patients may experience a fall in the serum folate concentration (Morgan et al 1987). This is associated with an increase in toxicity and symptoms. Supplementation with folinic acid (15 mg) or folic acid (5 mg) has demonstrated improvement in symptoms without affecting the efficacy of the methotrexate. Regimes vary; one suggested prescribes folic acid 5 mg on day 3, 4 and 5 (counting day of methotrexate administration as day 1). Some rheumatologists prescribe folate prophylactically, others wait to see if the folate levels fall or if symptoms such as mouth ulcers occur.

Azathioprine

Azathioprine is an immunosuppressant. Initially it gained recognition in the prevention of organ and tissue transplantation. This drug is referred to as a purine analogue that is thought to inhibit nucleic acid synthesis. It is thought to affect cell division by influencing the synthesis and function of ribonucleic acid (RNA) and deoxyribonucleic acid (DNA), resulting in cell death. Other purine analogues are 6-mercaptopurine and thioguanine but these agents are not commonly used in the rheumatic diseases.

Indications

- RA
- Psoriatic arthritis
- A variety of other autoimmune and collagen diseases
- For suppression of rejection in organ transplants.

Administration. Oral route only (Imuran) in rheumatic diseases, at a dose of 3 mg/kg body weight per day. Maintenance dose 1–3 mg/kg body weight daily.

If no response is apparent after 3 months, discontinuation of treatment should be considered.

Special precautions. Care should be taken with patients with liver and renal disease.

Cyclosporin

Cyclosporin was discovered in the early 1970s during work being carried out to produce anti-fungal agents. The usage of cyclosporin in the management of severe rheumatic conditions increased dramatically in the 1990s. Initially it was only considered as a suitable option for patients with severe refractory RA who had been unable to maintain remission with other disease modifying drugs. However, its use is becoming more common and cyclosporin is being used at a much earlier stage in disease management.

Cyclosporin is a potent immunosuppressant that has been shown to be very effective in preventing rejection of transplanted organs. The clinical outcome of the skin, heart, kidney, pancreas, bone and marrow have been greatly improved by the use of cyclosporin.

The mode of action is by inhibition of the production and utilisation of interleukin-2, a growth factor for lymphocytes. This effectively reduces the inflammatory response (Yocum et al 1988). Because it only influences specific immune responses it is referred to as a 'selective immunosuppressant'.

Indications.

- Severe active RA
- Psoriasis
- Atopic dermatitis
- Graft versus host disease.

Administration. Cyclosporin (Neoral) is available in oral capsules or solution. The taste of the liquid can be improved by dilution with orange juice, squash or apple juice. Grapefruit should not be taken as this affects the absorption of the drug. Neoral is taken on a daily dose basis that can be divided into two doses. Initially, 2.5 mg/kg body weight per day is given for the first 6 weeks. If there is no significant improvement, the dose can be increased to a maximum 4 mg/kg body weight per day if tolerated. If the response is inadequate after 3 months of maximum dose, the treatment should be discontinued. Some rheumatologists are combining cyclosporin with other disease modifying drugs if it has proved to be ineffective on its own, but these combinations have yet to be shown to be effective and safe.

Special precautions. Physical examination, including base line blood pressure and renal function should be carried out prior to the initiation of therapy (Table 12.2). Hypertension should be monitored throughout therapy and antihypertensive agents such as nifedipine should be given if necessary. If blood pressure remains elevated despite treatment, cyclosporin should be discontinued.

Avoid other drugs that are known to affect renal function. Use with caution in those patients who have hyperuricaemia or hyperkalaemia. Cyclosporin can affect clearance of steroids and non-steroidal anti-inflammatory drugs so great care should be taken monitoring the renal function of patients on these drugs. Vaccinations may be less effective and live vaccines should not be given.

A number of drugs interact with cyclosporin, including erythromycin, phenytoin, phenobarbitone and oral contraceptives.

Cyclophosphamide

In the past cyclophosphamide has been used in the management of malignant disease. More recently it has been successfully used as an immunosuppressant in other serious non-malignant conditions. Cyclophosphamide is classed as an alkylating agent which is capable of altering the structure and binding capacity of certain cells. This results in the abnormal linking of two cells that can block normal cell function. When this cellular effect influences the deoxyribonucleic acid in cells such as lymphocytes, the cells cannot divide properly and eventually die. This subsequently results in a degree of immunosuppression.

Cyclophosphamide is a very potent agent and it is only used in patients with refractory RA when all other agents have been unsuccessful.

Indications

- Polymyositis
- Vasculitis
- Systemic lupus erythematosus
- Glomerular kidney disease
- Malignant disease.

Administration. Administration is by the oral or intravenous route. There are several dose regimes and these vary according to individual rheumatologists, but typically the oral dose begins around 50–75 mg per day (Miller 1996).

Special precautions. Haemorrhagic cystitis is a common problem when giving cyclophosphamide. It is caused by a metabolite called acrolein. Prophylactic mesna, an agent that reacts specifically with acrolein, prevents this urothelial toxicity. Mesna is given simultaneously with cyclophosphamide, and further doses are given orally or intravenously 4 and 8 hours following treatment. The patient's fluid intake should be increased for 24–48 hours following intravenous cyclophosphamide.

Adverse reactions to disease modifying drugs. Cytotoxic, immunosuppressant agents have a higher and potentially more life threatening side effects profile than other disease modifying drugs. Table 12.2 includes the most common adverse reactions to second-line drugs and their monitoring requirements. However, it is not exhaustive and all adverse reactions should be noted and most require some form of action. It is strongly recommended that the reader refers to both local and national guidelines and other pharmacology texts for supplementary reading.

Table 12.2 shows only the haematological and urinary monitoring. The patient's well-being, compliance with the drug therapy and their disease activity are of equal importance.

Combination therapies

Induction of remission and the arresting of the inflammatory response is vital to reduce the long term effects of rheumatic diseases. Unfortunately, some patients fail to respond to even the most aggressive therapies. In an attempt to manage these refractory cases, combinations of disease modifying drugs are being prescribed. Cyclosporin and methotrexate have been used together, as have sulphasalazine and methotrexate. These are by no means the only combinations. Many randomised controlled trials are being conducted to assess efficacy and toxicity and that there is a strong potential for disease suppression.

DRUGS AND PREGNANCY

Ideally all drug therapy should be avoided during pregnancy and whilst the woman is breast feeding. However, in the real world this may not be possible. The first trimester is the most vulnerable time for the foetus when drug therapy can cause congenital malformations. The period from the third to the eleventh week poses the greatest risk. Preconception counselling and education are vital to ensure that couples are provided with as much information as possible, as some drugs such as methotrexate need to be stopped 6 months in advance of conception (see Ch. 7).

Table 12.3 outlines the implications for pregnant patients taking the most frequently prescribed medication in the rheumatic diseases.

FUTURE DEVELOPMENTS

Genetic research continues the quest to isolate a particular genetic pattern common to the rheumatoid patient population. If a genotype is found, the concept of genetic manipulation may prove effective in disease modification.

Table 12.3 Drug therapy in pregnancy

Class of drug	Comment
Analgesics	Aspirin can cause impaired platelet function. Dextropropoxyphene (found in co-proxamol) – can lead to foetal drug dependency (Rubin 1984). If an analgesic is required, paracetamol is the drug of choice.
Non-steroidal anti-inflammatory drugs	Can cause premature closure of the ductus arteriosus. Aspirin may increase the likelihood of minor malformations such as cleft palate, it can prolong gestation and labour and affect homeostasis in the neonate (Bleyer & Breckenridge 1970).
Corticosteroids	Dosage above 10 mgs daily may produce adrenal atrophy in the foetus. Cleft palate has been reported (Le Gallez 1988).
Sodium aurothiomalate (intramuscular gold)	No evidence of abnormality but not recommended (Le Gallez 1988). May be restarted late in pregnancy to influence activity following labour.
Auranofin (oral gold)	No reported adverse effects during pregnancy.
Antimalarial drugs	Not recommended as congenital deafness has been reported in neonates.
Penicillamine	Advice is conflicting, if benefit outweighs the risk to the foetus then the lowest possible dose is given (Richardson 1992).
Immunosuppressants (azathioprine, chlorambucil, cyclophosphamide, methotrexate)	All teratogenic when given in the first trimester of pregnancy.

Development of biological agents can provide anti-bodies against cells that are known to have a damaging and destructive effect on synovial tissue and cartilage. Work on anti CD4 antibody and anti-tumour necrosing factor (TNF) is thought to be promising, as is work on synthetically produced agents that can block the action of interleukins. Before the optimum therapy for rheumatic diseases can be found, a complete understanding of the current disease modifying drugs needs to be established. Large scale well-controlled trials should promote this understanding and aid a fuller exploration of the long term effects of these therapeutic options.

Monitoring disease modifying anti-rheumatic drugs

The provision of drug monitoring for rheumatoid patients is proving to be one of the most difficult elements of care provision. As units have expanded their client population, the need has increased for an adequate system for monitoring patients taking disease modifying anti-rheumatic drugs.

Because of the large number of disease modifying anti-rheumatic drugs in use and the diversity of current practice, a plethora of monitoring protocols are used and it is difficult to envisage uniformity of drug monitoring throughout the country. However, existing services could be enhanced, or in new units services could be established, by building on the experience and problem solving strategies of others.

Monitoring guidelines

It is apparent that throughout the UK there is great disparity in the monitoring of disease modifying anti-rheumatic drugs. This relates to the:

- Choice of essential investigations
- Intervals at which they should be performed
- Relevant actions to take if side effects occur.

The British Society of Rheumatology (BSR) recognised the problem and has produced National Guidelines based on current practice derived from local and regional protocols. These are 'core elements' that are intended to be modified for use at local level. Copies of these national guidelines are available to members of the British Society of Rheumatology, and nurses who are not members can ask a doctor to obtain them!

Each pharmaceutical company produces its own literature and this is similarly documented in the Data Compendium, MIMS and British National Formulary. The production of local guidelines must encompass information from all these sources to ensure safe and effective documents.

Nurses are the professionals who usually perform monitoring, but guidelines have often been devised without any nursing involvement. It is promising to see that individual units are developing their guidelines using a multidisciplinary team approach. This enables nurses to be actively involved in setting standards for patients that are safe and achievable, incorporating ideas gained from networking with colleagues in other units.

In many units the autonomy of the specialist nurse and rheumatology practitioner, has allowed them to establish nurse-led monitoring and this is now one of the prime elements of their job descriptions. Throughout the UK, many rheumatology nurses have single-handedly set up and managed monitoring systems. However, this has led to an enormous increase in patient uptake that has stretched single-handed resources beyond safe limits. A large proportion of the nurse's time is spent undertaking venepuncture and interpreting laboratory results, leaving little quality time to spend with the patient. In these circumstances nurses have become victims of their own success.

Fortunately for some the situation has been resolved with an increase in personnel, but other nurses find themselves trapped within roles they have created for themselves.

Shared care monitoring

Shared care monitoring refers to the joint provision of care between hospital and primary practice and in reality it is offered in many different settings. Many patients find this an excellent way to receive their monitoring and it is especially attractive if they live a distance from the hospital. An ideal situation is described in Chapter 16. Blood samples are usually obtained by the practice or district nurse and are either interpreted and actioned by the general practitioner, or sent to the hospital for the rheumatology staff.

The recent introduction in the UK of fund holding practices has raised the issue of responsibility; whose job is it to monitor the patient? Primary practices have argued that the purchase of a rheumatology service from the hospital should include the provision of a monitoring service. Hospital units reply by suggesting that as each practice has so few rheumatology patients, they could be monitored within the practice and this would:

- Be more convenient for the patient
- Ease the burden on the specialised staff in the rheumatology unit.

The latter would free specialised staff to utilise their time more productively, for instance undertaking more out-patient consultations, carrying out joint injections, counselling and educating the patient.

The question as to where the responsibility for monitoring lies remains unanswered in many cases. The debate will probably be settled amicably at local level. If not, national decisions will need to be made. As the patient's advocate, nurses must encourage the 'decision-makers' to keep the patient's well-being and their right to choose at the forefront of the debate.

Developing the relationship between primary and secondary care

Recent years have shown a growth in the sharing of information and experiences between practice nurses and hospital rheumatology staff (see Ch. 16). As rheumatology care provision has increased so has the number of patients presenting back to the general practice surgery for monitoring and advice. It became apparent to physicians and nurses alike that a liaison between hospital and primary practice would greatly benefit the patient. All too often patients return for their hospital consultations remarking that different information has being given at their doctor's surgery.

Practice and district nurses who are dealing with rheumatology patients should seek help from their more specialised nursing colleagues.

One solution, which has partially solved these problems, is for nurse specialists to hold seminars. These are usually well attended by community staff, practice nurses and physicians. It is not always feasible to offer such courses, but other methods to support practice nurses and community staff could include:

• **Provision of a helpline**

This should be manned by staff who are experts in drug monitoring. This can be time consuming but the use of an answering machine would avoid the need for a constant presence.

• **Produce a monitoring guideline booklet**

This could be circulated to all the general practitioner surgeries in the vicinity. This method has proved to be very helpful to many units and surgeries. A brief resume of the inflammatory diseases is sometimes incorporated and this has also been generally welcomed.

• **Good communication**

Ensure that lines of communication are maintained with the practice and that the practice is made aware that the patient needs to attend. Poor cooperation does not lend itself to a sympathetic care provision setting.

• **Networking**

Always attempt to network with other rheumatology nurses, especially when you or they are experiencing difficulties.

EDUCATING PATIENTS

Patients have a legal, ethical and moral right to information about their medication. The method, educational tools or learning settings employed will depend on individual resources and expertise. Any drug information literature should comply with:

• Standards
• Protocols
• Local guidelines.

This will ensure that legal obligations are met. Literature should also compliment the National Guidelines for 'Monitoring of Second-Line Drugs' produced by the British Society of Rheumatology.

There is a plethora of drug information literature produced for patients, but before handing it out give a verbal explanation and make sure that patients can understand the content (Hill 1997). This topic is discussed in Chapter 15. In the UK the Arthritis and Rheumatism Council has produced a variety of excellent drug sheets, that are free of charge and a number of rheumatology units have produced their own. A good example is shown in Chapter 8. There are also several booklets about disease management produced by agencies such as the Arthritis and Rheumatism Council and Arthritis Care. These are an ideal source of information for both inpatient and outpatients.

Therapy such as disease modifying drugs can have serious side effects that have profound repercussions for the patient. Unfortunately use of these drugs cannot be guaranteed to improve how the patient feels. It is clear that compliance may be affected if medication appears to be ineffective and makes the patient feel unwell. Compliance and a sense of confidence can be induced if effective education is given. Patient's demands are ever changing and nurses should be sensitive to their needs and strive to provide drug information tailored to them. For instance, some patients prefer to be told only the basic facts about their medication, as a full description is too heavy a burden for them to cope with. If this is the case, their wishes must be respected but clear details should be given how, where and when they can gain contact for further support. There are also many patients who desire to learn all that can be offered.

The economic and social implications of rheumatic diseases are vast. They are responsible for a large proportion of health care use, disability, social and psychological dysfunction. The lives of friends, families and loved ones can be dramatically affected. If the burden of disability for the individual patient and the health care system is to be reduced, drug therapy must be as effective as possible in the pre-damaged phase of their illness.

For true progress to be achieved, the patient must become an active participant in care and not a passive recipient of treatment. This means that patient education is a fundamental element in the management of rheumatic disease. Knowledge will enable them to truly make informed decisions and take full ownership of managing their lives whilst living with a rheumatic disease.

Action points for practice:

- Present a talk to your colleagues about monitoring disease modifying drugs. Reinforce this by producing a written package for individual reference.
- Design a poster about steroid therapy, demonstrating the various routes and potential side effects. This can be used as a visual teaching aid for the ward or rheumatology department.
- Write an essay outlining the use of non-steroidal anti-inflammatory drugs in the rheumatic diseases. List their side effects and discuss interventions that may alleviate them.

REFERENCES

Bleyer W A, Breckenridge R T 1970 Adverse drug reactions in new born. Journal of American Medical Association 213: 2049–2052

Bradley J D 1991 Comparison of an anti-inflammatory dose of ibuprofen, an analgesic dose of ibuprofen and acetaminophen in the treatment of patients with osteoarthritis of the knee. New England Journal of Medicine 325: 87–91

British National Formulary 1994 Drugs used in the treatment of musculoskeletal and joint disease. Pharmaceutical Press, London, ch10, p 377–397

Doherty M 1992 Rheumatology examination and injection techniques. W B Saunders, London, p 122

Durlington P N 1990 Secondary hyperlidaemia. British Medical Bulletin 46: 1005–1024

Emery P 1994 The optimal management of early rheumatoid disease: the key to preventing disability. British Journal of Rheumatology 33: 765–768

Ferraz M, Tugwell P, Goldsmith C et al 1990 Meta-analysis of sulphasalazine in ankylosing spondylitis. Journal of Rheumatology 17: 1482

Griffiths B, Emery P 1996 Today's management of rheumatoid arthritis. Prescriber 5 July 31–43

Harris K 1992 The role of prostaglandins in the control of renal function. British Journal of Anaesthetics 69: 233–235

Hill J 1997 A practical guide to patient education and information giving. Ballière's Clinical Rheumatology 11(1): 109–127

Hoppman R A 1991 Central nervous system side effects of non-steroidal anti-inflammatory drugs: aseptic meningitis, psychosis and cognitive dysfunction. Archives Internal Medicine 151: 1309–1313

Joyce P A 1989 D-Penicillamine pharmacokinetics and pharmacodynamics in rheumatoid arthritis. Pharmacology Therapies 42: 405

Johnson A G 1994 Do non-steroidal anti-inflammatory drugs affect blood pressure? Annals of Internal Medicine 121: 289–300

Justins D M 1996 Management strategies for chronic pain. Annals of the Rheumatic Diseases 55: 588–596

Kean E F, Forestier F, Kassam Y et al 1985 The history of gold therapy in rheumatoid diseases. Seminars in Arthritis Rheumatism 14: 180

Langman M J S, Weil J, Wainwright P et al 1994 Risks of bleeding peptic ulcer associated with individual non-steroidal anti-inflammatory agents. Lancet 343: 1075–1078

Le Gallez P 1988 Teratogenesis and drugs for rheumatic disease. Nursing Times 84(27): 41–44

Lipsky P E, Ziff M 1980 Inhibition of human helper T cell function in vitro by D-Penicillamine and copper sulphate. Journal of Clinical Investigations 65: 1069

Lukert B P, Raisz L G 1990 Glucocortoid induced osteoporosis, pathogenesis and management. Annals of Internal Medicine 112: 352–364

Martindale 1996 The extra pharmacopoeia. London Royal Pharmaceutical Society p 1017

Miller D R 1996 Pharmacological interventions. In:Wegener S T, Belza B L, Gall E P (eds) Clinical care in the rheumatic diseases. American College of Rheumatology, Atlanta, ch 11, p 68–69

Mitchell D M, Collins J V 1984 Do corticosteroids really alter mood? Postgraduate Medical Journal 60: 467–470

Morgan S L, Baggott J E, Altz-Smith M 1987 Folate status of the rheumatoid arthritis patients receiving long term low dose methotrexate therapy. Arthritis Rheumatism 30: 1348

Multi-Centre Trial Group 1973 Controlled trial of D-penicillamine in severe rheumatoid arthritis. Lancet 1: 275

O'Brien W M, Bagby G F 1985 Rare adverse reactions to non-steroidal anti-inflammatory drugs. Journal of Rheumatology 12: 13

O'Callaghan C A 1994 Renal disease and use of topical non-steroidal anti-inflammatory drugs. British Medical Journal 308: 110–111

Rashed S 1989 Effects of non-steroidal anti-inflammatory drugs on the course of rheumatoid arthritis. Lancet ii: 519–522

Richardson A 1992 Rheumatoid arthritis in pregnancy. Nursing Standard 6(45): 25–29

Rodnan G P, Benedek T G 1970 The early history of anti-rheumatic drugs. Arthritis Rheumatism 13: 145

Rubin C P 1984 Drugs in pregnancy and lactation. Medicine International 2: 307–310

Rynes R I 1993 Anti-malarials. In: Kelley W N (ed) Textbook of Rheumatology, 4th edn. W B Saunders, Philadelphia, ch 44, p 731–742

Scharf S L, Christophidis N 1995 Second line agents for rheumatoid arthritis. The Medical Journal of Australia 63(21): 215–218

Smith Pigg J, Webb Driscoll P, Caniff R 1985 Rheumatology nursing: a problem oriented approach. Wiley Medical, New York

Spiro H M 1983 Is the steroid ulcer a myth? New England Journal of Medicine 309: 45–47

Stricker B H C 1985 Acute hypersensitivity reactions to paracetamol. British Medical Journal 291: 938–939

Symmons D, Salmon M, Farr M et al 1988 Sulphasalazine treatment and lymphocyte function in patients with rheumatoid arthritis. Journal of Rheumatology 15: 575

Szczeklik A 1993 Antipyretic analgesics and the allergic patient. American Journal of Medicine 75: 82

Whittle B J R 1977 Mechanisms underlying gastric mucosal damage induced by indomethacin and bile salts and the action of prostaglandins. British Journal of Pharmacology 60: 455–460

Williams P, Gumpel M 1980 Procedures in practice. Aspiration and injection of joints. British Medical Journal 281: 990–992

Wolfe F 1990 50 years of antirheumatic therapy: The progress of rheumatoid arthritis. Journal of Rheumatology 17: 24

Wolkowitz O M, Rapaport M 1989 Long standing behavioral changes following prednisilone withdrawal. Journal of American Medical Association 261: 1731–1732

Yocum D E, Klippel J H, Wilder R L et al 1988 Cyclosporin A in severe, treatment-refractory rheumatoid arthritis using total lymphoid irradiation. Arthritis Rheumatism 31: 21

FURTHER READING

Kelly W N, Harris E D, Ruddy S, Sledge C B 1993 Textbook of Rheumatology, 4th edn vol I + II. W B Saunders, Philadelphia

Kumar P, Clark M 1994 Clinical Medicine, 3rd edn. Baillière Tindall, London

13

Complementary therapeutic interventions

Anne Cawthorn, Jane Billington

The aim of this chapter is to provide a better understanding of the complementary therapeutic interventions that may prove useful in the field of rheumatology. After reading this chapter you should be able to:

- Understand the issues related to implementing therapies
- Describe some of the benefits resulting from using therapies
- Discuss the role that counselling plays in relation to complementary therapies
- Demonstrate an understanding of some of the more popular therapies and be able to offer suggestions for their use.

The demand for complementary therapies has increased over the last decade and in response, nurses are introducing therapies into the care they give. It can be argued that they are attempting to return to the artistic side of nursing, sacrificed when they relinquished many of the more caring activities by aligning themselves to the more scientific medical model. These caring activities have now been demonstrated as having a part to play in the movement towards health, and this has resulted in nurses attempting to combine both art and science in an attempt to provide more holistic care.

The potential for using complementary therapies to enhance the quality of care is now recognised. Some nurses have already introduced them, whilst others are still considering this. However, whilst their potential benefits are not disputed, it is recommended that certain issues are addressed before implementing any therapy.

Vickers (1996) recommends that the following three

questions need answering before any therapy is implemented:

1. How should they be introduced into new settings?
2. How can they be used safely and competently?
3. How can they be used appropriately and effectively?

INTRODUCING THERAPIES

Before implementing any new therapy, the following steps should be taken. Initially, interested parties should be given information about the therapy, such as the philosophy underpinning it, relevant research findings and suggestions regarding its uses. If people do not understand what the therapy entails, a demonstration can be given. This is often the easiest way to convince the sceptics.

Secondly, consent must be obtained from the nurse manager, ward manager and each consultant. Also consent will be required from the patient before commencing any therapy. If a consultant refuses permission, their patients should not receive the therapy being offered. However, experience has shown that patients, or relatives, usually manage to persuade sceptical consultants, especially when other patients are benefiting from the therapies.

Other issues to be considered include:

- Which practitioner will carry out the therapy?
- How this will fit into their present role?
- Will they require training?
- What implications are there for time management?
- What costs are involved, for example for essential oils?
- How and when will the therapy be delivered?
- How can the safe and competent use of the therapy be ensured?

It is essential that any therapy offered should be undertaken by a competent practitioner. It is the manager's responsibility to find out whether the practitioner is both competent and adequately trained. Vickers (1996) suggests that training can be checked through the following enquiries. Initially, by investigating the validity of their course, by asking questions about where it was held, how many classroom hours it involved and how much supervised practice there was. These will need to be checked against the minimum recommended hours for each therapy. Where a manager is unsure of these details, they can be obtained from the complementary therapy regulating bodies such as the British Complementary Medical Association (BCMA), or individual bodies like the International Society of Professional Aromatherapists (ISPA). See Appendix 6 for useful addresses.

Finally, three further questions should be asked:

1. What does the therapist intend to do when practising?

2. How do they see their role?

These two questions are necessary to ensure that they will work in partnership with other members of the multidisciplinary team. It is often easier if the therapist is a nurse or health care professional, as they are already used to working as a member of the team. However, if an independent therapist is employed these issues will need to be addressed.

3. Are they aware of their limitations?

It is important that they are aware of what they can and cannot do.

MANAGEMENT OF THERAPIES IN DAY-TO-DAY PRACTICE

Before any therapy is introduced, a protocol and standards, will need to be in place. A good example is given on pages 216–222 in Price & Price (1995). These will need regular revision, to take account of any relevant research findings, as knowledge about using therapies in health care settings is growing rapidly. The efficacy of therapies will need to be monitored and some form of audit and evaluation will be required.

Finally, because this is a new discipline, it is important that there is support for the therapists, either through an informal reflective practice group, or through more formal clinical supervision sessions. This will enable the nurse to share experiences, either on a one to one basis or in a group. In this way both positive and negative aspects of giving therapies can be discussed, research findings can be evaluated and the results of clinical audit can be disseminated. Through this process, the practice of therapies should improve because of their close investigation. In addition the therapist can be supported, in what is a new aspect of care.

BENEFITS FROM USING COMPLEMENTARY THERAPIES

The benefits appear to come from a variety of sources. For example, the benefits of aromatherapy come from three areas:

1. Therapeutic effects of the essential oils
2. Benefits of touch and massage
3. Therapeutic relationship which develops between the patient and the therapist.

The first BMA Report (1986) was dismissive of therapies, stating that the benefits came merely from time, touch and compassion. Over the past 10 years it has been demonstrated that these are not the only benefits. However, what is more important, is that time, touch and compassion are now acknowledged as an important part of the healing process.

The 1993 BMA report was much more positive about the future of therapies. It also addressed the issue of what the therapies should be called, choosing the terms orthodox and non-orthodox in favour of the terms alternative and complementary. Orthodox medicine refers to anything which has been taught in medical training, which at the moment does not include therapies. There is still some confusion regarding complementary therapies and Peitroni (1996) suggests that the following model is one way of trying to understand them.

Group I

This group contains therapies which are a complete system of healing including:

- Acupuncture
- Homeopathy
- Osteopathy and chiropractic, naturopathy
- Herbal medicine
- Yoga.

The common feature of these therapies is that their practice is regulated in the same way that doctors are regulated and they have published ethical guidelines. In addition, most require a long training and the BMA Report (1993) was critical of health care professionals who practised them after short weekend courses. They also share some similarities with orthodox medicine in that they have a diagnostic, investigative and therapeutic base, some having been practised for centuries (Pietroni 1995).

Group 2

Group 2 includes diagnostic therapies:

- Iridology
- Kinesiology
- Biofeedback.

Group 3

This group includes therapeutic methods:

- Aromatherapy
- Massage

- Therapeutic touch
- Reflexology
- Bach flower remedies
- Hypnotherapy
- Spiritual healing.

In this group the therapists do not claim any diagnostic skills, but work in a therapeutic way to complement other areas of care.

Group 4

Group 4 are self-help measures:

- Breathing and relaxation techniques
- Meditation
- Visualisation
- Aerobics
- Autogenetic training
- The Alexander technique.

The aim of these therapies is to teach patients self-help techniques. In doing so, they learn more about themselves and how they contribute to their problems. These techniques are useful in helping with symptoms or for maintaining health and are useful as preventative measures.

CONTROL

A benefit of therapies is that they allow patients to regain control over what is happening to them. This is important for rheumatology patients who experience many changes, which have devastating effects on their quality of life. The literature shows that patients need to feel that they have some control over what is happening to them. This is especially true for chronically ill patients who lack control over the eventual outcome of their disease. Strauss (1984) found that patients do 'invisible work' whilst in hospital, in an effort to gain some control over what is happening to them. Increasing their sense of control allows patients to make changes regarding their situation.

This idea is supported by the work of Montbriand & Laing (1991) who investigated strategies employed by patients who were trying to retain some control over their care. They interviewed 75 patients on two surgical wards about their use of complementary therapies. Their findings revealed that although they were all receiving conventional treatments, 89% were also using complementary therapies, as a control strategy. In addition, the study identified that the chosen therapy closely corresponded with their locus of control. This facet of people's personality was originally referred to by Rotter (1966). He asserted that the amount of control people contributed to their health lay along a continuum. He postulated that the degree to which people perceived to their health outcomes varied depending on what they viewed as having an effect on their health. For example, people with a high internal locus of control subscribe to the theory that their own decisions and actions will directly affect their health. Conversely, those with a high external locus of control, believe that their health is determined by external factors such as fate, chance or powerful others such as doctors or their family. This was highlighted in a study by Montbriand & Laing (1991) who found that people with a high internal locus of control chose therapies in which they were more actively involved. Those with a high external locus of control chose therapies that required limited contribution on their part.

THERAPEUTIC RELATIONSHIP

An important aspect of complementary therapies is the therapeutic relationship that develops between the nurse and the patient. It has three components:

1. Intimacy
2. Partnership
3. Reciprocity.

Over recent years nurses have been encouraged to work in partnership with their patients. If developed properly, this partnership, should result in a tacit contract between them, with each having equal control over what is happening.

The therapeutic relationship is an important factor in the patient's recovery and can contribute in a movement towards healing. Peplau (1952) suggested that nursing is therapeutic because of the interpersonal process which transpires between the nurse and patient and which is achieved through both verbal and non-verbal communication. By using complementary therapies, the nurse is communicating acceptance of the patient. This can be therapeutic to patients who are struggling with a disabling illness and are attempting to cope with factors such as pain, fatigue and altered body image.

RESTORATION OF BALANCE

Another result of receiving therapies, is the restoration of balance or equilibrium. Pietroni & Pietroni (1996) remind us that 'disease or ill health arises as a result of a state of imbalance either from within the person or because of some external force'. Therefore, each

therapy in its own unique way, sets out to restore this imbalance.

TOUCH

Touch is an aspect of complementary therapies that is usually very therapeutic. It is one of the basic means of communication and can demonstrate warmth and affection and can create feelings of value, worth and ego integrity. Religious, cultural and sexual beliefs and attitudes influence the use of touch.

Nurses use touch for both therapeutic and technical reasons. Watson (1975) describes touch as being either:

• Instrumental

or

• Expressive.

Although patients normally receive a lot of touch, it is usually of the formal instrumental type, as opposed to the more spontaneous expressive touch. Rheumatology nursing requires much 'hands on' care and the use of instrumental and expressive touch may overlap. Where expressive touch is used deliberately, as in therapeutic massage and aromatherapy, it can prove to be very beneficial, contributing to the overall therapeutic results.

HOLISTIC ASSESSMENT

Therapies may vary in their effects and benefits, but one aspect common to all of them, is the holistic assessment. This focuses on everything, including physical, psychological, emotional, social and spiritual aspects, with its emphasis on the whole person, rather than on the symptom (Rankin-Box 1991). However, this approach is not unique to therapies, since many nurses who do not use therapies, use a holistic assessment.

Holistic assessment results in a relationship developing between the nurse and the patient in which they:

• Share power
• Information
• Responsibility.

In this way, patients are encouraged to be actively involved in their own recovery.

COUNSELLING AND HELPING

The response to therapy varies from patient to patient. For some, it may trigger the disclosure of their fears and anxieties, whilst others may just prefer to quietly enjoy the therapy. The therapist will need to be aware of this and facilitate the appropriate response. Quiet may mean enjoying silence, or it may involve using music to create a therapeutic environment. It is important to note that the use of music is personal to the patient. It may produce a feeling of calmness and tranquillity, but if the music or aroma evokes a painful memory, it can create a state of anxiety.

For the patients who prefer to talk throughout the therapy, conversations will occur on different levels. Many patients talk about general issues before relaxing and then quietly enjoying the therapy. Others have issues they wish to discuss such as diet or how to manage their stress. A holistic practitioner should be able to cope with these. However, if a patient requires more specialised help, there may be other members of the multidisciplinary team who are better qualified to give it. Examples of these are stress and anxiety management techniques which occupational therapists or psychologists often teach.

LISTENING SKILLS

Any therapist should have well developed listening skills to help patients who disclose information, which is triggered by the therapy. This is considered to be a prerequisite before commencing the ENB A49 Complementary Therapy courses. Many nurses find it beneficial to develop their counselling skills even further, in order to expand their practice.

Part of this developmental process is self awareness, which requires the nurse to know her prejudices, and most importantly, her limitations. Being self aware means that she understands her capabilities, but also knows when to refer the patient to others within the team, to a reputable therapist or to outside counselling agencies.

When nurses are providing therapies, they mainly use helping or counselling skills, as opposed to conducting actual counselling. Some authors separate the terms helping and counselling, whilst others use them simultaneously. However, their similarities lie at the core of the qualities required of the therapist:

- Empathy
- Warmth
- Genuineness.

Where the therapist and counsellor differ, is in the skills and techniques used by a trained counsellor and in the contract which the counsellor makes regarding the counselling goals. However, some therapists are trained counsellors and combine counselling with giving a therapy.

Having identified that listening is important it is

useful to look at what therapeutic listening involves. Van Ooijen & Charnock (1994) state that it has three phases:

1. Receiving and understanding
2. Communication of your understanding
3. An awareness in the other person that you have listened and understood.

To achieve this, the therapist must try to see things from the patient's frame of reference, by listening not only to what they are saying, but to how they are saying it. This requires attention to both verbal and non-verbal clues. The therapist will need to note if the two match, as occasionally the patient will say that they are all right, when their body language is saying just the opposite.

When using massage, a therapist is in a prime position to do this, as tension can easily be identified in the form of tense muscles. Common areas where tension is held are the neck and shoulders and lower back. These respond well to aromatherapy massage.

However, if the patient is saying that they are comfortable with the massage, but instinctively you feel this is not the case, it is useful to ask yourself the following questions:

- Is the therapeutic relationship right?
- Am I working in a partnership with the patient?
- Is the massage technique and pressure correct?
- Have their privacy and dignity been maintained?
- Is the use of music, silence, conversation or counselling skills appropriate?
- Is the patient comfortable with touch?
- Am I touching/massaging the right area?

When addressing the last two questions, it is important to note that although some people say they are comfortable with touch, in reality this is not always the case. If you sense that this is happening, you may want to try massaging other parts of the body as this sometimes resolves the problem. When this approach does not work, it may be more effective to change the therapy, as touch could have negative connotations relating to past experiences. These feelings could either be conscious or subconscious. A simple solution is to change to a non-touch therapy such as relaxation, which still provides the therapeutic relationship, but without the touch. However, this approach avoids, rather than addresses the underlying problem. It would be chosen when the patient is not aware, or denies that there is an underlying problem, where they do not want to look at the problem, or if time is limited. Most importantly, it would be used where the therapist lacks the skills to address the underlying problem.

Where it is appropriate to address the underlying problem, this can be done in two ways. Touch could be gradually introduced in a non threatening way, for example by using a simple holding technique such as Reiki (see page 244). This is undertaken with the patient fully clothed and often feels less invasive. Alternatively, massage can be performed with the clothes still on. Secondly, if the patient wants to address some of their underlying problems, they could be referred for appropriate counselling.

Other types of counselling which may prove beneficial as an adjunct to therapies are:

- Sexual counselling
- Bereavement counselling
- Transactional analysis (TA)
- Neuro-linguistic programming.

Sexual counselling is addressed in Chapter 6. It is important to note that in order to help patients cope with their sexuality we need to understand the nature of sexuality. Nurses often fail to acknowledge how broad it is, encompassing everything about being a man or a woman, including aspects such as:

- Body image
- Self esteem
- Self concept
- Self worth
- Gender
- Role.

If therapists work as holistic practitioners, sexuality should be an important aspect of the care they give.

Body image

One way of helping patients come to terms with their altered body image, is by massaging hands that have been deformed by rheumatoid arthritis (RA). It works through demonstrating an acceptance of them. An example where massage was useful for body image is illustrated in the case study in Box 13.1.

13.1 Case study   Massage for spinal curvature

John was a 43-year-old man with a long history of anky-losing spondylitis. He had a marked spinal curvature and massage could only be undertaken when he was sitting upright, leaning over the bed, supported by pillows. On completion of the massage John was asked to evaluate it. He replied by saying that what he enjoyed most was the touch. He went on to explain that I had touched him for

years, but this was the first time it had been just for him. This demonstrated how the use of expressive touch, could have a positive effect on the patient's body image.

NEURO-LINGUISTIC PROGRAMMING

Neuro-linguistic programming is an extremely effective tool for change. Its techniques are fast and very powerful, and it can be used in any situation for both simple problems and for more complex behavioural and emotional problems.

The neuro-linguistic programming practitioner gently focuses on what the patient wants to change. Using gentle questioning, they encourage the patient to become aware of how they have programmed themselves to respond in the way that they do. The patients are then encouraged to realise their own potential for change and to re-programme a more useful response. It is particularly useful for:

- Increasing communication skills
- Dealing with relationship problems
- Treating phobias, habits, nerves, panic attacks
- Helping to change limiting beliefs and feelings.

GRIEF AND LOSS

When using complementary therapies, it is important that the nurse is aware of issues surrounding grief and loss. Patients with long standing chronic diseases such as arthritis, may be trying to come to terms with varying degrees of loss. Each exacerbation of the disease may bring about further disability, resulting in loss of independence, status and role. As a result, the patient will need help and support over this difficult time.

Studies have identified that people go through a number of stages when faced with loss. A classic study undertaken by Kubler-Ross (1969) identified five stages:

1. Shock and denial
2. Anger
3. Bargaining
4. Depression
5. Acceptance.

These stages are helpful in highlighting what should be considered as normal behaviour. However, the model also has its critics. Buckman (1993) feels that patients do not necessarily go through stages, but rather that they demonstrate a range of emotions such as anger, blame, guilt and shame.

Worden (1984) suggests that in order to work through loss and successfully complete mourning there are four tasks that the person has to work through. The most important is working through the pain that the loss brings. Nurses can support and facilitate this by using therapies. Allowing the patient to grieve may involve encouraging them to express their emotions, which may involve them crying, expressing anger or working through feelings of guilt.

MASSAGE

Massage is a skill, formally used by nurses, but which fell out of favour until fairly recently. It can vary from a simple stroking technique, which is taught quite easily, to a more complex skill, requiring a lengthy training. Therapeutic massage involves manipulation of the soft tissues of the body and can relieve tension and increase relaxation. A massage has the effect of calming the mind, soothing the nerves and relaxing the body.

- It reduces pain and stiffness by relaxing tight, aching muscles.
- It reduces pain by stimulating large diameter fibres which has an effect on the gate control mechanism in the spinal cord (see Ch. 8).
- It nourishes tissues and assists in the removal of waste, through increases in blood and lymphatic circulation.
- It can lower the blood pressure, pulse and respiration rates.
- It promotes relaxation, if the massage is slow and soothing.
- It increases a feeling of wellbeing and helps with symptoms such as fatigue and depression, especially if the massage is slightly more stimulating.

Despite the contraindications to massage mentioned in most books, it is useful for problems associated with many rheumatological conditions. In practice, if great care is taken, there are few patients for whom massage is contraindicated. This can be achieved by modifying the massage to suit the patient, avoiding certain parts of the body. Generally only small areas are massaged such as back, neck and shoulder, hands, feet or face.

Massage is useful for back, neck and shoulder problems, including whiplash and shoulder injuries and has proved effective for headaches and migraine. Many arthritic problems respond well to massage, especially if it is very gentle and avoids pressure on swollen joints. However, if the patient has a temperature, or feels generally unwell, it is best avoided, and replaced with aromatherapy treatments, as they may be more therapeutic.

The UKCC (1993) recommends that nurses who practise any complementary therapy, practise at a level at which they are competent. This may allow them to use simple massage, but would require them to undertake a long course in order to use essential oils or perform a more therapeutic massage. If essential oils are to be used it is recommended that the nurse should have undertaken a long aromatherapy course which included blending the oils, and the chemistry of at least 40 oils.

AROMATHERAPY

Aromatherapy is an ancient healing art that has gained popularity recently, to become one of the most popular therapies both for nurses and patients. It involves the controlled use of essential oils, manufactured from plant materials, to promote healing and relaxation of the body, mind and emotions. The oils have a balancing effect on the mind and body. When analysing the research relating to aromatherapy, it is clear that in the UK, its practice is still in its infancy. This is in contrast with continental Europe where it is more widely accepted by doctors and where much more research has been undertaken. Research has demonstrated that the effects of touch and massage, benefit all age groups and are of particular importance in times of stress (Autton 1989).

The benefits of the therapy come from its variety of uses:

- Massage
- Baths
- Inhalations
- Compresses
- Creams
- Irrigations
- Mouthwashes
- Room fragrances.

Aromatherapy massage

Aromatherapy massage involves using a carrier oil, such as grapeseed or sweet almond oil. Concentrations of essential oils vary, but the lower dose of 1–1.5% which is 2–3 drops in 10 ml of oil, recommended by Price & Price (1995), is probably best suited to patients with rheumatic disease. The choice of essential oil is decided between the patient and the nurse, based on a number of factors. These are, patient's problems, any contraindications to certain oils, such as high blood pressure, epilepsy and allergies and the aroma of the blend. Oils which have proved useful for arthritis are:

- Lavender (*Lavendula angustafolia*)
- Roman chamomile (*Anthemis nobilis*)
- Lemon (*Citrus limonu*)
- Ginger (*Zingiber officinale*)
- Marjoram (*Origanum majorana*)
- Juniper berry (*Juniperus communis*)
- Black pepper (*Piper nigrum*)
- Rosemary (*Rosmarinus officinalis*)
- Eucalyptus (*Eucalyptus globulus*).

The nurse would use a combination of one or two of these, or she may choose alternatives to help with the patient's other problems.

Positioning the patient for massage is not always easy and is often dictated by what is comfortable. The optimum position is usually achieved by using pillows and many massages are performed with the patient sitting up resting on pillows. In addition to the requirements of the patient, it is important that the nurse finds a position, in which her back is not compromised.

Bathing

Essential oils can be useful in bathing, either in addition to massage, or as an alternative, when massage is not appropriate. Appropriate essential oils are those previously stated as being useful for arthritis. Alternatively, lavender, marjoram, Roman chamomile or sandalwood could be chosen to help with sleep problems.

After half filling the bath with warm water, 3–6 drops of essential oils are added and dispersed by agitating the water. The patient can relax in the bath for 10 to 20 minutes.

The guidelines regarding training and use of oils should still apply. Although their use in this application may appear simple, it should not be undertaken by staff who are not trained to use the essential oils. Care must be taken to watch for skin sensitivity, especially with ginger and black pepper and it is important that before submerging patients in a bath containing essential oils, a patch test is performed, to test for sensitivity (Price & Price 1995).

Inhalation

Inhalation is a simple, but effective way of using aromatherapy. The oils are absorbed through the nose and travel via the olfactory system to the limbic system in the brain. Inhalation can be used in one of two ways: one or two drops of essential oil are placed on a tissue

that can be placed on the pillow; alternatively, between three and six drops of oils are placed in a bowl of hot water. This is particularly effective in relieving congestion. Essential oils which may be useful are:

- Eucalyptus (*Eucalyptus globulus*)
- Benzoin (*Styrax benzoin*)
- Peppermint (*Mentha piperita*)
- Rosemary (*Rosmarinus officinalis*)
- Sandalwood (*Santalum album*)
- Frankincense (*Boswelia carter*).

Compress

A compress is particularly useful where massage is not suitable but where an inflamed joint or area of skin could benefit from the effects of the compress, combined with the therapeutic effects of the oils. Two oils that have proved useful due to their anti-inflammatory properties, are lavender and Roman chamomile. Again a patch test is recommended first and then two to three drops of oils added to one pint of either warm or cold water. This solution can also be used to irrigate an infected wound. These are useful due to the fact that all of the of the oils have antiseptic properties, some are antibacterial and others are antifungal or antiviral, (Price & Price 1995).

Creams

Creams are particularly useful where a skin condition is evident. Some skin conditions may be secondary to the disease, such as psoriasis or the butterfly rash associated with systemic lupus erythematosus. Others may be related to conditions such as athlete's foot. An aqueous cream is used as the base and two to three drops of essential oils added to each 10 ml of cream.

Mouthwash

This has two uses: to freshen the mouth; and when there is an infection of the mouth, gums or throat. In this case antifungal/antibacterial oils such as lemon, teatree (*Melaleuca alternifolia*) or peppermint should be used. Fill half a cup with warm water and add two to three drops of essential oils.

Room fragrance

This can be used to:

- Make a room smell nice
- Lift moods
- Neutralise an offensive smell.

Bear in mind that aromas are individual and so this form of aromatherapy should not be undertaken in wards or bays, just individual rooms.

Add five to six drops of essential oils to water and add it to an electric vaporiser.

13.2 Case study Baths for psoriasis

Jean was a 44-year-old woman with long-standing psoriatic arthritis. The psoriasis was over most of her body, but it was particularly problematic in the hairline and had a tendency to bleed. Baths using lavender and Roman chamomile took away the irritation from the body. Aqueous cream with the same oils dramatically improved the hairline.

13.3 Case study A variety of treatments

Sometimes it is useful to use a variety of methods, as illustrated by the following case study.

Linda was a 30-year-old woman who had been diagnosed as having systemic lupus erythematosus for the past 5 years. Her main problems were pain, fatigue, tension, anxiety, sleep problems, poor circulation, photosensitivity and a very marked butterfly rash.

A variety of treatments were used:

- Aqeuous cream with two drops of lavender and one drop of Roman chamomile to 10 ml of cream was applied daily to the rash. This allowed Linda to stop using her steroid cream.
- Weekly or fortnightly massage to back, arms and legs, to help relieve pain, tension and circulatory problems. The essential oils chosen were varied over time and a maximum of three were used together. Examples were eucalyptus, lavender, ylang ylang (*Canango odorata*), marjoram, sandalwood, black pepper and ginger.
- To help with anxiety and to support her whilst her beta-blockers were being reduced, neroli oil (*Citrus aurantium*) an anxiolytic oil was used.
- To support her at home, between treatments and to help her sleep problems, Linda was recommended to use essential oils in the bath.

This regime proved very effective and both her rheumatologist and her general practitioner were happy with the result. Before Linda received these treatments she experienced much pain and tension. Following them she required less analgesia and her quality of life was greatly improved.

HEALING

The human potential for transmitting energies is not new. Some societies take healing for granted, whilst in others healing is still considered to be one of the more 'fringe' complementary therapies. This situation is changing and there has been an increased interest in healing over recent years. Some nurses have introduced healing into their practice, although it is still considered to be in its infancy in the UK. By contrast, in the USA it is widely taught and practised and is now part of mainstream nursing. Delores Kreiger, who introduced it in 1974, has been instrumental in encouraging research into its effectiveness.

Confusion often arises over the names used to describe healing:

- Spiritual healing
- Faith healing
- Reiki
- Therapeutic touch.

Whilst the techniques vary slightly, they have many similarities. For each of them, the patient is fully clothed and is either lying on a couch or bed, or alternatively, sitting on a chair. The technique is non-invasive, involving either light touch or holding techniques. Alternatively the practitioner can work without touching the patient, as in therapeutic touch, with their hands hovering over the patient.

Sayer-Adams and Wright (1995) who teach therapeutic touch in England describe it as 'a consciously directed process of energy exchange during which the practitioner uses the hands as a focus to facilitate healing'. They see it is a contemporary interpretation of ancient healing practices and it is dependent upon the healer being able to channel these energies. Kreiger (1993) proposes that therapeutic touch can be useful in four areas:

1. To promote relaxation
2. To reduce pain
3. In treating psychosomatic illnesses
4. To increase wound healing.

Effectiveness in wound healing has been demonstrated through research Benor (1991), and an increase in callus formation of fractures has been evident on X-rays at two and a half weeks (Sayer-Adams & Wright 1995).

The benefits noted by Kreiger (1993) are relevant to rheumatology patients. Also the non-touch or the light holding techniques, may prove more acceptable to an anxious patient who has high levels of pain, than a more invasive or vigorous form of therapy.

Reiki

Reiki is another ancient form of healing which was rediscovered in the nineteenth century in Japan by a Dr Mikauuswi. Its uses are similar to those of therapeutic touch. A treatment takes between 20 minutes and 1 hour. The practitioner's hands are positioned either on or over the patient in specific areas (the chakras). Each person reacts in a different way, but the aim is to restore balance within the body. Following treatment, patients report pleasant feelings of security and a sense of peace and relaxation (Baginski & Sharamon 1988).

Anxiety management

Anxiety management can be used for patients who have been diagnosed as having clinical anxiety. Examples where it might be useful are panic attacks, specific phobias or where there are generalised social problems. It is not generally considered suitable for people with 'free floating anxiety' (an unrealistic feeling of impending disaster).

The therapist can either work one to one with a patient, or with a group. A cognitive behavioural approach is adopted in an effort to break the anxiety spiral. The overall aim is to facilitate the individual's own resources, so that they can be helped to overcome their fear, in a structured and supportive environment. This involves teaching the patient relaxation and breathing techniques. They are encouraged to understand the relationship between avoidance behaviour and the maintenance of phobia or panic and are involved in a programme of desensitisation.

These techniques can be used either independently or in conjunction with anxiolytic medication.

Stress management

Stress is part of all our lives. However, it is particularly evident when people are attempting to come to terms with a chronic illness and for whom the future is uncertain. The aim of stress management is to teach the individual how to:

- Reduce levels of stress
- Cope more effectively with stressors
- Learn to channel energy more positively.

Stress management can be taught on an individual basis or in a group.

The patients are taught to:

- Develop an insight into their stressors and the effects of these on the mind, body and behaviours

- Understand how their personality and personal beliefs may perpetuate stressful living
- Develop strategies for managing stress healthily.

Stress management training is appropriate for any patient who believes that his or her ill health may be caused by, or exacerbated by, stressful living. It is not appropriate for any patient who is suffering from panic attacks or clinical anxiety.

It can be seen that either stress or anxiety management techniques could be beneficial for certain patients with rheumatic disease. These might include those with chronic back pain, fibromyalgia, chronic fatigue syndrome and also all patients for whom suffering from a degenerative disease has increased their stress levels.

Bach flower remedies

By the time he died in 1939, Dr Edward Bach had developed 38 flower remedies, to treat every possible emotional state. These can be used separately or in combinations. When using flower remedies, the nurse is encouraged to focus on the person who has the disease and to ignore as far as possible, any physical symptoms. The remedies are selected according to the personality of the person and the aim is to transform negative thoughts and behaviour into positive ones (Ball 1996).

Remedies can be taken in two ways:

1. Place two drops of each chosen remedy into a glass of water and sip four times a day until the problem goes away
2. Place two drops into a bottle and fill up with 30 ml of mineral water. Keep it in the refrigerator and use four drops, four times a day.

In addition to the other remedies, Dr Bach developed a Rescue Remedy to use in a crisis. This is a mixture of five remedies:

1. Star of Bethlehem for shock
2. Rock Rose for terror
3. Impatiens for agitation
4. Cherry Plum to help with loss of self-control
5. Clematis for light-headedness.

In an emergency, four drops can be placed on the tongue, or rubbed onto the pulse points. Alternatively, four drops can be taken in a glass of water. Ball (1996) suggests that the remedies are completely safe, they mix well with other drugs, are free from side effects and it is not possible to overdose by using them.

Homeopathy

Homeopathy is considered to be a complete system of healing (Pietroni 1995). It has gained acceptance in the UK where it is one of the few complementary therapies, which has been available through the National Health Service. Homeopathy was developed by Dr Samuel Hanemann who observed that many of the treatments given to treat disease, actually cause symptoms similar to those produced by the disease itself. An example of this was observed when quinine was used to treat malaria. In high doses it caused the high temperature, sweats, and rigors experienced in a malarial attack. Hanemann then set about developing a system which required giving only very minute amounts of the treatment. This was based on the principle that 'like cures like'.

The homeopathic remedies are obtained from animal, mineral or plant extracts and are preserved in an alcohol solution which is then called 'the mother tincture'. This is the basis of the remedies and is diluted to form the various strengths. The remedies are effective at minute strengths because they are 'potentized' by a system of shaking called succession, which was developed by Hanemann. It is not fully understood how this works, but it is thought to affect the molecular structure of the liquid by leaving 'footprints' of the active ingredient on each molecule. This 'energetic memory' of the remedy is then left behind (Pietroni 1995).

Research into homeopathy has not been sufficiently conclusive to satisfy some sceptics who attribute its results purely to the placebo effect. However, this does not fully explain the results achieved by homeopathic veterinary surgeons, who successfully treat cattle with mastitis by adding remedies to their feed, or laboratory results which show the prevention of recurrent abortions in pigs (Pietroni 1995).

Chaitow (1995) reports variable results from several studies that have investigated the effects of Rhustox, in treating fibromyalgia.

ACUPUNCTURE IN RHEUMATOLOGY

The word acupuncture derives from the Latin *acus* meaning needle and *punctura* to puncture the skin. Acupuncture originated in China approximately 4000 years ago and has developed today into an intricate holistic approach to healing. It is a treatment that aims to diagnose illness, as well as aiding the body to restore a balance, which in turn promotes health.

History of acupuncture

It is uncertain how acupuncture originated in China.

One theory is that it was developed as a result of non-fatal arrow wounds that seemed to improve individuals' long-standing conditions. Others suggested that finger pressure over certain body points was observed to ease both physical and mental problems. The Chinese enhanced results by applying greater pressure, using stones and eventually pierced the skin using slivers of bamboo. Later they produced needles made from an array of metals including gold and silver. Today the majority of needles are produced from stainless steel.

The earliest records of acupuncture date back over 2000 years. It is thought that the earliest text was 'The Yellow Emperor's Classic of Internal Medicine' probably written between 300 and 100 BC, which described the fundamentals of Chinese medicine (Maciocia 1982, Maciocia 1993). However, it was not until many centuries later that acupuncture developed sufficiently to be utilised as a major treatment approach and gradually theories developed as to how it worked.

From the mid 1800s western medicine was introduced into China and rapidly became the dominant system of care and traditional acupuncture became marginalised. In 1949, with the formation of the People's Republic, Chinese medicine was at last given the opportunity to develop.

It was not until the 1960s that acupuncture spread from continental Europe to Britain where interest and education has flourished. The British Acupuncture Council was formed in 1995 to represent and govern professionally qualified traditional acupuncturists in all aspects of their work.

Traditional Chinese medicine approach to acupuncture

The Chinese propose that no person can separate themselves from their environment; that not only are they influenced by their surroundings but that they are an integral part of them. According to traditional law, everything in the universe, including human beings, shares a motivating energy called *qi* (pronounced chee). In translation the word qi means vital energy/force or subtle breath.

Yin/Yang

The theory of yin and yang is fundamental to oriental medicine (Fig. 13.1). Health is achieved by maintaining a balance between the yin and yang, the equal and opposite qualities of the qi. Literally the words yin and yang mean two banks of a river one in shade the other in sun. Thus shade, dampness and cold represent the

Figure 13.1 Diagrammatic representation of Yin-Yang principle.

Table 13.1 Examples of Yin-Yang correspondences

Yin	Yang
Night	Day
Cold	Hot
Shade	Brightness
Feminine	Masculine
Chronic	Acute
Gradual onset	Rapid onset
Fatigue	Restlessness
Pallor	Red face
Thirst	No thirst
Weak pulse	Full pulse
Loud voice, talks a lot	Weak voice, dislikes talking

character of yin whereas yang is akin to brightness and heat. They represent the concept of opposite stages in the cycles of life, which are dynamic and yet dependent on one another. It is thought that nothing in the world escapes this principle (Table 13.1).

Aspects of life can disturb the fine balance of yin-yang, disturb the flow of qi and result in disease or disharmony. These factors include emotional states such as anger, stress, grief and anxiety. A poor diet, which includes irregular meals, over or under eating, an excess of spicy, greasy, raw, salty or processed foods, is also detrimental. Weather conditions such as dampness, cold or wind may harm the qi together with a poor environment, hereditary factors, recreational drugs, infections and trauma.

Meridians

In individuals qi flows throughout the body but is concentrated along 14 major (12 are coupled) and 8 connecting channels or *Meridians*. Throughout the day and with the changes of the seasons the qi fluctuates but if it remains balanced, health will be maintained.

The main principle of acupuncture treatment is to restore the flow of the qi and the balance between the equal and opposite qualities of yin and yang. It achieves this by needling acupuncture points that lie along the meridians. There are approximately 800 acupoints and with appropriate needling the practi-

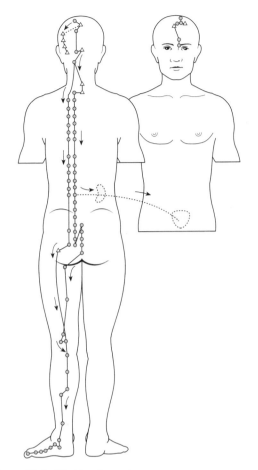

Figure 13.2 Bladder channels.

tioner is able to re-balance patients and thus enhance the body's self recuperation (Fig. 13.2).

The five elements

In addition to the theories of meridians and yin-yang the Chinese describe the inter-relating concept of the 'five elements':

1. Wood
2. Fire
3. Earth
4. Metal
5. Water.

They are each analogous with a system of correspondences which incorporate the meridians, major organs, seasons, emotions and even voice qualities. Each element is allied to a specific season, specific emotion and meridian (Table 13.2).

Table 13.2 The five element correspondences

Element	Wood	Fire	Earth	Metal	Water
Meridians	Gall bladder	Small intestine	Stomach	Lung	Bladder
	Liver	Heart	Spleen	Colon	Kidney
		Heart constrictor			
		Triple burner			
Season	Spring	Summer	Late summer	Autumn	Winter
Climate	Wind	Heat	Humidity	Dryness	Cold
Nourishes	Muscles	Blood vessels	Flesh	Skin	Bones
Sense	Sight	Speech	Taste	Smell	Hearing
Flavour	Sour	Bitter	Sweet	Pungent	Salt
Emotion	Aggression	Joy	Calmness	Sympathy	Caution
Excess emotion	Anger	Over-excitement	Depression	Grief	Fear
Voice	Shout	Laughter	Singing	Weeping	Groaning
Cereal	Wheat	Rice	Maize	Oats	Beans

These five elements relate profoundly to one another, so that when there is an imbalance within one element then there is a knock-on effect on the rest of the cycle causing disharmony within other elements. Eventually the discord will exhibit as either a physical or emotional condition associated with the errant elements within the cycle. Acupuncturists are trained to recognise the signs of imbalance associated with each element and are taught the approaches to redress the balance.

Western approach to acupuncture

The scientific opinion of acupuncture rejects the traditional theories of yin-yang, qi and the five elements. Instead it proposes that research findings support the theory that the release of endogenous opioids could mediate acupuncture analgesia. B-endorphin seems to be the major component in producing long lasting pain relief. Recently it has been proposed that the analgesic action of acupuncture could also be partly explained by the release of 5-HT from nerves stimulated by electro-acupuncture at 200 Hz. Acupuncture is also recognised as a 'potent anti-emetic', possibly acting by the same mechanism as ondansetron. It also has anti-depressant action, perhaps through altering 5-HT mobilisation in the brain (Starr 1994).

Melzack & Wall (1965) first put forward the 'gate theory' in order to explain various mechanisms for reducing pain (see Ch. 8). Acupuncture, along with other stimulatory techniques such as massage, heat, cold and transcutaneous nerve stimulation (TENS), are thought to help to close hypothetical gates in the spinal column which signal pain. It is suggested that acupuncture promotes the release of steroids which will particularly benefit the treatment of painful rhematological conditions.

The traditional Chinese diagnosis of rheumatological conditions

In Chinese medicine the term Bi syndrome accounts not only for rheumatological conditions but also for pain, aching and stiffness in muscles, joints, bones and tendons. The syndrome is generally thought to be caused by the blockage or obstruction in the circulation of qi and blood through the meridians. Conditions are thought to arise when the meridians are hindered by an external influence such as wind, cold and or dampness. This is why rheumatism and arthritis are more prevalent in cold damp environments according to oriental teaching. Although these external factors predominate they can also give rise to heat in the body which accounts for febrile conditions.

Five principle blockages are described in acupuncture, they are as follows:

- **Wandering Bi**

This is very much akin to rheumatoid arthritis (RA). The Chinese describe this obstruction as causing flitting pains which are widespread. Frequently there is fever and chills, the pulse is usually rapid and the tongue will have a yellow coating. Patients often react to windy conditions and changes in the barometric pressure.

- **Painful Bi**

Pain tends to be severe and restricted to specific joints. Warmth alleviates discomfort whereas cold aggravates this condition. The pulse is usually deep and wiry and the tongue will have a thin white coating.

• **Stationary Bi**

Pain is localised and does not move. It is associated with damp and it causes stiffness and swelling around joints. A damp environment or the approach of wet weather will exacerbate this condition. The tongue will appear swollen with a 'greasy' coating whereas the pulse will be moderate.

• **Heat Bi**

Heat is the predominant factor, which may have originated from the external influences of wind, cold or damp. One or several joints may be affected and inflammation and swelling will be evident. Pain is usually chronic and severe. The pulse is usually rapid and the tongue will have a yellow coating.

• **Boney Bi**

The prolonged lack of movement of blood produces phlegm which results in obstruction around joints causing swelling and degeneration with resulting pain.

TREATMENT OF RHEUMATOLOGICAL CONDITIONS

Treatment for all of the above syndromes is directed towards restoring a balance by opening the meridians to spread the qi and blood.

The traditional approach involves a detailed history taking which includes; feeling the pulses at the wrist, which gives considerable information to the practitioner about a patient's energy levels, examination of the tongue which is said to reflect what is happening throughout the patient's body. Once a diagnosis has been reached needles are inserted into appropriate meridian points which may be quite distant from the affected joints. Needling techniques are complex and sometimes a technique known a *moxibustion* is used, in which a dried herb or moxa is heated on or around needles.

13.4 Case study Acupuncture for rheumatoid arthritis

A 42-year-old woman presented with a 3-year history of RA. Initially her hands, wrists, feet, ankles, and elbows were affected and were hot, painful and swollen. As her condition developed some of her joints became deformed. On examination her tongue was red with a sticky yellow coating and her pulse was rapid.

The traditional diagnosis was Heat bi with phlegm obstructing the joints causing swelling and deformities. Treatment was aimed at reducing heat, clearing damp and removing obstructions from the channels. After only three treatments she experienced considerable improvement in pain, inflammation and swelling. She needed a further five sessions after which she required less medication and was able to walk much further without pain and use her hands more effectively.

Western acupuncture will focus on needling locally around affected joints and stimulating each needle either manually, by lifting and turning, until a heavy, tingling sensation is experienced or by attaching electrical acupuncture machines to the needles, which will enhance the production of endorphins. Treatment is aimed at relieving pain and does not recognise the theory of obstruction and blockages.

RESEARCH INTO ACUPUNCTURE

Acupuncture does not lend itself easily to controlled trials. Frequently, formula treatments are incorporated which do not fairly reflect traditional acupuncture. Often sham points are used, which when carefully examined turn out to be acupuncture non-meridial, extra points. Patients taking oral corticosteroids or who have had recent steroid injections will not respond well to acupuncture and usually require extra treatments. This is often not taken into account. Acupuncture does not always work immediately but may help the individual to slowly start to recuperate. All these factors make crossover studies difficult to assess (MacPherson & Blackwell 1994).

One study investigated knee pain in patients with RA (Man & Barger 1973). Twenty patients with pain in both knees were randomly allocated to two groups. Those in one group had a single steroid injection in one knee and in the other knee, a single electro-acupuncture treatment using only three points. Those in the second group also had one knee treated with a single steroid injection but the other knee had sham acupuncture. Pain, inflammation and range of movement were assessed before and after treatment by a physiotherapist who was unaware to which group patients had been assigned.

The results showed that in knees given the true acupuncture treatment, a 90% reduction in pain was noted, which lasted from 1–3 months, whereas for the knees which had the sham acupuncture only a 10% improvement in pain was noted and the effects lasted less than 10 hours.

Clinical research into acupuncture may need to be adapted and more carefully designed to take into account the traditional approach.

The treatment of RA, osteoarthritis (OA), fibromyalgia and many more conditions in rheumatology are still difficult to treat and not well understood by orthodox medicine. The Chinese, over thousands of years, have developed a holistic approach to health and disease, based on the subtle interplay between the opposing forces. This appears to enables them to successfully treat conditions that western medicine can only palliate. It is hoped that the future will see acupuncture and Chinese herbal medicine more readily considered and researched, so that patients may benefit from the best of western and eastern medical treatments.

REFLEXOLOGY IN RHEUMATOLOGY

Reflexology or Reflex Zone Therapy is a therapy in which the nerve endings of the feet are treated using precise compression massage. The zones of the feet that are treated are said to be connected to different parts of the body by a flow of energy. By treating the feet in this way the practitioner helps the body to re-balance and overcome ill health.

There is evidence that in India and China, massage and pressure treatments to the hands and feet were practised as much as 5000 years ago. Certainly in ancient Egypt primitive forms of this therapy were utilised. Paintings found in an Egyptian tomb depicted feet and hands being treated. The great Florentine sculptor, Cellini (1500–1571), was known to have used strong pressure to both his fingers and toes in order to relieve pain in other parts of his body, with great success.

An American ear, nose and throat surgeon, William Fitzgerald, who practised during the early 1900s, founded the therapy that we know today. He noticed that pressure applied to specific areas of the body, such as the nose, mouth and throat, led to a degree of local anaesthesia. This fired his interest and led him to test various parts of the body. He found that pressing over hands and feet also brought about analgesic results. By 1915, he was able to publish his principles of 'zone therapy' which mapped out various zones on the feet and the corresponding ten zones of the body (Fig. 13.3).

During the 1930s an American physiotherapist,

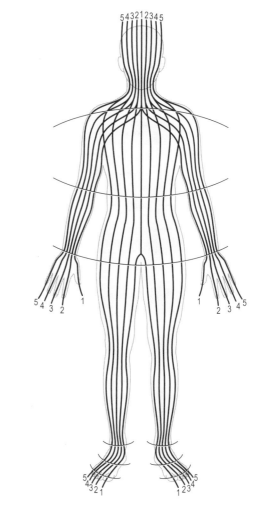

Figure 13.3 Ten zones of the body.

Eunice Ingham, developed Fitzgerald's principles and devised a precise approach to a therapy on the feet, which could be used to treat all parts of the body. She described her techniques in her book 'Stories the feet can tell' (Ingham 1992).

The zones of the body

Fitzgerald described the feet as being divided from heal to toe into ten fields, each of which corresponded to one of ten vertical body zones. For example the spine lies in the vertical body zone on the left and right of the body. It is reflected in body zone 1 of the feet, along the longitudinal arch of both feet (Hanne Marqardt 1983) (Fig. 13.4).

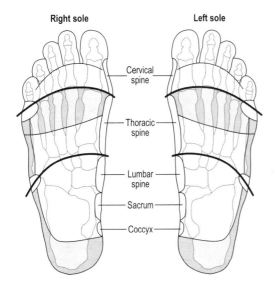

Right sole   **Left sole**

Cervical spine

Thoracic spine

Lumbar spine

Sacrum

Coccyx

Figure 13.4 The spinal column zones of the feet.

Treatment

Once the practitioner has taken a full history, the patient is made comfortable, either by lying down on a treatment couch or recliner chair. The feet are exposed and their appearance, tissue tone and general health is carefully noted.

Treatment involves firm but not painful compression strokes to the dorsum and plantar aspects of the feet, using the fingers and thumbs. The zones are often quite small, so the practitioner must be precise during the session. As the treatment progresses, certain zones may be tender reflecting an imbalance in this body area. Gentle compression treatment is applied to any affected zone.

Treatments must be tailored carefully to each individual, as responses can be dramatic. Seriously ill patients may not be able to tolerate a full treatment and the elderly and very young require a gentler approach.

Between treatments, patients may experience reactions such as:

- Increased nasal discharge
- Increased bowel movements
- Slightly offensive urine
- Skin problems
- Slight changes in the menstrual cycle.

This is a positive response that demonstrates that the body is starting to rebalance.

Reflexology is a simple easily learnt therapy that is ideally suited to nurse training. It has the potential to give symptom relief, ranging from pain relief to the management of constipation, stress and relaxation.

RESEARCH INTO REFLEXOLOGY AS APPLIED TO RHEUMATOLOGY

Research in reflex zone therapy is sparse. A limited study at the Hospital of Beijing College looked at its effect on acute low back pain in a group of teachers and office workers. Twenty patients, aged between 35 and 55 years, were given up to ten treatments but no other treatments or medication. All patients reported that the treatment effectively eliminated their pain and 25% had improvement after only one session. The remainder had improvement by the seventh session.

It can be seen from this chapter that therapeutic interventions have a role to play in enhancing the care given to rheumatology patients. Before implementing any therapy there are many factors that need addressing such as:

- Training
- Consent
- Safety
- Competency
- Efficacy
- Appropriateness.

The benefits resulting from using therapies come from a variety of sources. These are the holistic assessment, the therapeutic relationship, the restoration of control, the benefits from individual therapies (such as massage and essential oil) and, through offering time, touch and compassion. Each therapy works in a different way, but ultimately they all try to restore homeostasis within the person. The research basis for these therapies varies, but it is felt that nurses have a role to play in increasing the body of knowledge, through evaluation of the therapies as they use them.

Action points for practice:

- Describe what is meant by the terms Yin and Yang.
- In reflexology, how many vertical body zones are represented on the hands and feet?
- List the three phases involved in therapeutic listening.
- A 38-year-old male patient has psoriatic arthritis. Discuss the complementary therapies that may help him.

REFERENCES

Autton N 1989 Touch: An exploration. Longman, London.

Baginski B J, Sharamon S 1988 Reiki universal life energy. Life Rhythm, Germany

Ball S 1996 Healing the emotions. Holistic Nurses Association UK Centre Newsletter 3(4): 3

Benner P, Wrubel J 1989 The primacy of caring, stress and coping in health and illness. Addison Wesley, California

British Medical Association Report 1986 Report of the BMA Board of Science Working Party on alternative therapy. British Medical Association, Oxford University Press, Oxford

British Medical Association Report 1993 Complementary medicine: new approach to good practice. British Medical Association, Oxford University Press, Oxford

Buckman R 1993 How to break bad news: a guide for health care professionals. Macmillan, London

Chaitow L 1995 Fibromyalgia: what causes it, how it feels and what to do about it. Thorsons, London

Giovanni M 1994 The practice of Chinese medicine. Churchill Livingstone, Edinburgh

Ingham E D 1992 Stories the feet can tell through reflexology and stories the feet have told through reflexology. Ingham Publishing Corporation, London

Kreiger D 1993 The therapeutic touch: how to use your hands to help or heal. Prentice Hall, New York

Kubler-Ross E 1969 Living with death and dying. Souvenir Press, London

Maciocia G 1982 History of acupuncture. Journal of Chinese Medicine 9: 9–15

Maciocia G 1993 The foundations of Chinese medicine: a comprehensive text for acupuncturists and herbalists. Churchill Livingstone, New York

Macpherson H, Blackwell R 1994 Rheumatoid arthritis and Chinese medicine – a review. European Journal of Oriental Medicine1(3): 17–29

Man S C, Brager F D 1973 Preliminary clinical study of acupuncture in rheumatoid arthritis with painful knee. Arthritis and Rheumatism 16(4): 558–559

Marquardt H 1983 Reflex zone therapy of the feet. Thorsons, London

Melzack R, Wall P D 1965 Pain mechanisms: a new theory. Science 150: 971–978

Montbriand M J, Laing G P 1991 Alternative health care as a control strategy. Journal of Advanced Nursing 16: 325–332

Nursing Times Special Issue 1993 Complementary Therapy Autumn 90–95

Peplau H 1952 Interpersonal relations in nursing. G P Putman's, New York

Pietroni P 1995 The family guide to alternative health care. C L B Publishing, Godalming

Pietroni P, Pietroni C 1996 Innovations in community care and primary health: the Marylebone experiment. Churchill Livingstone, Edinburgh

Price S, Price L 1995 Aromatherapy for health care professionals. Churchill Livingstone, London

Rankin-Box D 1991 Proceed with caution. Nursing Times 87(45): 34–36

Rankin-Box D 1995 The nurses' handbook of complementary therapies. Acupuncture. Churchill Livingstone, Edinburgh

Rotter J B 1966 Generalised expectations for internal control versus external control reinforcements. Psychological Monographs 80: 1

Sayer-Adams J, Wright S 1995 The theory and practice of therapeutic touch. Churchill Livingstone, Edinburgh

Starr M 1994 5HT: the story so far. Acupuncture in Medicine 12(2): 100–102

Strauss A L 1984 Chronic illness and the quality of life. Mosby, St. Louis

UKCC 1993 Code of professional conduct. UKCC, London

Van Ooijen E , Charnock A 1994 Sexuality and patient care. Chapman Hall, London

Vickers A 1996 Massage and aromatherapy: a guide for health care professionals. Chapman Hall, London

Watson W H 1975 The meaning of touch. Geriatric Nursing Journal of Communication 25: 104–110

Wells C, Nown G 1993 In pain: a self help guide for chronic pain sufferers. Optima ch 9, p 197–199

Worden W J 1984 Grief counselling and grief therapy, 2nd edn. Routledge, London

FURTHER READING

O'Connor J, Bensky D 1985 Acupuncture a comprehensive text. Shanghai College of Traditional Medicine. Eastland Press, Seattle

Ellis N 1994 Acupuncture in clinical practice – a guide for health professionals. Chapman Hall, London

Maciocia G 1993 The foundations of Chinese medicine: a comprehensive text for acupuncturists and herbalists. Churchill Livingstone, New York

McMahon R, Pearson A. 1991 Nursing as therapy. Churchill Livingstone, Edinburgh

Ross J 1995 Acupuncture point combinations – the key to clinical success. Churchill Livingstone, Edinburgh

14

Surgical interventions

Catherine Sturdy

The aim of this chapter is to enable the nurse to support and care for the patient who has a rheumatic disease and is undergoing surgery. After reading this chapter you should be able to:

- **Discuss the reasons for surgical intervention in the care of a patient with rheumatic disease, and some of the problems that may be encountered**
- **Describe the specific care required by the patient with inflammatory joint disease undergoing joint surgery**
- **Describe the particular nursing assessments and care required by the patient, perioperatively**
- **Discuss the difficulties the patient faces during rehabilitation**
- **Understand the importance of multiprofessional team care.**

Surgical intervention is part of the total care of the patient with inflammatory joint disease. Thanks to the many advances in orthopaedic surgery techniques, particularly in the field of joint replacement, it is no longer regarded as the last resort when all medical treatment has failed. However, in 1983, an American orthopaedic surgeon, Mack Clayton was quoted as saying,

'For the future course of rheumatoid arthritis I have more faith in rheumatology than I do in surgery. I don't think we rheumatoid arthritis surgeons are going to be in the rheumatoid arthritis business forever, because I expect rheumatologists to find ways to control the disease. Perhaps in our lifetime we'll even see it cured!'(Fuller 1983).

Until that happens, surgery continues to have a great deal to offer.

Following total joint replacement patients with degenerative arthritis may return to near normal function, with little deterioration over time, but the patient with rheumatoid arthritis (RA) has a systemic, chronic disease which will continue to progress even after surgery. This patient will require ongoing support from all members of the multiprofessional team, particularly as a programme of surgery is often in prospect (Figgie 1994).

AIMS OF SURGICAL INTERVENTION

The primary aims of surgical procedures in rheumatology care are:

- Reduction of pain
- Improvement of function
- Maintenance of function
- Correction of deformity
- Prevention of further deformity
- Cosmesis
- Maintenance of independence.

The goal of any intervention is that the patient should be enabled to experience the best possible quality of life. Certain surgical procedures need to be carried out as a matter of urgency; for example repair of ruptured tendons in the wrist or fusion and decompression of subluxed cervical vertebrae when causing neurological symptoms. Most other surgery is elective. Although surgical intervention has a number of objectives, its main aims are reduction of pain and improvement and maintenance of function, including increased mobility and the preservation and improvement of the ability to carry out activities of living. Each patient has individual requirements and expectations and this is illustrated by a letter to a consultant from the husband of a patient with RA, awaiting knee surgery:

'She is growing more and more demoralised and frustrated by her growing immobility. She has reached the stage when she can barely walk across the room. The agony of rising from sitting to standing position is so severe that she spends most of her days and nights seated in one place and moves about as little as possible.

She is only 48 and has too many things to do that are all worth doing to resign herself to a static and useless inertia. She feels very strongly that any operation, device or regimen which offers a prospect of restoring some of her lost mobility is to be pursued now even if there is a risk of it proving detrimental or less effective than one would hope'. (Reproduced with permission)

Body image

The effect on a person's self image of the appearance of a deformed joint should not be underestimated. As Smith Pigg et al (1985) describes, 'signs of the disease or its treatment are evidence that the person is different. People who are different run the risk of interference in their interaction with others. The chronically ill, whose condition or treatment is visible, run the risk of frightening or repelling others'.

Ageing is a natural process for us all, but the grieving and adaptation to ageing and reduction of function that for most people takes place over a lifetime, can be compressed into a few years for a person with RA. (Maycock 1988). The effects of disease on body image are discussed in depth in Chapter 6.

The mere existence of a deformity is not necessarily an indication for surgery and when surgical intervention is discussed a compromise may have to be reached. Some believe that 'Cosmesis should not be considered as an important indication, although it is usually improved by increased function' (Short & Palmer 1994).

In decreasing order of importance, the aims of surgery according to Souter (1979) should be:

- Relief of pain
- Restoration of function
- Prevention of further damage
- Cosmetic improvement.

Because of this, it is imperative that patients are fully involved, and that their views are listened to, at all stages of decision making. They must have all relevant information and support, to avoid false expectations and for them to gain maximum benefit from surgery.

COMMON SURGICAL PROCEDURES

This section gives an overview of some of the surgical procedures available to people with inflammatory joint disease. The most common are:

- Arthroscopy
- Synovectomy
- Debridement
- Tenosynovectomy
- Release of contracture
- Osteotomy
- Arthroplasty
- Total arthroplasty/joint replacement
- Arthrodesis.

Arthroscopy

An arthroscopy is primarily an investigative procedure offering an opportunity to see clearly how the inside of a joint is affected by disease. Biopsies of synovial tissue may be taken. Further intervention can be planned from the information obtained. The washing out of the joint during the procedure can produce benefit by removing small loose bodies. Certain synovectomies and debridements can be performed by arthroscopic means.

Synovectomy

Synovectomy is indicated where there is excessive proliferation of synovium within one or two affected joints, but is rarely carried out if many joints are affected. It is particularly beneficial when the excess synovium is causing pain, but there is still adequate cartilage and movement in the joint.

Surgical synovectomy of the knee has been shown to provide effective pain relief in up to 70% of patients 10 years after their operation (Clayton 1963). It preserves the patient's own joint and although it may not prevent progression of disease in the joint, it does not preclude further intervention, such as total joint replacement, at a later date.

Debridement

Debridement of osteophytes may be performed as part of the above procedure. This will be at a later stage of the disease, and is not as effective in weight bearing joints as in the elbow and wrist, for example.

Tenosynovectomy

The synovium around the tendon sheath can become inflamed. Tenosynovectomy at the wrist is usually very successful at relieving pain, increasing function and preventing tendon ruptures (see Table 14.1).

Post-operative pain relief and physiotherapy are essential to enable the patient to gain full advantage from these procedures.

Release of contracture

Release of contracture is usually part of an arthroplasty procedure, but it can be used to relieve fixed flexion deformities of knees, and certain finger deformities.

Osteotomy

In osteotomy, the bone is divided near the joint and realigned. This can be useful, particularly in the knee, when the disease has 'burnt out' leaving a deformed joint. In this way, the abnormal stresses through the

Table 14.1 Rating of common elective procedures for rheumatoid arthritis. Clayton 1992 (with permission).

Procedure	Rating
Total hip arthroplasty	95
Forefoot reconstruction	90
Total knee arthroplasty	90
MCP thumb fusion	90
Dorsal wrist reconstruction (synovectomy, tenosynovectomy, excision of distal ulna)	85
Flexor tenosynovectomy of hand or wrist	85
Total shoulder arthroplasty	85
Elbow synovectomy	85
Triple arthrodesis (or talonavicular arthrodesis)	85
Total wrist arthroplasty	80
Total elbow arthroplasty	80
MCP arthroplasty	80
Wrist fusion	80
Knee synovectomy	75
Ankle fusion	75
MCP synovectomy	70
PIP synovectomy/arthroplasty/fusion	70
Hip (salvage) girdlestone	60
Knee (salvage) fusion	60
Total ankle	NR

Note: In general, procedures rated 80 and above are best for patient and surgeon. Ratings are based on a 100 point scale according to the following category/point scale:

Pain relief	40
Function	20
Prevention	10
Cosmetic	10
Complications	10
Longevity	10

lower limb, and consequent pain, can be relieved (See Fig. 14.1). This procedure is also frequently used as part of reconstructive surgery of the foot.

Arthroplasty

The term 'arthroplasty' implies a refashioning of the joint. This is performed by excision of part of the joint or by partially or totally replacing the joint with a prosthesis.

Excision arthroplasty involves the removal of the end of the bone in the affected joint. It is particularly useful in the forefoot, elbow and wrist. Occasionally silicone implants are used in addition, particularly in the small joints of the hand. These can greatly improve the cosmetic appearance, but careful assessment is essential to ensure that function is not compromised.

The most successful *total joint arthroplasties* are hip and knee replacements (Table 14.1). Figures 14.2 and

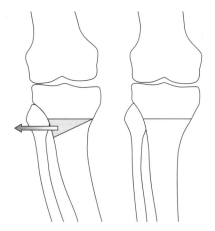

Figure 14.1 Diagrammatic representation of how a below knee osteotomy can aid realignment.

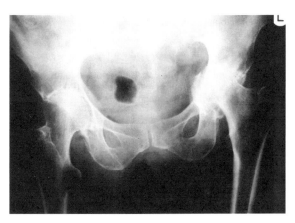

A

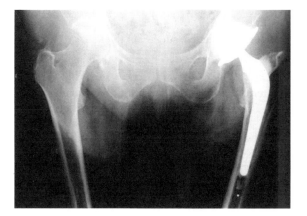

B

Figure 14.2 Total arthroplasty of the hip.
(A) Disease of the hip caused by RA. (B) The same hip following insertion of a Charnley prosthesis.

14.3 illustrate the damage that can be caused to hips and knees by RA, and the change in their appearance following total arthroplasty. These X-ray pictures are of the same patient.

Arthrodesis

An arthrodesis is the surgical fusion of a joint and is used to fix a badly affected, painful joint in a useful position. Movement in the joint or group of joints is lost, but this disadvantage can be far outweighed by the resulting relief of pain and improvement in func-

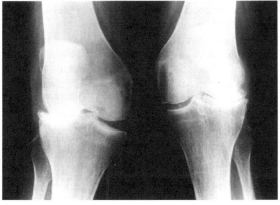

A

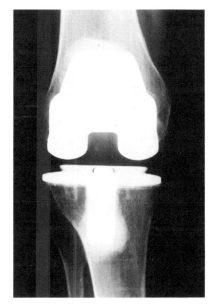

B

Figure 14.3 Total knee arthroplasty.
(A) Knees affected by RA. (B) Right knee with the Insall Burnstein knee prosthesis inserted.

tion. It is most frequently performed in the hind foot, wrist and thumb.

The success of an arthrodesis depends on adequate fusion, which is not always easy to obtain particularly when there is a degree of osteoporosis.

A careful assessment of the patient's requirements and expectations is essential.

A combination of several of the above procedures may be employed.

SURGERY TO THE LOWER LIMB

Because of the multi-joint involvement that is experienced by many patients with RA, decisions about the order in which surgery is carried out are crucial. For a person with severe pain in their knee or hip, it may be difficult to understand why surgery to the foot is being recommended in the first instance. It is daunting for a patient to be faced with a programme of surgery and it is essential that they are a partner in decision making and are given all the relevant information and support.

Ideally, the joint that is giving the patient the most problems should be attended to first. However, in order to obtain the maximum benefit from any lower limb surgery, and to protect a hip or knee prosthesis from loosening and eventual failure, it is essential that the mechanical axis is restored as far as possible. For example, if there is a valgus deformity at the knee, a new hip joint would be subjected to abnormal wear which would shorten its life. In this case it may be necessary to consider knee surgery first, even though the hip may be causing the most pain.

Following surgery, it is probable that mobilisation will be difficult because of upper limb involvement. Because of this, it may be necessary to inject shoulders or elbows with steroids prior to surgery and to prepare adapted walking aids, such as the 'pulpit frame' (Fig. 14.4). This four wheeled padded rollator frame has an upholstered pad shaped to the body, enabling the patient to gain maximum support.

The foot and ankle

Surgery to the foot and ankle is aimed at reducing pain and the restoration of the architecture, so that gait is restored to as near normal as possible. Before foot surgery is undertaken it is necessary to ensure that the peripheral circulation is adequate, particularly when the patient has vasculitic problems.

For patients with rheumatoid disease, the most frequent deformities of the foot are:

• Hallux valgus

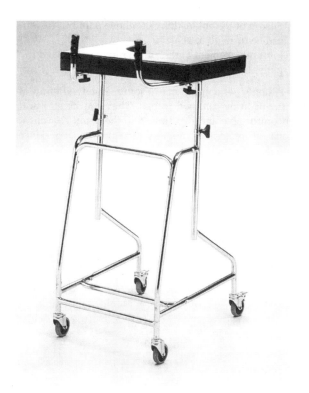

Figure 14.4 A pulpit frame (from Days Medical with permission).

• Bunions
• Depressed / subluxed metatarsal heads.

Many patients with subluxed metatarsal heads report a sensation of 'walking on pebbles'. Simple orthotic supports within well-fitting shoes, often with a deep toe box, along with physiotherapy exercises to maintain flexibility, are all useful. The patient should be given advice on how to care for the feet, with particular attention paid to skin integrity. If surgery is required, the smallest abrasion caused by rubbing against an ill fitting shoe, can be a focus of infection and cause cancellation of planned surgery. This is illustrated in Case Study 2 at the end of this chapter.

Procedures commonly employed in the foot and ankle include:

• Simple bunionectomy
• Realignment of the metatarsophalangeal joints
• Resection of metatarsal heads
• Open reduction of metatarsophalangeal dislocations: fixation is often maintained by a Kirschner wire for up to 6 weeks post operatively
• Triple arthrodesis: fusion of the talo-calcaneal, talonavicular and calcanocuboid joints

• Fusion of the ankle: this can relieve pain but fusion can be difficult to achieve
• Joint replacement at the ankle: rarely performed in patients with inflammatory disease.

Patients who have many joints involved, find it difficult to be confined to bed. They can be stiff and uncomfortable and in addition to the usual complications of restricted mobility, frequently experience additional problems with skin integrity. Early standing and walking may produce extra swelling in an operated foot/ankle but this must be regarded as a necessary trade-off for the overall well-being of that patient (Hurwitz 1994).

The knee

Arthroscopy

In addition to being employed for diagnostic purposes, arthroscopy can provide the opportunity to perform synovectomy, and to wash out any debris from the knee joint.

Synovectomy

Synovectomy will provide effective pain relief, particularly if the joint retains a reasonable range of movement. Any debris can be removed from the joint at the same time. Early movement after surgery is imperative, often with the use of a Continuous Passive Motion machine. Manipulation under anaesthetic may be required if the flexion achieved after a week is less than 70°.

Total knee arthroplasty

Historically, total knee arthroplasty had a lower rate of success than total replacement of the hip (Harburn 1989). However, later studies showed the success rate of the knee procedure to be equal or greater than that of total hip arthroplasty. This was attributed to better understanding of the biomechanics of the knee and to improved design and variety of implants (Huo & Galloway 1994).

In the past, there has been a reluctance to use this procedure on younger patients. This was based on the assumption that the implant would be liable to premature failure, because of the higher stresses likely to be imposed on it by a younger person. However, young people with generalised joint disease are not likely to stress a new joint in the same way as a fit person, and so many surgeons are now carrying out total knee arthroplasty on younger age groups.

The main indications for this type of surgery are relief of pain, where there is loss of function and joint cartilage, and when these combine to affect the patient's way of life. In common with the total arthroplasty of any joint, the procedure is contraindicated if any infection is present.

The hip

Up to a third of patients with RA develop hip involvement. As the disease in the hip progresses, it is not only movement that is painful, resting by sitting in a chair and eventually lying in bed bring no relief. Sleep is disturbed, activities of living become restricted and painful movement makes self care difficult. The attrition of constant pain has a deep psychological effect and the impact of hip disease on a rheumatoid patient can be devastating (Clayton 1992).

Patients with juvenile chronic arthritis tend not to complain of such pain, but hold their hips in a position of comfort. In time, this leads to fixed flexion deformities at the hip that may require surgical intervention.

The patient with an osteoarthritic hip responds very well to hip replacement, particularly as it is often the main or only affected joint.

Hip involvement is present in up to 38% of patients with ankylosing spondylitis. The hip can become ankylosed in a position that makes mobility painful and difficult.

Osteonecrosis of the femoral head can occur in systemic lupus erythematosus, or following long term treatment with steroids. In these cases, total arthroplasty may eventually be required.

Synovectomies, tenotomies and osteotomies can all be used at various stages of hip disease. However, if all non invasive therapies have had little impact, the treatment of choice for a patient with disabling pain is a total hip replacement, an operation with a very high rate of success (Table 14.1).

There are several prostheses available. Details can be found in orthopaedic textbooks (see Further Reading).

SURGERY TO THE UPPER LIMB

Lower limb surgery is usually carried out before upper limb surgery. However, the joints of the upper limbs may be so badly affected, that following lower limb surgery the patient would be unable to mobilise, even with adapted walking aids or intra-articular injections.

In such cases surgery to the upper limbs may be required first. However the use of walking aids can produce stresses on sometimes delicate upper limb prostheses, which can lead to problems of loosening and failure.

All the upper limb joints are interdependent and a full upper limb functional assessment is required before surgery is considered.

The hand and wrist

A pain free and stable wrist is essential for optimal hand function. Unfortunately up to 90% of patients with RA will eventually have wrist involvement, with pain, swelling and deformity, compounding the difficulties they already experience with daily activities.

Synovectomy

Early synovectomy, particularly when the articular cartilage is still intact, can be of great benefit.

Carpal tunnel syndrome

The pain caused by compression of the median nerve as it passes, with the flexor tendons, through the carpal tunnel at the wrist can be relatively disabling, particularly when it affects both wrists. The symptoms can vary from mild tingling on the palmar aspects of the thumb and first three fingers, to loss of motor function and intense pain which disrupts sleep. The compression can be relieved by surgery, and according to Nakano (1994) is one of the most successful operations that can be performed on the hand. Carpal tunnel decompression is often carried out under local anaesthetic, with the patient only needing to be hospitalised for a day. However, as always, careful assessment of other problems and home circumstances is essential.

Ruptured tendons

Many tendons, particularly those with a large range of motion, run through a tendon sheath lined with tissue. The inflammatory process can lead to this tissue becoming thickened and roughened, thus preventing the free movement of the tendon. In addition, the surrounding bony structure can become altered, and surfaces may lose their smoothness due to cartilage damage and osteophyte formation. These factors can contribute to rupture of the tendon. Tenosynovectomy can be employed to remove the thickened tissue, and bony prominences can be surgically removed if they are seriously compromising the free movement of the tendon. If tendon rupture occurs, repair and/or transfer are performed to restore function.

Fusion of the wrist

If a wrist fusion is considered, particularly if both wrists are involved, careful assessment has to be carried out to ensure that any existing independence is not compromised. For example the patient should not become more dependent for hygiene or nutrition needs, or be less able to use walking aids. The position of fusion needs to be carefully planned, considering the patient's needs and wishes.

Hands

The hand is often the first area to be affected by RA and very early in the disease, erosive damage can occur on the joint surfaces.

The psychological and functional problems caused by deformed hands cannot be overestimated. Our hands are constantly on view to others and to ourselves. They help us to communicate. They are not only essential for daily living activities but also in our leisure pursuits. Deformed hands are an ever present, visible and painful reminder of disease, both to the person affected and to those with whom they come into contact. Even the touch of greeting or comfort can cause distress.

Common deformities of the hand include:

- Ulnar drift, caused by damage at the metacarpophalangeal joints aggravated by normal activities (Fig. 2.16)
- Swan neck deformities (Fig. 2.18)
- Boutonniere deformities (Fig. 2.17).

Again, the main aim of surgical intervention is to maintain and improve function, and to relieve pain. Interventions range from synovectomy, tendon transfers, silastic implants, to fusion of the affected joint.

Hand surgery is a speciality in itself. The hand therapist, with particular skills in dynamic splinting, is an essential member of the team. As always, it is imperative that the patient fully understands the implications of the surgery, and the hard work that is going to be involved afterwards!

The elbow

The elbow is another area where synovectomy, often combined with excision of the radial head, is a useful procedure if carried out early enough. Arthrodesis is usually used only as a salvage operation, as it drastically restricts function.

Assessment of the shoulder is essential when considering elbow replacement surgery. There needs to be adequate rotation at the shoulder in order to avoid placing abnormal stresses on the delicate hinge joint at the elbow.

Elbow replacements are becoming increasingly successful with the improvement of implant design and surgical technique. Clayton (1992) gives this procedure a rating of 80 (Table 14.1) and Kraay et al (1994), reported that out of 86 total elbow replacements in patients with RA, 92% of the operations were still considered successful after 3 years, and 90% after 5 years.

Wound healing can be a problem as there is only a small amount of soft tissue covering the elbow joint. The post-operative splint needs to be well padded, and if the patient uses a walking aid, for example a gutter frame, this may need to be adapted until the wound is fully healed.

Successful surgery will lead to pain relief and improvement of function. However some extension may be lost, and patients are advised not to lift heavy loads with outstretched arms, since this can lead to excessive wear on the new, delicate joint.

The shoulder

The relief of pain is the main indication for shoulder replacement. Surgeons often advise against arthroplasty when relief of pain is not the primary objective. Although improvement of movement may follow, this cannot be guaranteed, because of damage already caused to the joint by the disease process, and to the rotator cuff in particular.

Another determining factor is the patient's willingness to undergo a long rehabilitation. It may be a year before full benefit is obtained.

Shoulder replacement can be painful compared with other joint replacements, and typically causes considerable pain in the first 24 hours. For this reason, pain management is particularly important in the immediate post-operative period (Follman 1988).

The care of a patient undergoing shoulder arthroplasty is further explored in Case Study 1 on page 264.

Surgery to the spine

In RA, the principal involvement of the spine occurs in the cervical region. Up to 80% of patients can have some degree of damage, but only a small percentage require surgery. Severe pain, instability and neurological deficit are danger signs. Atlantoaxial subluxation can lead to cord and brain stem compression, vertebral artery insufficiency and sudden death.

The success of spinal fusion depends on the extent of neurological involvement at the time of surgery. Boden & Bohlman (1994) quote 87% early death or failure in patients with severe neurological involvement, but 80% success rate when patients have less severe involvement.

Wedge osteotomy of the spine is occasionally performed in patients with ankylosing spondylitis. This intervention may be useful if a patient's day to day function is becoming impaired because of increasing kyphosis (hump back). Problems that can be improved include loss of peripheral and forward vision and difficulties in swallowing liquids.

PLANNING SURGERY FOR THE PATIENT WITH RHEUMATOID DISEASE

This section will consider problems that may be encountered, preparations required, and the involvement of each member of the team, with particular emphasis on the role of the nurses. It is not intended to be a detailed examination of general orthopaedic nursing care, but an indication of the specific needs of the rheumatoid patient.

Patients with systemic rheumatic disease face multiple problems in preparing for surgery. For surgery to be safe and successful, the patient must be supported by the expertise of all members of the multiprofessional team. This is illustrated later in this chapter in Case Study 2, page 268.

Whenever possible, the joint that should be dealt with first is the one causing the patient the greatest problem. However, the appropriate programme of surgery may require careful planning. The patient's physical and psychological well being must be considered, as should their motivation and ability to undergo often rigorous rehabilitation. Although there are basic ideals for programming surgery, each patient is an individual, both in disease pattern and personal wishes and therefore needs to be individually assessed.

The combined clinic

Ideally, planning for surgery starts at a clinic appointment with the rheumatologist, the orthopaedic surgeon and members of the multiprofessional team, at which the patient has the opportunity to ask questions and express wishes and anxieties. This clinic would include:

- Rheumatologist
- Orthopaedic surgeon
- Nurse

- Physiotherapist
- Occupational therapist.

The rheumatologist knows the patient's disease history and status, current medication and potential medical problems. The orthopaedic surgeon will discuss the feasibility of surgical options, considering such things as existing damage and bone stock. This provides the opportunity to determine whether any special, custom made, prostheses are required. A decision may be taken to perform surgery urgently if, for example a tendon rupture is imminent. It may be necessary to admit the patient early, prior to surgery, so that fixed flexion deformities can be reduced, to ensure that the best possible results are obtained from surgery. The nurse is present to:

- Commence preoperative education
- Reinforce explanations
- Provide psychological support
- Offer advocacy if required.

The therapists will commence their assessments and plan for rehabilitation. Current function is assessed, as well as how projected surgery will alter function. The patient's requirements are taken into account.

Patients with progressive joint disease should be operated on as soon as possible, once the need for surgical intervention has been identified. The longer they have to wait, the greater the likelihood of added problems.

The pre-assessment clinic

Patients admitted for elective surgery experience more anxiety than those admitted for surgery as an emergency (Cochran 1984). There is a significant relationship between stress factors, emotional stress and RA disease activity (Crosby 1988).

The patient is usually invited to attend the pre-assessment clinic approximately 2 weeks prior to planned surgery. Attending the clinic has several benefits both for the patient and the service (Bond & Barton 1994). It provides an opportunity to allay fears and anxieties, to commence or continue education and to assess whether the patient is free from infection and medically fit for an anaesthetic and surgery. Problems, such as urinary tract infections, that would otherwise result in a last minute cancellation can be rectified. If surgery has to be postponed, it gives time to arrange for theatre time to be utilised for someone else on the waiting list, thus avoiding the waste of expensive resources. An assessment can also be made as to how soon the patient needs to be admitted prior to surgery

to rectify problems such as a low haemoglobin or to modify any treatment. Plans for rehabilitation and discharge can also be commenced.

Admission

Not all patients undergoing surgery have the advantage of attending combined and pre-assessment clinics, or of being admitted to a specialist rheumatology unit. However, for those that do, some assessments and preparations may be started prior to admission. Whichever model of nursing is used, the admission assessment needs to keep discharge planning in mind from the beginning and to take account of the following:

- Psychological state
- Educational needs
- Fatigue.
- Pain
- Skin integrity.

Psychological state

The anxieties experienced by a person being admitted for surgery are well documented elsewhere (Holloway & Hall 1992).

Patients who have experienced successful surgical interventions in the past, and have benefited by relief of pain and improvement of function may be less apprehensive about subsequent admissions for operation (Coffey 1991). Similarly, someone who has coped successfully with hospital admission in the past is more likely to perceive themselves as being able to cope again (Clarke 1984). However the converse is also true and unfortunate experiences in the past can colour future expectations, as can the knowledge that the forthcoming operation may not be the final one.

A high degree of motivation is required. The patient will have to face a potentially long and difficult rehabilitation period, made more difficult by problems in other joints, caused by the disease. No matter how skilful the surgeon and how good the care and support given by the multiprofessional team, the patient takes a major part of the responsibility for a successful outcome. The patient is the senior partner in the procedure and not a passive recipient of care.

Educational needs

Education is an important factor in the process of empowering the patient and encouraging them to be a partner and to feel in control. However, surgical intervention initially involves a period when the patient is not in control. In this situation, it is desirable to use education to place the patient in a position of cognitive control, as explained in Chapter 7. All members of the team should give explanations of what this episode entails.

The patient needs to understand the procedures in order to join with the team in setting achievable goals and this not possible if they do not understand or have the relevant knowledge. This is particularly important when a patient with RA is nursed on a general orthopaedic ward. Here they are likely to be surrounded by patients who do not have systemic illness and who seem to rehabilitate post-operatively far more quickly and easily. Unless they understand the reasons, it is very easy for them to become despondent and frustrated in such a situation.

The relatives should be included in any information giving. The patient will require additional help and support on discharge and those at home often experience higher levels of stress and anxiety than the patients themselves.

Any verbal explanations should be backed up by written information. The use of joint models and prostheses, pictures and X-rays are all helpful, as is talking with someone who has undergone a similar procedure successfully.

Fatigue

When the fatigue experienced by patients with RA is compounded by anxiety about forthcoming surgery, it may be necessary to admit the patient early, to ensure that she is rested and prepared for surgery. Fatigue can be assessed using the tools shown in Tables 9.3 and 9.4. Rehabilitation activities may need to be programmed to match the patient's characteristics. For example, some patients find they have more energy early in the day, so physiotherapy should be carried out early, when the patient is most able to cooperate fully.

Pain

Pain levels should be assessed by use of a daily diary card (Fig. 8.4) or a body map (Fig. 4.2). This will highlight problems in joints that may be further stressed during rehabilitation. These may benefit from intraarticular injections of steroid prior to surgery.

The treatment of post-operative pain should be discussed with the patient. Patient controlled analgesia allows the patient to receive effective pain relief exactly when it is needed. It is self administered and consists of a pre-set amount of analgesia in a pre-filled syringe and pump mechanism. However if this method is to be used by a patient with RA, a practise run is advisable. Patients with decreased hand function may not be able to press buttons attached to their wrist because they have neither the dexterity nor the strength. It may be necessary to use a blowpipe to activate the patient controlled analgesia equipment. Whichever method is chosen, the patient needs to have confidence that she can access the pain relief mechanism and pain should be assessed by use of the tools outlined in Chapter 4.

Concern is often expressed that during fasting and immediately post-operatively, anti-inflammatory medication may be missed. Whenever possible, this treatment should be continued by injection or suppository.

Skin integrity

This section gives a brief description of the relevance of skin integrity during surgical intervention. A more detailed discussion of the problems of skin integrity, experienced by patients with rheumatoid disease is included in Chapter 10.

An assessment should be made of current pressure area risk. A pressure-relieving mattress or low air loss bed may be required. The operating theatre staff should be informed where there is high risk and if possible a pressure-relieving mattress used on the operating table. When the Waterlow scale (Waterlow 1983) is used for post-operative reassessment, 10 risk points should be added to the existing score if the patient is having lower limb surgery and is on the operating table for 2 hours or more.

The presence of vasculitic problems and nodules must be noted. Areas of broken skin are a potential focus for infection and present a high risk, particularly if a prosthesis is to be inserted. Few surgeons are prepared to operate in the presence of ulcers.

During replacement surgery of the hip and knee joints, disarticulation of the joint requires a considerable amount of force. The lower limbs need to be checked for bruising pre- and post-operatively. A bruise caused by a surgeon's thumb can later break down into an ulcer that is very difficult to heal. Wrapping the lower leg in a pressure absorbent material such as 'Velband' can afford some protection during surgery.

Lifting and handling

Lifting and handling can pose a major problem. Patients with RA should be discouraged from using a 'monkey pole'. Even if there is no current upper limb involvement the potential for damage exists. Sliding sheets, handling slings and mechanical aids can be utilised if necessary. If a mechanical hoist is used, slings lined with sheepskin should be used in preference to canvas slings, because they are less likely to cause trauma to frail skin. If aids are to be used post-operatively, practising their use before surgery will build confidence.

Investigations and observations

The patient with systemic rheumatoid disease should be in the optimum physical condition to withstand surgery. An admission for surgery is an opportunity for a full assessment of disease status by all members of the team. The routine preparations for theatre for a patient undergoing orthopaedic surgery can be found in the Further Reading list on page 271.

Baseline observations

A raised temperature can indicate a 'flare' of disease or an infection. There may be an underlying cardiac condition, indicated by irregular pulse. Respiration problems can include chest infection, involvement of costal joints or damage caused by medication such as methotrexate. The blood pressure may be raised, not only through anxiety and pain, but also as a side effect of some non-steroidal medications or steroids.

Some routine investigations are usually undertaken.

- Investigation of disease activity is carried out by checking C-reactive protein, plasma viscosity or erythrocyte sedimentation rate and rheumatoid factor.
- The cause of a low haemoglobin must be investigated and blood transfusion may be required prior to surgery.
- Urinary tract infections are not unusual in patients with restricted mobility, particularly if there is a reluctance to take an adequate fluid intake because of difficulties in getting to the toilet. A mid-stream specimen of urine should be collected for microscopy, culture and sensitivity.
- Swabs must be taken from any broken areas of skin.
- In addition to chest X-ray and any X-rays required by the surgeon, the anaesthetist may require an X-ray of the cervical spine, particularly if the patient has any history or symptoms of cervical spine involvement. A cervical collar may need to be worn to theatre.
- Blood must be taken for grouping and cross matching, since a patient with rheumatoid disease often requires extra replacement of blood post-operatively.

- Any previous embolitic problems should be noted and a decision made whether anticoagulant therapy is required.
- Doppler studies may be required to ensure that the circulation is adequate prior to lower limb surgery, particularly if the patient has impaired circulation or vasculitic problems.
- Analysis of the synovial fluid may be required if there is any suspicion of infection.

Medication

Patients on steroid therapy will require steroid cover for surgery because the normal mechanism of steroid secretion is suppressed as a result of their abnormally high plasma levels (see Ch. 12). Increased doses are required so that the body can cope with a major stressor such as surgery. Hydrocortisone is administered intramuscularly or intravenously in the peri-operative period. The dose prescribed will depend on the amount of oral steroid the patient normally takes, and the length of time they have been taking it. Most surgeons now prescribe prophylactic antibiotic cover for any patient undergoing joint replacement surgery. This cover is particularly important for the immuno-suppressed patient. Opinions differ as to whether the low dose methotrexate therapy used in the treatment of RA and psoriatic arthritis has any detrimental effect on post-operative healing.

Therapist's assessments

The therapists should continue assessing the patient and planning for after the operation. The physiotherapist should explain and encourage the patient to practise deep breathing and circulatory exercises. The occupational therapist should reassess functional abilities and plan any extra facilities that may be required on discharge.

Post-operative care

It is not possible to devise a standard plan of care. The specifics of post-operative care will depend on the site of surgery and the individual patient's pattern of disease and joint involvement.

For routine orthopaedic post-operative care, see Further Reading list. However there are several specific areas of concern when caring for the patient with inflammatory joint disease following surgery.

- Routine observations of temperature, pulse, respiration and blood pressure are carried out. Further blood transfusion may be necessary, depending on the blood loss during operation and the patient's post-operative haemoglobin. Intubation may have been difficult, and it may be necessary to continue to nurse the patient in a cervical collar in the immediate post-operative period.

- The neurocardiovascular status of the affected limb is checked regularly and compared with that of the unaffected limb. This is particularly important when a nerve block has been used as part of the anaesthetic procedure, for example a subclavian block during upper limb surgery. The patient may be unaware of any problems in the anaesthetised limb.

- If patient controlled analgesia is being used, its safety and effectiveness are checked according to protocol. Although a pre-operative trial might have been successful the patient may be unable to use the system effectively post-operatively, and it will then be necessary to resort to nurse administered intramuscular analgesia until the patient feels that oral analgesia is adequate.

- Skin integrity is reassessed and any appropriate action taken, such as extra protection for vulnerable pressure areas. Not only is the wound checked, but all the skin is checked for any bruising which may have occurred during the passage through theatre. Any wound drains are usually removed at 24 hours post-surgery. The timing of the removal of skin closures varies with the site of surgery, however clips and sutures need to be removed with great caution, particularly where the skin and underlying tissues are of poor quality.

- Positioning for comfort can present a major problem. Other joints may be stiff and painful, particularly after a period without anti-inflammatory medication and one or two hours under anaesthetic when joints may have been moved into unaccustomed positions. Passive and active exercises are encouraged as soon as possible, without compromising the operated joint. Any splints must be well fitting and may need extra padding. If an upper limb requires elevating, care must be taken to ensure that surrounding joints are not placed under undue stress.

- Extra assistance may be required with eating and drinking. Where there is already limited movement, the added restrictions of surgery, intravenous infusions and drains can limit independence even further.

- Assistance will probably be required for moving, elimination and hygiene needs. As mentioned earlier, the use of a monkey pole should be discouraged.

- The patient with inflammatory joint disease and multiple joint involvement will not make such rapid progress in the post-operative period as the person with one affected joint. Reassurance may be needed that the caring team understands this, especially when the patient is nursed on a general orthopaedic ward. Here the patient may observe people who have had similar operations and appear to be making a rapid recovery.

The care of a patient undergoing shoulder replacement surgery is outlined in Case Study 14.1.

Discharge planning

Planning for discharge is a multiprofessional activity that should take place throughout the patient's stay. Many patients with chronic disease will have an existing comprehensive package of care, and so adaptations and equipment may already be in the home. However these will need to be reassessed as requirements may be altered by surgical intervention. An example of a multiprofessional discharge planning checklist is illustrated in Appendix 4. To facilitate 'seamless care' as envisaged in Chapter 16, close liaison with the primary care team is essential.

Case Study 14.1 A patient undergoing total shoulder replacement

In this example, Roper's model is used as the basis for assessing and planning care (Roper et al 1990).

David is 60 years old and lives in a bungalow with his wife who is fit and well. He was made redundant 2 years ago. He has had RA for 20 years, and during the past 5 years both his knees and hips have been replaced. The same team carried out all his previous surgery, and, after much effort on his part, he has gained benefit both in relief of pain and improvement of function.

His main complaint now is of severe pain in his right shoulder. He is right handed and is finding that many of his activities are becoming restricted (Fig. 14.5). Swimming and walking with the dog, two of the leisure activities that he has come to enjoy since his previous surgery, are becoming increasingly difficult and painful.

His disease appears to be well controlled on:

- Methotrexate 10 mg weekly
- Folic acid supplement of 5 mg daily on 2 days per week
- SR Diclofenac 75 mg twice daily

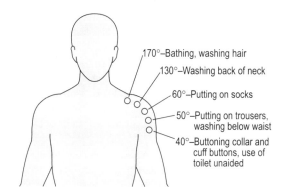

170°–Bathing, washing hair

130°–Washing back of neck

60°–Putting on socks

50°–Putting on trousers, washing below waist

40°–Buttoning collar and cuff buttons, use of toilet unaided

Figure 14.5 The range of shoulder movement necessary to perform activities of daily living.

• Co-proxamol, two tablets when required, up to eight per day.

However, he needs increasing amounts of analgesia to control the pain in his shoulder. This is a disappointment to him, as his knees and hips are now virtually pain free.

Physiotherapy, application of heat and cold and complementary measures have been to no avail. X-ray of the shoulder shows a joint damaged by the disease, although on examination, the rotator cuff appears intact.

The team occupational therapist has been involved in previous episodes of care, knows the domestic situation well and is aware of how the bungalow is equipped with aids such as tap turners, raised chairs and toilet seats.

After consultation with his rheumatologist and orthopaedic surgeon, David is admitted for total shoulder replacement.

Pre-operative assessment by the medical team showed no major medical problems or signs of infection and his disease was quiescent. Upper limb assessment demonstrated existing disease but no major damage in his elbow, wrist or hand.

Nursing assessment

The following abbreviations are used:

(A) = Actual problem
(P) = Potential problem
(N) = No problem

Maintaining a safe environment (A)

Being right handed, David experiences problems reaching objects. At home he has everything he needs in a position suitable for him. He is about to undergo surgery for which he will need a general anaesthetic. He will be unable to maintain his own safety.

Communicating (A)

Although he has had previous successful surgical interventions, he still communicates anxiety about the forthcoming operation. He wears a hearing aid.

Breathing (P)

A recent chest X-ray showed no chest problems. He smokes between 5 and 10 cigarettes daily. He will probably be having a subclavian block, and there is a very slight risk of pneumothorax post-operatively.

Eating and drinking (A)

Because of the pain in his shoulder, he has problems cutting up food and lifting a full cup or glass to his mouth. He is not very adept with his left hand.

Eliminating (A)

David feels that his increased analgesia intake is causing constipation. He is also very anxious that he will experience difficulties with elimination post-operatively. He is unable to use a urinal in bed and finds bedpans very difficult and embarrassing to use. However, he has never had problems with micturition.

Dressing and cleansing (A)

Washing and dressing have become increasingly difficult. He uses a shower at home and manages with minimal assistance from his wife. His skin is intact.

Mobilising (P)

David is aware that mobilising will need to be restricted prior to theatre, following his premedication. He does not use walking aids. The physiotherapist has discussed post-operative mobilisation with him.

Controlling body temperature (N)

Temperature on admission is normal. He expresses no problems with controlling body temperature and does not feel that the ambient temperature has any effect on his arthritis.

Working and playing (N)

He is looking forward to resuming his normal activities. He has brought books and magazines, a personal stereo and some favourite tapes, and does not feel boredom will be a problem during his hospital stay.

Expressing sexuality/body image (P)

David expresses no problems, although he does ask how soon he will be able to resume sexual activity after his operation.

Sleeping (A)

The pain in his shoulder has disturbed his sleep pattern and he finds it difficult to find a comfortable position in bed. He is anxious that he will not be able to sleep the night prior to surgery.

Dying (P)

David expresses slight anxiety about the anaesthetic, but his fears are allayed by the fact that he has had four previous anaesthetics.

Plan of care

1. The function of the right arm is restricted.
- Ensure that the locker and nurse call system are within reach on the left side of the bed.
- Check that he feels safe within the ward environment, particularly in the toilet and bathroom areas.
2. A general anaesthetic will be required for a surgical procedure.
- Discuss with him the reasons for fasting pre-operatively.
- Ensure that his cervical spine has been checked, and that all pre-operative assessments have been carried out.
- Explain a cervical collar is to be worn to theatre and ensure that it fits correctly.
3. David is anxious about the forthcoming operation.
- Explore with him the reasons for his anxiety.
- Explain the procedure thoroughly using a model shoulder and prosthesis.
- If possible, introduce him to a patient who has had a similar operation.
- Liaise with the therapists to ensure that he and his wife know what to expect during the rehabilitation period and on discharge.
- Discuss what assistance he may need on discharge, demonstrating the use of the sling and body strap if that is to be used.
- Discuss strategies for coping with post-operative pain with him.

- Offer patient controlled analgesia and if he is in agreement, experiment to determine the best method of delivery.
- Inform the operating theatre staff that he wears a hearing aid and would like to wear it until he is anaesthetised.
4. There is a potential for breathing problems post-operatively.
- Reinforce deep breathing exercises taught by the physiotherapist.
- Advise him to inform his nurse immediately if he has pain in his chest or breathing difficulties after his operation.
- Discourage him from smoking prior to his operation and offer support and encouragement to stop smoking completely.
5. David's ability to eat and drink is restricted by pain in his shoulder, and will be more so immediately following surgery.
- Offer assistance to cut up food and ensure that everything is within reach at meal times.
- If he is embarrassed because he feels he is a 'messy eater' ensure that he has privacy at mealtimes if he wishes.
- Liaise with the occupational therapist about the use of a non-slip mat, special plate or cutlery to enable him to eat with one hand.
- Ensure that cups and glasses are manageable and not too heavy or too full.
6. David has a tendency to constipation.
- Discuss diet with him.
- Ensure that he has his bowels well open prior to surgery.
7. He is anxious about elimination post-operatively.
- Reassure him that post-operatively, he will be able to stand, with help if necessary, to urinate and will be helped out to the toilet as soon as he is able.
8. David experiences difficulties with hygiene and personal care.
- If required, assist him to shower, observing for any lesions, nodules or signs of pressure.
- Complete pressure area risk assessment.
- Ensuring privacy, assist him to prepare for theatre.
9. David is anxious that resumption of sexual activity may be a problem after his operation.
- Allow time and privacy to discuss this.
- If possible, introduce David to another male patient who has had a similar procedure.
- Encourage David to discuss this with the physiotherapist.
- Provide opportunity for David's wife to discuss this, if this is their wish.

10. His sleep pattern is disturbed by pain.
• Review his analgesic regime in the days before surgery.
• Discuss with the medical team, the possibility of night sedation pre-operatively.
• Explore ways of finding a comfortable position in which he can rest and be as pain free as possible.

On the evening prior to surgery, the anaesthetist visits David and the pre-medication is prescribed. He is not due to go to theatre until 12 noon, and so he may have his anti-inflammatory drug at 6am with tea and toast. He is prepared for theatre in the routine way, assisted to shower and helped into his theatre gown. The pre-operative preparations are checked, the pre-medication administered and he is advised not to get out of bed. The screens are drawn to allow him to rest, and the call bell is placed close to his left hand should he require anything.

The nurse caring for him accompanies him to the anaesthetic room.

Post-operative period

After recovering from his anaesthetic David is returned to the ward.

He has had a Neer Total Shoulder prosthesis inserted (Fig. 14.6) and has a vacuumed wound drain in situ. Fluid loss during surgery was minimal, however the intravenous fluids continue slowly to maintain hydration and venous access, should it be required.

His right arm is supported in a sling with a body strap. Temperature, pulse, respiration and blood pressure reading are recorded hourly initially reducing to 4 hourly.

Until the effects of the subclavian block have worn off hourly recordings are made of:

• Colour
• Sensation
• Movement
• Warmth
• Radial pulse.

Any impairment not related to the block could indicate a dislocation of the new prosthesis. Loss of sensation in the little and ring fingers could indicate ulnar nerve impairment, possibly caused by pressure of the sling over the elbow. If adjustment of the sling does not correct the problem, the medical staff should be informed immediately.

Post-operative reassessment of the plan of care

1. David's right arm is held close to his body, immobilised in a sling incorporating a body strap.

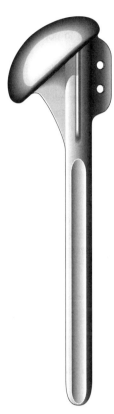

Figure 14.6 Neer total shoulder prosthesis (with kind permission of 3M Health Care Ltd).

3. Initially David does not experience much pain in the operated shoulder, but as the effect of the subclavian block begins to wear off, he describes pain in his shoulder, although his lower arm remains numb. The pain radiates across his neck. He has elected to use patient controlled analgesia and the button is placed near his left hand. As he becomes accustomed to using it, he finds it effective and uses it for the first 12 post-operative hours.

Sitting up in bed, well supported by pillows helps relieve his pain. The smallest change in position can be effective and he finds the most comfortable position is with a pillow underneath his right forearm, the hand slightly higher than the elbow. A film dressing and padding cover the surgical wound. An ice pack applied to the site also brings relief.

Intramuscular morphine 10 mg is required at 6 hourly intervals for the next 24 hours, but after this time David reports that his pain is adequately controlled by his oral Co-proxamol.

He is assisted to get out of bed and mobilise as soon as possible, thus reducing the risk of stiffness and pain in his other joints.

4. He experiences no breathing problems post-operatively but is encouraged to continue his deep breathing exercises.

5. David has an intravenous infusion for the first 24 hours. He feels nauseous and vomiting can exacerbate the shoulder pain, so anti-emetics are prescribed and given with effect. He then tolerates fluids and is feeling hungry by lunch time on the day after surgery, when he manages a slice of toast!

6 & 7. On the evening of the day of surgery, he is assisted to stand by his bed to use a urinal. By the following morning he is able to go out to the toilet with assistance.

8. Assistance is required with hygiene. The body strap is loosened with care to enable axillary hygiene and to check the skin underneath. The physiotherapist advises when the strap and sling may be removed completely for showering.

Pressure areas are reassessed, particularly his heels, following his time on the operating table.

Wound care

David has a drain in situ, which is removed after 24 hours as there is minimal drainage. The bulky padding is removed from the wound that is left covered by a transparent film dressing. When asked if he finds it unacceptable to have the wound visible, he says not, but would prefer it covered when he has visitors. Clips will be removed at 12–14 days. There have been no problems with wound healing following previous surgical interventions.

The physiotherapist commences the rehabilitation regime from the first post-operative day. She informs the nurse what time she will be working with David so that analgesic cover is ensured. A check X-ray is performed.

On the first day, his arm remains in the sling but in a resting position. Simple maintenance exercises are carried out; hand, wrist and forearm movements, cervical spine and elbow movements. David is involved from the start in the process. These simple gentle exercises are not excessively painful, particularly with analgesic cover, and his confidence is boosted.

Once the drain is removed on the second day, pendular exercises are commenced. David is shown how to lean forward, letting his arm hang freely. Starting with small movements he swings his arm forwards and backwards, from side to side and in a circular motion, repeating each movement five times. He gradually builds up to doing this four times a day. The physiotherapist assists him to elevate his arm, and gradually as the pain decreases he is able to perform his own assisted elevation exercises, lying supine, with the use of a pulley. After a week, he starts active exercises to increase his range of movement and control. He can now manage without his sling during the day, but still finds it helpful at night.

He is discharged home after 10 days. His wound clips are still in situ and the community nurse has been requested to check these in 3 days and remove them if the wound is healed completely. He has an outpatients' appointment with the orthopaedic and rheumatology team in 2 weeks. The physiotherapist gives him a programme of exercises, and will continue to see him regularly as an outpatient.

Both he and his wife feel confident that they will manage well at home. They have a contact number for the ward should they have any anxieties. They understand that it will be several months before David feels the full benefit of his surgery, indeed he may continue to notice improvement over the next year. However he is already noticing a reduction in pain, and is determined that the surgery will be a success. He has been given written instructions to remind him that he must not drive a car for at least 6 weeks, but he could start doing light gardening in 2 months. He should undertake no heavy work for 6 months. He has also been advised to take care when walking his dog, holding the lead in the left hand. Even small dogs can pull! David is enjoying his hydrotherapy and is hoping to resume swimming regularly when the physiotherapist advises.

David had an uneventful episode of treatment. His disease was quiescent at the time, and he had no underlying medical problems. He was well motivated, and had confidence in the team and himself.

Case Study 14.2 Patient awaiting bilateral total knee replacement

This example illustrates some of the problems that can be experienced in planning surgery for a patient with rheumatoid disease.

Mrs P is 48-year-old Indian woman who is married to an Englishman; they have two daughters. She is articulate and artistic and is a successful photographer. Her mother had severe and aggressive RA; indeed she was wheelchair orientated towards the end of her life. A rheumatologist had originally seen Mrs P 5 years prior to the present episode, when she was diagnosed and treatment commenced.

The rheumatologist wrote to the general practitioner 'This patient has deteriorated enormously since I last saw her 5 years ago. At that time she had rather scattered rheumatoid disease that she seemed to cope with, and I think that the problem is that she has continued to struggle without showing or complaining how bad she is. She now has a widespread polyarticular active rheumatoid and is dependant on her two teenage daughters'.

Her inflammatory indices were raised, and her rheumatoid factor titre was 1:1280. Her disease-modifying drug was hydroxychloroquine, which was clearly now ineffective. A plan was made to admit her urgently, administer a 'pulse' of steroid, and change her disease-modifying drug.

It was 6 weeks before Mrs P was admitted. She had an exhibition organised that she had put a lot of work into and did not wish to let herself or others down. When she was finally admitted she was already beginning to develop flexion deformities in her knees. She had subluxed metacarpophalangeal joints and ulnar deviation. All members of the team were involved in her care:

- Joint protection strategies were reinforced
- 'Flotron' therapy was used in an attempt to reduce the flexion deformities of her knees
- Pacing of activities was discussed
- Pain control strategies were explored
- Sulphasalazine therapy was commenced
- Mrs P began to build up a relationship with the team.

Shortly after discharge, she developed a rash and the sulphasalazine was discontinued. She had been planning to visit India to see her family for several months and was unwilling to start a new drug until after her return. On her return, azathiaprine was commenced. This was effective treatment for over a year. She was seen regularly in outpatients where it was noted that although her knees were deteriorating she was 'coping' but perhaps presenting, once again, a better picture than the truth. Two months after the last recorded outpatient visit, her husband wrote to the rheumatologist in desperation (see patient letter page 254).

Mrs P was referred to the orthopaedic surgeons and attended a combined clinic. Plans were made to perform bilateral total knee replacements. Whilst awaiting surgery, she had a cerebral bleed. An aneurysm was 'clipped' and she returned to the rheumatology unit for rehabilitation. She was hypertensive and because she was leucopenic, azathiaprine was discontinued. It was eventually reinstated but at a subsequent outpatient visit it was concluded that this therapy was ineffective. A small dose of oral steroid was prescribed.

Eventually a year after surgery was planned, Mrs P was admitted for the procedure. At this time it was noted that apart from her knees, her worst problems were, her shoulders, elbows, fingers, neck and hips. However, because she was still hypertensive, and in view of her recent history, surgery was cancelled. Another date was planned 3 months hence. Her hypertension was well controlled whilst at home.

On readmission her main anxiety was that the surgery would be cancelled again. By now she knew the case team well and expressed little anxiety about the surgery itself. Her blood pressure was within acceptable limits. Routine preparations were made for surgery and she appeared relaxed and philosophic on the evening prior to operation.

On the morning of surgery her blood pressure was again slightly elevated. She was prepared for theatre in as calm and unhurried a manner as possible and rested on her bed listening to soothing music. However, on the anaesthetist's advice, surgery was cancelled. She was then referred to the cardiologists.

Eventually her blood pressure appeared to be under control again and 6 months later she was readmitted. Mrs P had a small ulcer on her toe, which had only occurred the previous week, caused by friction against her shoe! She understood the importance of skin integrity and freedom of any source of infection. She arrived for admission looking very anxious, but did not really believe that such a small lesion could lead to the operation being cancelled again. However the surgeon decided it would be unwise to proceed.

During the following 3 months, Mrs P needed all the support the team could offer her. She was seen at regular intervals, both to ensure that the ulcer was healing, and to give her the opportunity for psychological support. Eventually, 2 years after the surgery was first proposed, Mrs P had successful bilateral total knee replacements.

She has gained freedom from pain in her knees and regained her optimism, She also stands approximately 9 cm taller.

Mrs P will require further surgery and it is hoped that future episodes will not be so eventful.

Surgical intervention is part of the overall care of the person with rheumatic disease. It is not a 'last resort' and can have a major impact on quality of life through relief of pain and maintenance and improvement of function.

A variety of interventions are available at all stages of joint disease. Techniques and prostheses have improved, and total joint arthroplasties are now very successful. Youth is no longer such a determining factor against intervention.

In addition to the meticulous and specialist nursing care required by any patient undergoing orthopaedic surgery, patients with rheumatoid disease have special needs. They may have systemic disease and are more likely to have underlying medical problems. They may be facing a programme of surgery, and do not have the security of knowing that a forthcoming operation is going to solve all their problems.

Pain relief and skin integrity give particular cause for concern.

Difficulties with mobilisation after surgery can be compounded by pain in other affected joints. Rehabilitation can be a long and difficult process, and it is essential that the patient has the motivation and support to achieve the best possible result.

Every patient is an individual and has an individual pattern of disease, needs and wishes; the multiprofessional team must work in partnership with the patient and family.

Action points for practice:

- Mrs Jones, a 35-year-old secretary, has RA which is causing pain, deformity and loss of function in her hands and wrists. Consider what surgical options are available to her and discuss the support you, as part of the multiprofessional team, could offer in the decision-making process, leading to surgical intervention.
- Jane is a 45-year-old patient with RA. She has had aggressive disease for many years and is wheelchair orientated due to major destruction in her knees, which now do not cause pain at rest. Her first husband deserted her early in the course of her disease. Her second husband married her when she was already wheelchair orientated and devotes himself to caring for her. A year after successful bilateral knee arthroplasties she still spends much of her time in her wheelchair and consequently the improved function obtained in her knees is deteriorating. Discuss whether Jane was a suitable candidate for total knee arthroplasties.
- Mrs P in Case Study 2, now requires surgery to her left elbow, possibly a total arthroplasty. She now has fixed flexion in that joint, in addition to constant pain on movement. Consider how the nurse and the multiprofessional team will be involved in preparing her for surgery. Plan her care during the peri-operative period using a model of your choice.

REFERENCES

Boden S, Bohlman H 1994 Orthopaedic management of the spine in rheumatic disease. In: Klippel J H, Dieppe P A (ed) Rheumatology. Mosby, St Louis Sect 8, ch 27, p 5

Bond D, Barton K 1994 Patient assessment before surgery. Nursing Standard 8(29): 23–28

Clarke M 1984 The constructs of stress and coping as a rationale for nursing activity. Journal of Advanced Nursing 9: 267–275

Clayton M 1963 Surgery of the lower extremity in RA. Journal of Bone and Joint Surgery 45: 1517–1536

Clayton M 1992 Generalised surgical principles and procedures. In: Clayton M, Smyth C (eds) Surgery for rheumatoid arthritis. Churchill Livingstone, New York ch 7, p 83

Cochran R M 1984 Psychological preparation of patients for surgical procedures. Patient Education & Counselling 5: 153–158

Coffey M 1991 Total knee replacement. Nursing Times 87(36): 37–38

Crosby L J 1988 Stress factors, emotional stress and rheumatoid disease activity. Journal of Advanced Nursing 10: 1852–1854

Figgie M 1994 Introduction to the surgical treatment of rheumatic disease. In: Klippel J H, Dieppe P A (ed) Rheumatology. Mosby, St Louis, Sect 8, ch 20, p 1

Follman D A 1988 Nursing care concerns in total shoulder replacements. Orthopaedic Nursing 7: 3

Fuller E 1983 When RA requires surgical management. Patient Care 17: 73–94

Harburn R 1989 Total knee arthroplasty and revision. Canadian Operating Room Nursing Journal 7(1): 4–12

Huo M, Galloway M 1994 Orthopaedic management of the knee in rheumatic disease. In: Klippel J H, Dieppe P A (ed) Rheumatology. Mosby, St Louis, Sect 8, ch 25, p 5

Holloway B, Hall J 1992 Planning for a more comfortable stay. Professional Nurse 7(6): 372–374

Hurwitz S 1994 Orthopaedic management of the foot and ankle in rheumatic disease. In: Klippel J H, Dieppe P A (ed) Rheumatology. Mosby. St Louis, Sect 8, ch 26, p 6

Kraay M J, Figgie M P, Inglis A E, Wolfe S W, Ranawat C S 1994 Primary semiconstrained total elbow arthroplasty. Survival analysis of 113 consecutive cases. Journal of Bone and Joint Surgery-British 76(4): 636–640

Maycock J 1988 The image of rheumatic disease. In: Salter M

(ed) Altered body image – the nurses' role. John Wiley, Chichester, ch9, p118

Nakano K K 1994 Entrapment neuropathies and related disorders. In: Sledge C B, Harris E D, Ruddy S, Kelley W N (eds) Arthritis surgery, Saunders, Philadelphia, ch 33, p 622–623

Roper N, Logan W W, Tierney A J 1990 The elements of nursing. Churchill Livingstone, Edinburgh

Short W, Palmer R 1994 Orthopaedic management of the hand and wrist. In: Klippel J H, Dieppe P A (ed) Rheumatology. Mosby, St Louis, Sect 8, ch 23, p2

Smith-Pigg J, Webb Driscoll P, Caniff R 1985 Rheumatology nursing a problem oriented approach. John Wiley, New York, ch 13, p 284

Souter W A 1979 Planning treatment of the rheumatoid hand. Hand 11: 3

Waterlow J 1983 A risk assessment card. Nursing Times 81(48): 49–55

FURTHER READING

Davis P 1994 Nursing the orthopaedic patient. Churchill Livingstone, Edinburgh

Wilson Barnett J 1978 Stress in hospital. Churchill Livingstone, Edinburgh

15

Patient education

Jackie Hill

Patient education (PE) is an essential component in the management of rheumatic disease. It should be regarded as an enhancer of other therapies that can dramatically improve the patient's life. After reading this chapter you should be able to:

- Discuss the need for patient education
- Underpin practice with an appropriate theoretical educational model
- Select the most suitable method of delivering patient education
- Choose pertinent topics for inclusion in a patient education programme
- Discuss the merits of written literature, audio-visual and computer assisted learning
- Assess the effectiveness of a patient education programme.

When patients are first told that they have one of the more serious rheumatic diseases, they are often frightened, despondent and anxious. This is not really surprising, as the image is one of disability, deformity, pain, psychological and social dysfunction, and a reduced quality of life. Although there have been many advances in the treatment of these diseases, disorders such as rheumatoid arthritis (RA) are unpredictable, and the most severe cases continue to result in increased mortality (Pincus & Callahan 1989).

PE has a wide ranging role in the management of rheumatic disease and its effects have been shown to bring about:

- Increases in knowledge
- Changes in behaviours
- Increased physical function
- Increased psychosocial health.

A DEFINITION OF PE

PE is any set of planned educational activities designed to improve patients' health behaviours and through this their health status and ultimately their longterm outcome. A task force of the National Arthritis Advisory Board in the United States has recently developed a set of standards for arthritis patient education, and has defined PE as: 'organized learning experiences designed to facilitate voluntary adoption of behaviours or belief conducive to health. It is a set of planned educational activities that are separate from clinical patient care. The activities of a patient education program must be designed to attain goals the patient has participated in formulating. The primary focus of these activities includes acquisition of information, skills, beliefs and attitudes which impact on health status, quality of life, and possibly health care utilization' (Burckhardt 1994).

The process of PE can be represented schematically as shown in Figure 15.1. PE is not a treatment per se. It should be regarded as a treatment enhancer, magnifying the effects of standard treatments by persuading patients to adhere more closely to or adopt actions that are believed to be beneficial. The ultimate success or failure in terms of health status or longterm outcome will remain dependent upon the inherent effectiveness of the treatment employed.

Theories and models

Theories and models do not tell us what to do or how

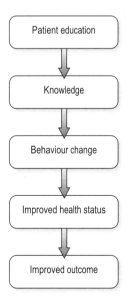

Figure 15.1 The process of patient education.

to do things. They do however guide our practice, and the most successful PE programmes are underpinned by a combination of theories and models (Lorig 1996).

Originally, the traditional biomedical model was used. This assumes that disease can be completely explained by disordered physiology and biology. For some diseases it has worked well, but the biomedical model is not really suitable for chronic diseases and many health professionals now discount its use and follow a more pragmatic approach.

The learning and teaching theory developed to pass knowledge to children has also been tried, but it is inappropriate when teaching adults. A more interactive, didactic style is more successful when working with mixed ability adult groups (Lorig et al 1987). Patients are usually adults whose experience is one of their major resources. In general, they do not accept advice unless it is justifiable and makes sense to them. This was highlighted in one study where only six out of 32 patients took the number of drugs prescribed by their General Practitioners. The other 26 compared their perceptions of the potential side effects and efficacy with their symptoms, and made a judgement on the required dosage. The study recommended a shift of emphasis from didactic programmes to more informal methods of PE (Donovan et al 1989).

The respect, intimacy and reciprocity required to bond the nurse/patient relationship, will enable the nurse to perceive the patient as a person with his or her own knowledge, belief values and experience. These must be incorporated into any system of care, including PE programmes.

Models and theories are discussed in Chapter 5, but an overview is given here of those most commonly used in PE. They are based on producing changes in behaviour and include the:

- Health belief model
- Learned helplessness theory
- Stress and coping theory
- Self efficacy theory.

Health belief model

The health belief model was originally postulated to explain the lack of uptake of tuberculosis screening (Becker 1974), and it is one of the oldest and most widely used health education models. It is based on the person's perception of a combination of the:

- Perceived threat

plus

- Expectations of benefit.

Before they change their behaviour, patients evaluate the perceived threat by weighing up their susceptibility to, and the severity of the danger. Lorig (1996) uses AIDS as a good example. AIDS is perceived as a severe disease. However, there are many different beliefs about susceptibility and safe sex will only be practised by those who believe themselves to be susceptible.

Severity and susceptibility, are only parts of the model. The equation is not complete without expectation. Patients must also believe that:

- A new behaviour will be beneficial
- They are capable of carrying out the behaviour change
- The costs of change do not outweigh the benefits.

Learned helplessness theory

Seligman (1975) developed the learned helplessness theory following research on dogs. These animals learned that whatever their response to electric shocks, they received further shocks and subsequently they became unresponsive and helpless. This work has evolved and has been adapted to human behaviour. The individual comes to believe that their actions have no effect on eventual outcome. They do not believe they can control their disease and expect to fail in their endeavours; they become passive and unresponsive to behavioural change. This state is known as 'learned helplessness' and it is characterised by lack of:

- Motivation
- Cognition
- Action.

A patient with severe RA who has tried many disease-modifying drugs that have caused side effects or failed to provide efficacy, may expect all drugs to fail. They tend to stop trying to overcome their problems and become non-compliant with their treatments. A typical response is 'Why bother, what difference does it make?'

Stress and coping theory

Any chronic, incurable disease will cause stress and coping deficits. One of the key elements of nursing is to help patients to cope with their illness (Wilson Barnett 1984) and so stress and coping theory are relevant to rheumatological PE. There are many different coping theories, but one of the most useful focuses on the work by Lazarus & Folkman (1984). This theory has particular merit as it has practical application, works well alongside self efficacy theory and it is recommended by respected authors (Lorig 1996, Newbold 1996).

Coping has been described as 'a set of cognitive and behavioural responses to events perceived as stressful' (Lazarus & Folkman 1984). They also suggest that 'persons are constantly changing cognitions and behaviour efforts to manage specific external and/or internal demands that are appraised as taxing or exceeding the person's resources'.

This is a cognitive appraisal model that is in keeping with the concept of PE. It features:

- Problem focused coping
- Emotion focused coping.

In problem focused coping, the acquisition of knowledge results in the belief that the stressor is controllable and its effect can be modified, avoided or minimised. Emotion focused coping is based on the elimination of undesirable emotions which follow on from the experience of the stressor (Auerbach 1989).

Stress and coping strategies should be incorporated into PE programmes, but it must be borne in mind that each patient is different and what works for one may not work for another. Strategies need to be tried, their effectiveness assessed and if they are not successful, new methods explored. There is a substantial literature on coping (Lazarus & Folkman 1984) that can guide nurses on how to provide a variety of the most fitting options in their PE programmes.

Self efficacy theory

PE is based on the premise that patients should be active collaborators in their care and have the knowledge and skills to manage their disease. Self efficacy is an essential component of this complex scenario, as it refers to a person's confidence in their ability to perform a specific task or achieve a certain objective (Bandura 1977). If a person exhibits high self efficacy in the face of a stressor, they will be more likely to carry out constructive coping behaviours and maintain a positive sense of well-being.

In a recent study, changes in self efficacy following a stress management programme were associated with depression, pain, health status and disease activity. Enhanced self efficacy was related to a reduction in symptoms. Self efficacy theory is discussed in more detail in Chapter 5.

Many theories can be applied to PE, with their origins in the fields of adult education, communication, sociology and psychology. Each has something to offer and perhaps the most successful programmes are those which incorporate something from each.

STARTING THE PE PROCESS

The question of the 'best time' to start the educational process has yet to be resolved. It may be that the greatest reduction in disability can be achieved by intensive intervention at an early stage of the disease, and learning coping skills shortly after diagnosis will help patients for the rest of their lives (DeVellis & Blalock 1993). However, there are problems with this approach. Soon after being told their diagnosis, patients commonly undergo a period of grief or bereavement reaction, leading to a period of 'denial'. Trying to educate them under these conditions can be counter-productive and lead to further depression (Donovan et al 1989). Counselling sessions would be more helpful than PE at this stage.

When the patient starts to ask questions about their disease and treatments, it is a sign that they have begun to accept their diagnosis and the process of PE can begin.

THE AIMS OF PE

The aim of PE is to maintain or improve the patient's health status. Unfortunately, simply adding to their stock of knowledge does not do this. Some studies have shown that PE can change behaviour and increase health status, but the literature is not consistent (Lorig et al 1987). Even when behaviour changes occur, these actions do not automatically lead to changes in health status.

Effective self management relies upon the patient's willingness to cooperate and their ability to comply with self care activities, and so PE is a combined effort between the multidisciplinary team, the patient and their partner/carer (Fig. 15.2). This can be difficult as disease activity can vary dramatically from day to day

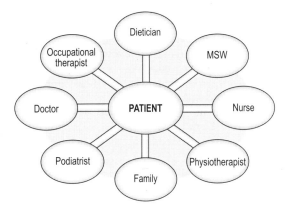

Figure 15.2 Typical multidisciplinary patient education team.

and so it is important that patients can tailor their therapies accordingly (Hill 1995). They need to be able to:

- Vary their drug usage according to their symptoms
- Employ coping strategies
- Regulate their daily exercise programmes
- Plan rest/activity periods.

THE EFFECTS OF PE

There are many claims for the overall 'effectiveness' of PE, but few have defined this term. A PE programme can be considered to be effective if it brings benefits that are additional to the existing treatments (Hill 1997), and a recent 45 study literature review estimated that the addition of PE to conventional rheumatology care brought about a 15–30% betterment (Hirano et al 1994).

A second proposal is that PE should achieve benefits comparable to those resulting from conventional therapy but with fewer side effects or at a lower cost (DeVellis & Blalock 1993) and a number of studies have shown that PE is successful at:

- Increasing knowledge
- Changing behaviour
- Improving physical and psychological health status.

Increases in knowledge

The acquisition of knowledge depends on a number of variables, such as:

- The skills of the teacher
- The content of the programme
- The receptiveness of the patient.

When these variables are favourable, PE can indeed increase the patient's knowledge in a number of areas. This was demonstrated in a study in which patients attending a nursing clinic were taught about:

- Disease aetiology
- Drugs and how to take them
- Exercise
- Joint protection
- Pain control
- Coping strategies.

After 6 months, patients were tested for increases in knowledge, compared to week 0 using the Patient Knowledge Questionnaire (Hill et al 1991). They had increased their scores significantly and this knowledge was further enhanced at 12 months from entry (Hill et al 1994).

Another study evaluated the effectiveness of educating patients during their routine outpatient visit. It was found that overall knowledge of diagnosis and treatment was high at 86%. Knowledge of the use and likely effects of drugs ranged from 52–92%, but many patients were unaware of the side effects of drugs and how to avoid them (Mahumed et al 1995).

Further evidence is obtained from a literature review of 34 studies which measured changes in knowledge, in which 94% attained increases (Lorig et al, 1987). There is of course a difference between knowing something and acting upon it. For instance, many people know that smoking causes a wide range of health-related problems, but they continue to smoke. However, in the context of chronic diseases, knowledge is an essential precursor to behavioural change and can bridge the gap between knowing and doing.

Behaviour changes

The literature review undertaken by Lorig et al (1987), showed that PE can change behaviour patterns to a large extent. They report increases of:

- 79% in the practice of exercise
- 33% in the practice of joint protection
- 86% in the practice of relaxation.

Hawley (1995) used 'effect size' to compare treatment and control groups. This is a rigorous, standardised measure of change advocated and described by Kazis et al (1989). In the 34 studies scrutinised, self-management behaviours such as compliance with exercise and coping skills improved following PE.

Improving physical and psychological health status

The more serious rheumatic diseases are capable of causing pain and swelling, stiffness, joint deformity and fatigue, which inevitably lead to a deficit in mobility, energy and everyday skills. These symptoms and ensuing shortcomings leave the patient feeling frustrated and inadequate which causes anxiety and depression. Weiner (1975) terms this the 'burden of arthritis'. Although medication, physical modalities and surgery can help to alleviate some of the problems, they are rarely the whole answer. PE however, has been shown to be a beneficial therapy in that it can increase both physical and psychological status. The strongest evidence is provided by the technique of meta-analysis, in which data from a number of similarly conducted studies are analysed together to provide a more robust statistical analysis.

This is the type of study undertaken by Mullen et al (1987) who investigated the data from 15 studies on the effects of PE on disability, pain and depression. Ten studies were on patients with RA, four RA/osteoarthritis (OA), and one on OA alone. The results showed that compared with the control groups, treatment groups had a reduction of:

- 22% in their depression
- 16% in their pain
- 8% in their disability.

The reduction in pain following the PE programmes was similar to that experienced by patients following the ingestion of non-steroidal anti-inflammatory drugs, and it is suggested that PE has an independent effect and is therefore a distinct modality. PE can contribute to the health status of those patients with arthritis and when given in addition to other treatments provides a cumulative effect.

Long-term efficacy

The chronic nature and lack of cure for many rheumatic diseases necessitates the assessment of long-term efficacy of treatments. However, there is a paucity of research in this area.

A 20-month follow-up study showed that patients experienced a slight decline in functional ability but retained their decrease in pain, depression and physician visits (Lorig & Holman 1989).

Another study assessed the effect of PE 4 years after completion. This included patients with RA, OA and other forms of arthritis. It was shown that the PE group maintained:

- 15% to 20% reductions in pain
- Made fewer visits to the physician
- Maintained their belief in their ability to cope.

However, their disability increased over the 4 years, and improvement in depression was not maintained (Lorig et al 1993).

A controlled study which revisited patients 12 months after completion of the initial PE programme reported maintained improvement in knowledge, self reported health behaviour and disability scores (Lindroth et al 1989). A further follow-up to this study was undertaken at 5 years (Lindroth et al 1995). The improvement in performing exercise and joint protection seen at 12 months did not persist, but those patients who had been in the PE group had more contact with their rheumatologists, physiotherapists and occupational therapists. They developed an increased sense of control and coping from 12 months to 5 years, resulting in a reduction in the problems they reported.

PLANNING A PE PROGRAMME

There are a number of considerations to be taken into account when planning a PE programme, for instance the physical condition of the patients who will be attending and the learning environment. Patients are usually in pain that will shorten their attention span, and they are also prone to inactivity stiffness. Those who have only recently been diagnosed are often confused about their illness and can be anxious and depressed. It is difficult to master new facts when there are physical distractions or if the environment is not conducive to learning. To overcome these problems make sure that you plan:

- Easy access to the learning environment
- A comfortable temperature
- Short teaching sessions
- Use of appropriate seating
- Exercise breaks
- Some refreshment to allow patients to take their drugs.

No matter how much thought is put into the practical arrangements, it will be to no avail if the content is not seen as relevant to the individual patient. When planning the composition of a PE programme it should be borne in mind that patients are usually adults with their own beliefs and knowledge base. Adults are self directing individuals with their own experiences; any information proffered should make sense to them and appear to be justifiable. For instance, when deciding whether or not to take drug therapy, they compare the potential efficacy and side effects with the severity of their symptoms and act accordingly.

Content of a PE programme

PE is a complex process and the success of the programme depends heavily on the quality of the planning (Taal et al 1996). The most effective programmes will need to include the elements shown in Figure 15.3, and it is a good idea to start PE programmes with tasks that patients are sure they can achieve. The most successful PE programmes are those which endeavour to fulfil the aspirations of both patients and health professionals, so begin by getting patients to write down their own goals in a form of contract with themselves.

There may be differences of opinion about what is necessary to include in a PE programme, and this was highlighted in an evaluation of the Arthritis and

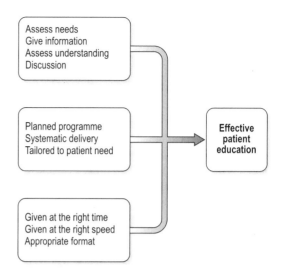

Figure 15.3 Requirements for effective patient education.

Rheumatism Council's patient literature. Some doctors thought that giving the patients too much information could lead to undue anxiety and stress. The patients interviewed wanted more detailed information about:

- Their condition
- Treatments and drugs
- Self management
- Dietary guidance
- Exercise
- Practical tips
- Communication skills.

There are many PE programmes running throughout the UK and they typically contain the topics shown in Table 15.1.

Methods of delivery

PE can be delivered in a number of ways; for instance formal or informal sessions can be introduced into either the inpatient or outpatient department. The programme can be taught by health professionals or lay persons and the sessions can be given on a one to one basis or to a group. Each has advantages and disadvantages and each patient will have their own preference. However they are taught, it is important that the patients are provided with feedback about their performance, being careful to stress the most positive aspects first.

Opportunity education

Educating patients about their disease and treatments

Table 15.1 Topics normally included in a PE programme

Topic	Typical content
Disease process	Aetiology, symptoms, blood tests
Drug therapy	Effects, side effects, usage
Exercise	Effects, how and when to do, assessing effects
Joint protection	What it is, use of splints, life style alterations
Fatigue	Causes, energy conservation
Pain control	Drug therapy, relaxation, distraction etc.
Coping	Practical strategies, self efficacy, contracting
Diet	Effects on health, fatigue
Relaxation	What it is, how it works, how to do it
Complementary therapies	Acupuncture, aromatherapy, massage
Communication	Talking to doctors and health professionals
Self help	Self efficacy, voluntary organisations
Goal setting	How to set achievable targets and reach them

is one of the primary functions of the rheumatology nurse and so every encounter with the patient should be treated as an opportunity to teach ((Daltroy & Liang 1988). It is common for short encounters to take place at:

- The patient's bedside
- In outpatient clinics
- In general practitioner surgeries.

These so called '30 second interventions' can yield positive results in the hands of a skilled practitioner. For instance a patient who is given a new drug can be asked a simple question such as, 'when are you going to take you tablets?' This will highlight any problems, such as whether they will take it with food or not. The skilled practitioner can also direct the conversation to include possible side effects and interactions with other drugs. The patient will have gained valuable knowledge and the consultation will have taken little longer than normal.

One to one PE

One to one teaching is very labour intensive which makes it the most costly. However, is considered by some to be the most effective way of imparting information as it can be tailored to each individual's needs (Tucker & Kirwan 1989). Because it is costly, programmes must be well-planned and the following items should be carefully thought about:

- The time needed to produce and deliver the programme

- What is going to be taught
- How is it going to be taught
- Documenting what has been taught
- Assessing the effectiveness of the programme
- The cost of the programme.

PE programmes need to be accessible to the patient. Those patients whose routine clinic consultation includes a PE session as part of their normal management find this easiest and most convenient, and research has shown it to be practical and effective (Mahumed et al 1995).

One of the most significant aspects of one to one teaching is its flexibility. The educator can avoid a rigid format and can include topics that are important to the patient. The timing of introduction of the subject matter can also be varied according to the patients needs. The skilled teacher can also manipulate the session to include their own agenda alongside that of the patients. For instance, if the patient wants to talk about pain and the educator wishes to teach drug therapy, an explanation of the effect of drug therapy on pain will meet both needs.

A number of studies have demonstrated that individualised PE programmes are more effective than routinised programmes (Lorish et al 1985, Neuberger et al 1993) and wherever possible this format should be used.

Group teaching

A number of hospitals and community bases teach groups of patients through structured PE programmes. Health professionals usually undertake teaching, but it is becoming more common for lay teachers, who have some arthritic problem to become teachers. This inspires some of the attendees, as the lay teachers act as very positive role models.

Group teaching has several advantages. Firstly it is comparatively cheap compared to one to one programmes. Some also believe that it is a more effective method of teaching patients skills, such as joint protection and exercise. It has a further advantage to some patients who value meeting others with the same illness and who gain benefit from sharing their experiences and meeting other patients socially.

There are of course negative aspects. Attendees will have different knowledge bases and levels of skill, which makes it difficult for the educator to meet everyone's needs. Some patients find it difficult or expensive to attend sessions and others find it daunting to express their problems verbally for fear of failure or criticism.

The Arthritis Self Management Programme (ASMP)

This is a community-based programme that began in 1978 in the USA. The underlying theoretical basis is the patient's belief that s/he can affect the consequences of their disease (self efficacy). It is believed that perceived self efficacy is a significant determinant of human functioning that operates partially independently of underlying skills. The ASMP was pioneered by Lorig and her colleagues and was the first arthritis PE programme to utilise lay teachers. Over the years the programme has been adapted as experience and research results have emerged. For instance the programmes now use pairs of teachers comprising one professional and one lay teacher rather than lay teachers alone. The lay teachers are accepted by both patients and professionals and have proved as effective as professionals in their teaching (Lorig et al 1986).

Changes have been made to the content and methodology (Lorig & Gonzalez 1992) and at present it is usually taught as 6 × 2 hour sessions over a period of months. The format remains the same in that patients with RA, OA or other forms of arthritis are taught in mixed groups.

The programme focuses on:

• Utilising information
• Problem solving
• Symptom management
• Use of coping skills.

The topics taught in the ASMP are similar to those listed in Table 15.1, but they are taught using the techniques shown in Box 15.1.

Box 15.1   Techniques taught in the ASMP
• Contracting • Feedback • Goal setting • Guided imagery • Principles of self help • Visualisation.

The ASMP has been very well researched in the USA. A controlled study on the effectiveness of the programme (Lorig et al 1985) showed a significant improvement in:

• Patient knowledge
• The practice of self management behaviours
• Pain.

The programme has become extensively used in the USA and has been adapted by other teams (Lindroth et al 1989, Taal et al 1993, Davis et al 1994) for use in Australia, New Zealand and Europe. The ASMP has been anglicised for use in Britain and its effects are currently being researched.

LEARNING AIDS

There are a number of techniques that can be used to enhance teaching and aid the learning process. Some, such as reiteration, are straightforward but nonetheless need to be thought about and incorporated into the programme. Others, for instance written material, needs careful research and piloting on the intended recipients.

Verbal information

Most patient teaching is presented verbally, but patients along with the rest of us, tend to forget a great deal of what they are told. A study from a rheumatology outpatient clinic (Anderson et al 1979) showed that patients who attended the clinic for the first time recalled about 40% of the information they were given. This figure is in broad agreement with much of the published literature.

When giving information follow some simple guidelines:

• Present the most salient points first.

This is because we remember best what we are told first.

• Consider the patient's priorities.

They will recall most easily what *they* consider to be most important.

• Do not bombard them with facts.

Most people only remember the first four or five items presented to them.

• Give written back-up.

Oral information is easily forgotten. Written information should always be provided as a supplement. The patient can then take this material home and digest it at their leisure. They can then share it with their families/partners and use it as an aide memoire in the future.

Written information

Patients themselves feel they need written information (Donovan & Blake 1992) and there is some evidence to support its effectiveness. Twenty patients with RA increased their knowledge after reading information, but when the literature was combined with lectures, the knowledge gain was significantly greater (Vignos et al 1976).

A number of professional organisations produce some excellent patient literature. They include:

• Arthritis Care
• Arthritis and Rheumatism Council
• Arthritis Foundation
• Pharmaceutical companies.

Many hospitals, wards and those that organise PE programmes, prefer to produce their own literature. Producing useful written material is more difficult that it appears at first sight and unless the material can be read and understood by those for whom it is intended, will prove to be an expensive but useless exercise.

Writing material for patients

The purpose of written information is to inform and empower the patient and so it must be:

• Informative
• Accurate
• Understandable.

Unfortunately, medically-based literature is difficult to write, as the terminology is inherently alien to the general public. Some authors have tried to address this problem (Boyd 1987) and the following guidelines can help to make the content more user friendly.

• Use lay terminology – knee cap rather than patella, persistent rather than chronic
• Simple sentence structure
• Use one or two syllable words wherever possible
• Limit the number of words using three or more syllables
• Write in short paragraphs
• Personalise the material with words like I, we, us
• Use positive not negative language
• Start with the aims of the material
• Use a question and answer format
• Include what the patients want to know as well as what they need to know.

Readability

Having written the material it is important to assess whether it is easy to read (Arthur 1995) and unfortunately this is one stage that is often left out. The readability of a document refers to the reader's ability to decipher the text (Meade & Smith 1991). The need for assessing readability was highlighted in a recent study (J Hill, personal communication, 1996), on 100 patients with RA who were attending an outpatient clinic.

Twelve percent had difficulty with their reading and so drug information leaflets about penicillamine, supplied from the clinic, were re-written to be easy or fairly easy to read. This was achieved without altering the information they contained and patients exhibited significant increases in their knowledge of their drug.

Assessing readability. Ease of readability depends on the structure of the sentence and the length of the words used, and there are a number of formulae that can be used to estimate how difficult a leaflet is to read. They are based on the:

• Number of syllables per word
• Number of words in each sentence.

The Flesch Reading Index (Flesch, 1948), the Dale-Chall Formula (Dale & Chall, 1948) and the SMOG Grading (McLaughlin, 1969); SMOG standing for 'simple measure of gobbledygook', are the most commonly used. There is a highly positive correlation amongst formulae and so the best advice is to use what you have available. Some word processor packages now include formulae, for instance Word for Windows incorporates the Flesch Index which makes it possible to assess material as it is composed. It should be noted that most of these formulae have been developed for use with the English language and because of the differences in grammatical construction they are not suitable for use with other languages.

Although they are useful, reading ease formulae are only tools, they do not assess:

• Good writing
• The accuracy of information
• The lay-out of the material.

An example of an information sheet is shown in Box 15.2.

Design of the material

Layout of the material is another important aspect. A well-thought out design will encourage the patient to read it. There are a number of considerations such as:

• Typeface
• Type size
• Colour of the paper
• Size of the leaflet.

The typeface should be clear, plain, and visible; a sans-serif font is attractive and easy to read. Once you have chosen the typeface, do not try to make headings or words stand out by adding a different one. Try using larger letters of the same typeface or use bold or italics.

Box 15.2 Penicillamine Information Sheet

What is penicillamine?
Penicillamine is one of a group of drugs known as slow acting anti-rheumatic drugs. It is a tablet, and is thought to slow down the arthritis. It should help to stop joint damage and lessen pain and stiffness. Penicillamine is not an antibiotic.

How does it work?
It works by slowly building up in the body until the proper level is reached.

How long will it take to work?
It takes 10–12 weeks before you start to feel better. Sometimes it takes even longer.

What dose will I take?
Penicillamine is started at a small dose and slowly built up as follows:

> 125 mg a day for 2 weeks
> 250 mg a day for 2 weeks
> 375 mg a day for 2 weeks
> 500 mg a day as your normal dose.

A few people need a higher dose than 500 mg a day.

When should I take the tablets?
A full day's tablets are usually taken all together as one dose. You can take them at any time of day. You should take them when your stomach is empty and so it is best about 1 hour before food or 1 1/2 hours after food.

How long can I stay on the tablets?
As long as you have no bad side effects, you can stay on them as long as they are helping the arthritis. Some people have been taking them for many years.

Are there any side effects?
A few people get side effects. This usually happens at the start of treatment, but it can happen even if you have been taking it for many years. Side effects can be:

- Upset stomach or feeling sick
- A nasty taste or loss of taste (it slowly returns to normal)

- Rash or itching
- Mouth ulcers
- Large bruises caused by changes in the clotting cells (platelets) in the blood
- Sore throat and fever caused by changes in white cells that fight infections
- Protein in the urine caused by changes in the kidneys.

Remember, only a few people get side effects

What should I do if I get side effects?
You should tell your doctor or nurse straight away.

Do I need to have special tests because of my tablets?
Yes, blood tests every **2 weeks** for the first 8 weeks then **once a month**. This is to check that the blood can clot properly and that the white cells can fight infections. If your GP checks your blood, phone the surgery and ask if your blood tests are normal. If there are any problems you may have to stop the tablets for a while until the blood goes back to normal.
Test your **urine once a week** because the tablets can affect your kidneys. This test is very easy but you must be shown what to look for. If the test shows any protein, **don't panic!** Phone your doctor or nurse and they will tell you what to do. Sometimes you have to stop taking the tablets for a while and sometimes the dose needs changing. Once this is done, the urine usually goes back to normal.

Can I take other medicines with my penicillamine?
Yes, it mixes with most other tablets such as your painkillers and anti-inflammatories. You should leave a **3-hour gap** between your iron and penicillamine and a **2-hour gap** between antacid indigestion remedies and your penicillamine. If you don't do this, the penicillamine will not work as well.

Is penicillamine safe in pregnancy?
No. If you want to have a baby you should come off your penicillamine well before you get pregnant. Discuss this with your doctor, nurse or pharmacist.

The size of the type should not be too small; 12 point or larger is ideal and eye span should be approximately 60 or 70 characters in length. Capital letters are more difficult to read, so use lower case with plenty of 'white' space between lines.

Coloured paper can be eye catching, but beware of using colours such as yellow on white as this is difficult to read.

Finally, consider how easy the document will be to handle. If it is produced to be stored in a folder then A4 is fine, but if it is a single pamphlet A5 or ⅓ A4 is better.

An example of written PE information is shown in Appendix 5.

Each of us learns in different way, some may find it easier to read, others to watch and some to listen. It is therefore important to offer patients a variety of different modalities.

Audiocassettes

Audiocassettes provide written information in verbal format and are invaluable for those patients who have difficulty reading or are blind or partially sighted. Many people use them to practise relaxation techniques or distraction therapy, but there is no reason why information about drug therapy, pain control or other modules of a PE programme cannot be dictated onto a tape.

Videos

Although written and audio formats are both excellent ways of exchanging facts, skills such as exercise and methods of joint protection are easier to demonstrate on a video. They are particularly valuable for those people who have difficulty with reading, but they should be considered as a part of a PE programme rather than a substitute for it. Many voluntarily funded organisations such as the Arthritis and Rheumatism Council and Arthritis Care produce excellent videos for patients. Their value is greatly enhanced if they come with an explanatory booklet, as is the case with a programme on medications that has been well received by patients (Clayson et al 1994).

Videos can be used in almost any setting; group sessions, one to one, wards, outpatient clinics or in the home.

Computer assisted learning

Developments in computer technology have the potential to make enormous strides in methods of delivering patient information, and computer assisted learning has been advocated as a way of empowering the patient rather than the educator, and therefore a positive move in the direction of self care (Luker & Caress 1989).

Advances in personal computer technology offer the possibility of patients having access to expert systems. Expert systems allow individuals to interrogate the computer for the information that they require. Explanations are provided in text, computer graphics and sound format. Many people now have access to the internet, and again this gives access to information from all over the world at the touch (well almost) of a switch.

Research carried out in the mid-1980s in the USA, assessed the effect of a computer based education lesson for patients with RA (Wetstone et al 1985). It covered ten main topics including:

• Aetiology of the disease
• Dietary advice
• Exercise regimes
• Joint protection techniques
• Medications
• Other treatments.

Patients were able to access the topics of their choice in any order, and review them at will. When compared with a matched control group, the computer educated group was shown to have enjoyed the lesson and improved significantly in a number of areas. They had:

• Gained more knowledge than the controls
• Improved their outlook on life
• Were more hopeful of a good prognosis
• Reported an increase in their use of behaviours such as joint protection.

Expert systems allow PE to be genuinely patient-centred and self directed and are therefore to be encouraged.

Action points for practice:

• Describe two theoretical models that you consider to be appropriate for use in a PE programme.
• Write a drug information leaflet that will be easily understood by your patients.
• Write a list of topics that would be suitable for inclusion in a PE programme for patients with systemic lupus erythematosus.
• Describe ways of assessing the effectiveness of a PE programme.
• Carry out a literature search on the effects and side effects of PE, discuss the merits and problems associated with such programmes.

REFERENCES

Anderson J L, Dodman S, Copelman M, Fleming A 1979 Patient information recall in a rheumatology clinic. Rheumatology and Rehabilitation 18: 18–22
Arthur V A M 1995 Written patient information: a review of the literature. Journal of Advanced Nursing 21: 1081–1086
Auerbach S M 1989 Stress management and coping research in the health care setting: an overview and methodological commentary. Journal of Consulting and Clinical Psychology 57(3): 388–395

Bandura A 1977 Self-efficacy: toward a unifying theory of behavioural change. Psychological Review 84: 191–215
Becker M 1974 The health belief model and personal health behaviour. Health Education Monographs 2: 236
Boyd M D 1987 A guide to writing effective education materials. Nursing Management 18(7): 56–57
Burckhardt C S 1994 Arthritis and musculoskeletal patient education standards. Arthritis Care and Research 7: 1–4
Clayson M, Cole A, Phillips P 1994 Medication for arthritis –

an educational package for patients. Scandinavian Journal of Rheumatology (suppl 97) Ab 113

Dale E, Chall J S 1948 A formula for predicting readability. Educational Research Bulletin 27: 11–20

Daltroy L H, Liang M H 1988 Patient education in the rheumatic diseases: a research agenda. Arthritis Care and Research 1: 161–169

Davis P, Busch A, Lowe J C et al 1994 Evaluation of a rheumatoid arthritis patient education program: impact on knowledge and self-efficacy. Patient Education and Counseling 24: 55–61

DeVellis R F, Blalock S J 1993 Psychological and educational interventions to reduce arthritis disability. Baillière's Clinical Rheumatology 7: 397–416

Donovan J L, Blake D 1992 Patient compliance: deviance or reasoned decision making? Social Science Medicine 34: 507–513

Donovan J L, Blake D R, Fleming G 1989 The patient is not a blank sheet: lay beliefs and their relevance to patient education. British Journal of Rheumatology 28: 58–61

Flesch R 1948 A new readability yardstick. Journal of Applied Psychology 32: 221–233

Hawley D 1995 Psycho-educational interventions in the treatment of arthritis. Baillière's Clinical Rheumatology 9: 803–823

Hill J 1997 A practical guide to patient education and information giving. Baillière's Clinical Rheumatology 11(1): 109–127

Hill J 1995 Patient education in rheumatic disease. Nursing Standard 9: 25–28

Hill J, Bird H A, Harmer R, Wright V, Lawton C 1994 An evaluation of the effectiveness, safety and acceptability of a nurse practitioner in a rheumatology outpatient clinic. British Journal of Rheumatology 33: 283–288

Hill J, Bird H A, Hopkins R, Lawton C, Wright V 1991 The development and use of a patient knowledge questionnaire in rheumatoid arthritis. British Journal of Rheumatology 30: 45–49

Hirano P C, Laurent D D, Lorig K 1994 Arthritis patient education studies, 1987–1991: a review of the literature. Patient Education and Counseling 24: 9–54

Kazis L E, Anderson J J, Meenan R F 1989 Effect sizes for interpreting changes in health status. Medical Care 27: S178–S189

Lazarus R S, Folkman S 1984 Stress appraisal and coping. Springer, New York

Lindroth Y, Bauman A, Barnes C, McCredie M, Brookes P M 1989 A controlled evaluation of arthritis education. British Journal of Rheumatology 28: 7–12

Lindroth Y, Bauman A, Brookes P M, Priestley D 1995 A 5-year follow-up of a controlled trial of an arthritis education programme. British Journal of Rheumatology 34: 647–652

Lorig K 1996 Patient Education a Practical Approach, 2nd edn. Sage, Thousand Oaks

Lorig K, Feigenbaum P, Regan C, Ung C, Holman H R 1986 A comparison of lay-taught and professional-taught arthritis self-management courses. The Journal of Rheumatology 13: 763–767

Lorig K, Gonzalez V 1992 The integration of theory with practice: a 12-year case study. Health Education Quarterly 19: 355–368

Lorig K, Holman H R 1989 Long-term outcomes of an arthritis self-management study: effects of reinforcement efforts. Social Science Medicine 29: 221–224

Lorig K, Konkol L, Gonzalez V 1987 Arthritis patient education: a review of the literature. Patient Education and Counseling 10: 207–252

Lorig K, Lubeck D, Kraines R G, Seleznick M, Holman H R 1985 Outcomes of self-help education for patients with arthritis. Arthritis and Rheumatism 28: 680–685

Lorig K, Mazonson P D, Holman H R 1993 Evidence suggesting that health education for self-management in patients with chronic arthritis has sustained health benefits while reducing health care costs. Arthritis Rheumatism 36: 439–446

Lorish C D, Parker J, Brown S 1985 Effective patient education: a quasi-experimental study comparing an individualized strategy with a routinized strategy. Arthritis and Rheumatism 28: 1289–1297

Luker K, Caress A 1989 Rethinking patient education. Journal of Advanced Nursing 14: 711–718

McLaughlin H 1969 SMOG grading – a new readability formula. Journal of Reading 12: 639–646

Mahmud T, Comer M, Roberts K, Berry H, Scott D L 1995 Clinical implications of patients' knowledge. Clinical Rheumatology 14: 627–630

Meade C D, Smith C F 1991 Readability formulas: caution and criteria. Patient Education and Counseling 17: 153–158

Mullen P A, Laville E A, Biddle A K, Lorig K 1987 Efficacy of psychoeducational interventions of pain, depression, and disability in people with arthritis: a meta-analysis. Journal of Rheumatology 14: 33–39

Neuberger G B, Smith K V, Black S O, Hassanein R 1993 Promoting self-care in clients with arthritis. Arthritis Care and Research 6: 141–148

Newbold D 1996 Coping with rheumatoid arthritis. How can specialist nurses influence it and promote better outcomes? Journal of Clinical Nursing 5: 373–380

Pincus T, Callahan L F 1989 Reassessment of twelve traditional paradigms concerning the diagnosis, prevalence, morbidity and mortality of rheumatoid arthritis. Scandinavian Journal of Rheumatology 79: 67–95

Seligman M 1975 Helplessness: on depression, development and death. W H Freeman, San Fransisco

Taal E, Rasker J J, Wiegman O 1996 Patient education and self-management in the rheumatic diseases: a self efficacy approach. Arthritis Care and Research 9(3): 229–238

Taal E, Riemsma R P, Brus H L M, Seydel E R, Rasker J J, Weigman O 1993 Group education for patients with rheumatoid arthritis. Patient Education and Counseling 20: 177–187

Tucker M, Kirwan J R 1989 Does patient education in rheumatoid arthritis have therapeutic potential? Annals of the Rheumatic Disease 50: 422–428

Vignos P J, Parker W T, Thompson H M 1976 Evaluation of a clinic education programme for patients with RA. Journal of Rheumatology 3: 155–165

Wetstone S L, Sheehan J, Votaw R G et al 1985 Evaluation of a computer based education lesson for patients with rheumatoid arthritis. The Journal of Rheumatology 12: 907–912

Wiener C L 1975 The burden of rheumatoid arthritis: tolerating the uncertainty. Society of Science and Medicine 9: 97–104

Wilson Barnett J 1984 Key functions in nursing: the fourth Winifred Raphael memorial lecture. RCN, London

FURTHER READING

Glanz R, Rimer B, Lewis F 1990 Health behavior and health education: theory, research, and practice. Jossey-Bass, San Francisco

Ley P 1992 Communicating with patients: improving communication, satisfaction and compliance. Chapman Hall, London

16

Seamless care

Lynne Dargie, Jane Proctor

The aim of this chapter is to promote an awareness of the need within the community, for adequate support mechanisms for rheumatology patients, to complement the specialist care provided by hospitals. After reading this chapter you should then be able to:

- Analyse the need for seamless care in the light of demographic trends, epidemiological factors and current financial resources
- Discuss the factors necessary to implement effective shared-care schemes
- Describe how such a scheme may be set up
- Explain the potential advantages of shared-care
- Discuss the contribution made by the nurse in meeting the needs of rheumatology patients in the community.

Orton (1994) states that 'demographic trends, changing patterns of illness and the rising cost of health care, all point to primary care as the key to the provision of effective health care services in the future'. Changes in the National Health Service in the United Kingdom have directed a large proportion of health care provision to the community sector; to general practitioners and associated community health services (NHS Management Executive 1991). In view of these changes, close interprofessional communication and collaboration between hospital rheumatology departments and primary health care teams is necessary if the development of a seamless rheumatology service is to be achieved. This combined approach can be difficult to implement, but could offer those with a rheumatic disease a cost-effective quality service, with greater accessibility.

THE SCOPE OF THE PROBLEM

General practitioner consultations

In 1991–1992, 15% of the population of the UK consulted a general practitioner with a disease of the musculoskeletal system. This was a rise of 2% since 1981–1982. The consultations showed a marked increase in the incidence of osteoarthritis (OA) whilst the rates for rheumatoid arthritis (RA) had declined (Charlton et al 1995). The majority of these patients are seen in general practice and do not require referral to hospital. Consequently they rely on the primary health care team to provide the relevant specialist advice and support. If the primary health care team does not possess the necessary knowledge, patients with a rheumatic disease will be denied the benefits of appropriate treatment and education.

Research has highlighted some of the consequent problems. In one study, a proportion of general practitioners overprescribed non-steroidal anti-inflammatory drugs and underprescribed analgesics when treating patients with OA. Physiotherapy and local steroid injections were also underused (Davis & Suarez-Almazor 1995). Another study of 249 patients with RA, found that only 65% of patients taking disease modifying anti-rheumatic drugs were receiving the ideal monitoring regime from their surgery (Helliwell & O'Hara 1995).

Patients have their own beliefs about rheumatic diseases. In a study of patients who are over 65 years and have arthritic symptoms, many believed that no therapies would be effective and that even quite severe symptoms were normal for their age. Consequently they thought that they were untreatable (Vetter et al 1990). However, in present day society, many patients want to know more about their illness and methods of self-management and the general practitioner can be left feeling somewhat frustrated if he is insufficiently knowledgeable to offer such support (Fig. 16.1.).

Outpatient consultations

In the UK, between 1988 and 1992 there was a 33% increase in consultations with rheumatologists. This was accompanied by a 22% increase in waiting time from referral, to new patient consultation (Kirwan 1994).

Having waited, sometimes for long periods to see a consultant, patients often face travelling and parking difficulties which can pose problems for the more disabled. The frustrations that this causes, coupled with the patient's anxiety and the doctor having to rush the consultation, can create considerable barriers to communication (Haslock 1987).

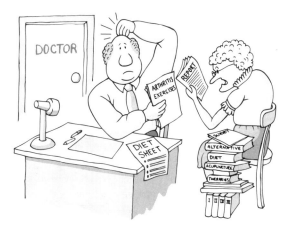

Figure 16.1 Cartoon. (By kind permission of Dr William Bird.)

Education is not always available, partly due to time constraints but perhaps due also to inadequate ability and the unwillingness of some rheumatologists to impart such knowledge.

ASPECTS OF EXISTING SERVICES

Primary health care team

A survey undertaken in 'Which' magazine (Consumer Association 1992) found that the two top concerns of patients were:

• How long they had to sit in the waiting room
• The length of time it took to get an appointment.

These difficulties have been overcome with notable success in primary health care (Hasler 1994).

In addition, most patients prefer to see the same doctor and such personal, continuous care is linked with patient satisfaction (Freeman & Richards 1993, Hjortdahl & Laerum 1992). The general practitioner and other primary health care team members, such as the practice nurse, district nurse and health visitor, have such a one to one relationship with their patients. Because of this they have the opportunity to have:

• Knowledge of the patient's physical, psychological, financial and social needs
• The ability to visit the patient at home
• The ability to make referrals to community health services such as physiotherapy, occupational therapy, social services and the voluntary sector.

Primary prevention of many rheumatic disorders may not be possible, but with increased knowledge, primary health care team members may be able to assist in early diagnosis and treatment, anticipate required support for patients and carers and encourage the promotion of self help (Knox 1987).

Hospital rheumatology team

Hospital rheumatology teams are able to offer the specialist knowledge and support that is required by patients with the more serious conditions. Hospitals have facilities for more detailed clinical assessment, investigation and treatment than is possible in the community, coupled with increased accessibility to other professionals such as occupational therapists and physiotherapists who may have specialised in the field of rheumatology.

The employment of increasing numbers of rheumatology nurse specialists has enhanced patient education and provided the opportunity for coordinated activity between primary and secondary healthcare (Maycock 1990).

The need for musculoskeletal services is likely to increase during the next decade. This is in part due to the increasing numbers of the very elderly and in part due to the development of surgical techniques and the growth of public expectation (Horbury 1995). Failure to increase resources for a speciality that is already underresourced will result in the further restriction of access to care and makes the quest for developing new ways to manage the interface between primary and secondary care that much more urgent (Kirwan 1994).

THE ADVENT OF A SEAMLESS SERVICE

Shared-care is a clinically effective, cost-effective initiative that is acceptable to patients and general practitioners and allows more patients to receive specialist advice. In this context, shared-care can be defined as 'the joint participation of general practitioners and hospital consultants in the planned delivery of care for patients with a chronic condition, informed by an enhanced information exchange over and above routine discharge and referral letters' (Hickman et al 1994). Such a concept will allow the most appropriate care to be provided within the most appropriate setting, providing scope for joint initiatives to be undertaken (Barrett & Tomes 1992).

THE PRINCIPLES OF GOOD SHARED-CARE

Dargie & Proctor (1993, 1994) and Orton (1994) have suggested that there are a number of underlying principles that require consideration if shared-care schemes are to be effective (Box 16.1).

Box 16.1 The principles of good outpatient shared-care

- Identifying health needs at a local level
- Increased investment into primary care
- Full utilisation and development of multidisciplinary skills
- Effective joint planning initiatives.

Adapted from Dargie & Proctor (1993, 1994), and Orton (1994), with permission.

Identifying health needs at a local level

In the UK, current government policy has geared the health services to provide health care that is more responsive to local need. Consideration of the health and social data of a locality is a prerequisite to effective health care planning and future resource allocation (Tinson 1995). Collation of local data regarding the morbidity of musculoskeletal disease and the social, political and environmental factors that affect the health of patients can ensure that a need for improved local services is assessed. However, it is important that the data collected is used in conjunction with the needs expressed by the individual patients, whose pain and disability can result in a vast array of problems. Aims and objectives of care can then be designed to meet the identified needs of the population. Strategies and resources can be planned and utilised more effectively and the data can contribute evidence of the need for change. A study of urban patients with rheumatic disease, (Liebman et al 1986), found that the top ten expressions of need were:

- Help with understanding medications
- Explanations of special exercises
- Provision of an arthritis doctor
- Explanations of their type of arthritis
- Podiatric care
- Reading materials about arthritis
- Help with household chores
- Self help support groups
- Provision of canes and crutches
- Someone to talk to about things that make them nervous.

Increased investment in primary care

The development of any shared-care initiative requires an increase in resources and at the time of writing there is a lack of financial incentive for general practitioners to set up shared-care initiatives in rheumatology. In the UK, diabetic, asthma and hypertension clinics in general practice entitle general practitioners to receive financial reimbursements. By contrast, initiatives in rheumatology receive no remuneration despite the fact that rheumatic disorders are second only to cardiovascular disease in producing severe disability. Orton (1994) recognises that under present funding arrangements, rheumatology specialists running practice-based clinics are disadvantaged. This arises because consultants are seeing, in the community, patients who would otherwise be using hospital outpatient services. As a consequence, the number of hospital referrals is reduced and the consultant spends less time at the hospital, both of which affect hospital funding.

There is a growing recognition that the current and future demand for musculoskeletal services is likely to exceed available resources and strategies are being devised which recognise the need to invest in joint initiatives between primary and secondary care (Horbury 1995). Proposals aimed at providing a more efficient, effective service to cope with future demand include:

- Provision of care close to home
- Deriving benefit from self management interventions
- Teams of specialists trained in different disciplines working together
- Increased investment outside hospitals
- A more systematic approach to incorporating research results into practice
- Promotion of collaboration rather than competition.

Full utilisation and development of multidisciplinary skills

If the challenges presented by the provision of future health care are to be met, 'doctors, nurses and managers need to recognise each other's talents, integrate their work and forge new relationships' (Hasler 1994). Although hospital rheumatology specialists are considered as part of the secondary health care team, there is no reason why elements of such a concept should not be utilised across the health care boundaries, as this can be advantageous to the patient.

Rheumatologists and general practitioners

General practitioners possess a wide body of comprehensive medical skills that can benefit patients in the surgery or home setting. They are also able to go beyond the confines of diagnosing and treating illness, possessing an enhanced ability to deal with their patients' psychological and social problems (Branch 1994). However they are generalists and not necessarily qualified to provide the specialist care required by rheumatology patients.

The great majority of general practitioners acknowledge the need for postgraduate education in rheumatology, and 50% would welcome education in practical skills. The provision of sufficient knowledge and skills will both enhance patient care and help to prevent unnecessary referrals to the rheumatologist, of patients with non-inflammatory musculoskeletal disorders (Blaaw et al 1995).

Shared-care offers the opportunity for mutual professional education between primary and secondary health professionals in rheumatology. This may occur through regular meetings to discuss topics, primary health care team members sitting in on hospital outpatient clinics, clinical assistantships where general practitioners work alongside consultant rheumatologists and the provision of study days. The distance learning diploma in Primary Care Rheumatology devised by the Primary Care Rheumatology Society and Bath University is one such initiative for general practitioners.

Rheumatology nurse specialist

The rheumatology nurse specialist, with her extended rheumatology skills, aims to facilitate the highest possible standards of care to rheumatology patients in conjunction with all members of the caring team (Sturdy 1992, unpublished work). Rheumatology nurse specialists have achieved improved outcomes through their supportive educational approach to patients (Grahame & West 1996). Such skills and knowledge are invaluable assets that could be utilised by general practitioners and community nurses, providing a point of contact in dealing with particular patient problems in the community.

However rheumatology nurse specialists are in short supply. In some areas of the UK there is only one for an entire county and in other areas, none at all. It would therefore seem unlikely that such a limited resource could participate in both hospital activities and in the development of many community initiatives. In one area of the UK, this problem has been addressed by employing a senior lecturer/consultant in community rheumatology who is supported by a community rheumatology sister (Hay & Schollam 1994 unpublished work). The following was achieved within a year of implementation:

- Receipt of over 200 referrals from primary and secondary care sources
- Twenty-five to thirty-five home visits made per month

- Two drug monitoring clinics established in the community
- Coordination of 40 patients' individual drug therapy regimes
- Helpline established for use by patients and primary health care teams
- Two patient education groups developed in the community
- Education meetings devised for primary health care staff
- Provision of a central information centre for community services.

These activities are an indication of the benefits to both patients and the primary and secondary health care teams and it is suggested that this model could be implemented in many more areas of the country.

Practice nurses

In recent years the role of the practice nurse has moved away from its traditional image of undertaking tasks delegated by a general practitioner and has expanded, particularly in the areas of health promotion and ill health prevention.

Hyde (1995) has described the present day practice nurse as:

- Raising health consciousness
- Teaching
- Providing therapeutic nursing care
- Acting as patient advocate
- Practising anticipatory care.

In some areas, practice nurses are also taking on the additional role of nurse practitioner, a role that enables them to make initial assessments and diagnoses (Hasler 1994). Current government legislation in the UK is encouraging practice nurses to utilise and develop their skills in many new areas of health care and their involvement in the management, follow up and education of rheumatology patients could therefore be a natural progression.

District nurses

The district nurse possesses the essential skills that enable patients to be cared for in their own environment, with the aim of achieving maximum levels of independence and comfort. Patients and their carers are encouraged and assisted to make informed choices about their health care needs within the context of their own lifestyles (Nottingham Health Authority 1990). District nurses are able to plan and provide for episodic and continuing programmes of care for the acutely ill or chronically sick. In addition, they are able to provide subsequent care involving:

- The organisation of community resources, both professional and voluntary
- Ensure continuity of care between the hospital and the home
- Promote health, rehabilitation and counselling
- Ensure quality of care is maintained.

The current attributes of district nurses, in caring for patients with rheumatic diseases, would be enhanced by increasing their knowledge base (Hill 1986). In the UK, the development of English National Board courses in rheumatology nursing and the Royal College of Nursing Rheumatology Nursing Forum have provided such opportunities for expanding the knowledge base of some nurses.

Health visitors

It is frequently believed that health visitors work predominantly with children aged 5 and under, providing assessments and preventative care. However, their role is increasingly extending to all age groups, imparting the skills of health promotion and ill health prevention, involving public health education and community participation in activities. They have a wide knowledge of resources available to deal with health and welfare problems and possess particular skills in counselling and advising. Patients, particularly with chronic rheumatic disease may incur complex problems that affect the whole family unit, or the patient may be a child. Further development of the existing skills of the health visitor could be an invaluable resource in such situations.

Combined care

Many patients prefer to see a nurse at regular intervals rather than a doctor only occasionally (Bird 1985). It has also been shown that compared with consultant-run arthritis clinics, nurse-run clinics, can result in significant improvement in patients' levels of knowledge, satisfaction and symptoms (Hill 1991, Hill et al 1994). The further development and combined utilisation of nursing skills in rheumatology across the primary/secondary care boundaries can therefore be justified by the enhanced patient care it provides.

Effective planning of combined initiatives

Effective combined initiatives will not evolve without

meticulous planning. Barrett & Tomes (1992) believe that to achieve a smooth transition between primary and secondary care both entities must operate as one. This requires close cooperation, excellent communication and the development of common systems.

Protocols and guidelines

Protocols and clinical guidelines can provide written details of care to be administered in specific situations. Such research-based guidelines are thought to help decision making through the documentation of standardised care. The quality of care can then be maintained, hence patient outcomes improved (Mansfield 1995). Shared management protocols for rheumatic diseases may outline:

- Service aims
- Clinic formats
- Individual roles
- Clinical assessment criteria
- Investigations
- Education
- Monitoring regimes for disease modifying drugs
- Local resources
- Liaison methods
- Re-referral criteria
- Methods of audit.

The use of such protocols and clinical guidelines could assist the primary health care team members, who may be less knowledgeable regarding rheumatic disease, to maintain a continuity of quality care. However, in a study of attitudes and behaviours of clinicians towards clinical guidelines, it was found that 64% of clinicians did not use guidelines because they were poorly developed and 49% because they were impractical (Mansfield 1995). Therefore, it has been suggested that if protocols and guidelines are to be utilised effectively, they should reflect local require-ments and needs rather than being regimentally structured (Barrett & Tomes 1992).

SHARED-CARE SCHEMES

In their examination of shared-care schemes Hickman et al (1994) devised a taxonomy (Table 16.1) of such initiatives partly to create awareness of different schemes that may be appropriate to different settings and to encourage their development.

Community clinics

Community clinics are classified as the provision of a clinic within the general practice, attended by a hospital specialist. Orton (1994) suggests that without the involvement of the primary health care team members, such a clinic could be viewed as being 're-located', with very little improvement in the quality of care given. However, there is the opportunity for integrated teamwork, with the consultant or rheumatology nurse specialist encouraging the development of skills by the primary health care team.

Various arthritis clinic initiatives have arisen. These range from drug monitoring clinics specifically for patients with RA, to the clinic such as that discussed in detail later in this chapter, which caters for all types of rheumatoid disease.

Basic model

Shared-care via the basic model is described as communication by letter or standardised record sheet, to exchange information between the hospital and the general practitioner. Because of its regularity, it is viewed as an extension of normal communication. However, unless a shared-care coordinator is available to monitor the process, it may not be possible to identify when letters or sheets do not arrive at the expected time (Hickman et al 1994).

Table 16.1 A taxonomy of shared-care schemes for chronic disease (adapted from Hickman, Drummond & Grimshaw (1994) by kind permission of Oxford University Press)

Classification	Description
Community clinics	Clinics run in general practice by hospital specialist and/or primary health care team
Basic model	Liaison through regular letters or standardised record sheets
Liaison model	Primary health care teams and specialist health teams have regular patient discussions/meetings
Shared-care record card	Agreed data and results recorded on a card transferred by patient between surgery and hospital
Computer-assisted shared-care	Data is entered onto central hospital computer by participants, examined by consultant, with letters and recommendations for further care sent to GP
Electronic mail	A common database with multi-access ports, available to hospital and primary health care teams

Liaison model

In the liaison model of shared-care, regular meetings are held between the hospital team and the general practitioner to discuss the care of individual patients. This may involve the development of joint management plans and guidelines and/or the initiation of jointly held clinics.

Shared-care record card

The shared-care, co-op or liaison card or booklet allows the systematic recording of data, which can be carried by the patient between their general practice and hospital appointments. Transfer of such valuable information could prevent tests being repeated and provides an up-to-date picture of a patient's health status.

Shared appointments may be pre-planned through re-referral criteria or be unplanned depending on the patient's condition.

Computer-assisted shared-care

Jointly agreed data is collected by the hospital and general practitioner and entered onto a central hospital computer. The hospital consultant examines the results of each hospital visit and updates the computerised patient record. Letters with advice and recommendations are then sent back to the general practitioner. Coordinating staff are alert to any breaks in the circle of information exchange, giving appropriate recommendations where required.

Electronic mail

This consists of a common database, where the health professionals involved in shared-care can enter agreed data, so that information is then accessible to all participants. The data can be entered either straight onto the computer or sent by electronic mail. Such a system could be linked to other databases in hospital or general practice, to supply additional information, for example on pathology, patient administration, or general practice administration (Hickman et al (1994).

PROFILE OF A COMMUNITY-BASED ARTHRITIS CLINIC

The following account is based on the experience gained in establishing and running a community based arthritis clinic founded on a partnership between the local community health centre and local hospital (Fig. 16.2).

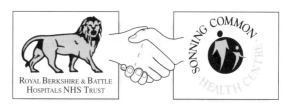

Figure 16.2 The partnership required to establish a community based arthritis clinic (by kind permission of the Royal Berkshire & Battle Hospitals NHS Trust and The Sonning Common Health Centre).

In 1992 a need was identified for improved monitoring, education and support of people with arthritis, in the locality of Sonning Common near Reading in the south of England. After 9 months' initial planning, the innovation of a community-based arthritis clinic emerged. The aim was to:

• Respond to the needs of the local population
• Encourage other practices to set up similar shared-care initiatives.

The locality

The clinic is based in a health centre located in a large village, situated in semi-rural surroundings. The majority of the population and that of the surrounding small villages are served by the health centre, which has 7600 registered patients. The Battle Hospital in Reading is 8 miles away and accommodates a rheumatology department. Public transport between the two is limited and despite it being a fairly affluent area, 17% of the population do not have a car and rely on public transport to attend the hospital.

The village itself exhibits a highly developed community spirit, endeavouring to provide many voluntary organisations to meet the villagers' needs. Funds were raised to purchase a local minibus, volunteers driving people to their essential destinations in return for a donation towards fuel costs.

The Sonning Common Health Centre is a fund-holding practice that endeavours to be pro-active in meeting the needs of its population. It had supported a move to provide a satellite rheumatology clinic at the local community hospital. However, clinic visits still involved a 6 mile journey, particularly disadvantaging the elderly, disabled and those on low incomes. Its other initiatives include a wide range of health promotion and screening facilities, a private minibus service, its own dispensary and prescription delivery service to outlying villages.

The primary health care team consists of:

- Two full-time and three part-time general practitioners
- Three part-time practice nurses
- One practice manager
- Fifteen support staff
- One dispensary auxiliary
- One full-time and one part-time health visitor
- One full-time and one part-time district nurse
- One part-time community staff nurse
- Two part-time auxiliaries.

Identifying the need

Analysis of the community profile revealed the difficulties encountered by patients with musculoskeletal disease when attending hospital outpatient appointments. For those who did manage to attend the hospital, there was a restricted time appointment with the consultant or his assistant, but little or no education. This was partly due to the time constraints and partly due to the lack of a rheumatology nurse specialist. It was also found that many patients were attending the hospital for routine monitoring of their drugs, which could quite easily have been carried out at the health centre.

Within the community, there was a local Arthritis and Rheumatism Council representative for support, but nobody within the primary health care team had specialist knowledge of musculoskeletal disorders. Consequently, patients who wanted to know more about their illness and to be able to self-manage their disease were likely to be issued with a prescription for a non-steroidal anti-inflammatory drug, as the only response to their painful illness.

These existing problems were contributing towards unnecessary hospital referrals which resulted in longer hospital waiting lists and caused travelling difficulties for patients. This was coupled with a poor community health support mechanism that resulted in some inappropriate treatment responses and little scope for patient participation in managing their own illness. It was therefore decided at a primary health care team meeting to address some of these problems by initiating a nurse-run arthritis clinic. The skills of a general practitioner, practice and district nurse would be utilised and developed in close collaboration with the local hospital consultant rheumatologist, a private physiotherapist and an Arthritis and Rheumatism Council representative.

Aims of the arthritis clinic (Dargie & Proctor 1993) were to:

- Provide an easily accessible service for the assessment, support, education and monitoring of arthritis patients and their families tailored to individual needs.
- Help patients to participate in preventing the deterioration of their condition, maintain its stability and cope with its effects on their day to day life.
- Utilise the resources available in the local community.
- Develop a specialist arthritis resource for patients and fellow team members.
- Strengthen the links between the community and the local hospital rheumatology department.
- Encourage other practices to set up similar initiatives.

Setting up a community-based arthritis clinic

Literature search. In the absence of a rheumatology nurse specialist in the area, a literature search of other nurse-run arthritis clinics was undertaken. This revealed many hospital-based clinics, but if any clinics existed in the community, nobody had written about them. However, valuable facts, ideas and contacts were gathered from the available literature, providing a foundation upon which adaptations could be made to incorporate the needs of the local community.

Identification of local and national resources

A number of resources were identified that would prove valuable in setting up such an initiative. The hospital possessed a specialist rheumatology resource of doctors, allied health professionals and an extensive rheumatology library; the primary health care team members involved in setting up the clinic also had some knowledge of rheumatology. This enabled both parties to utilise and share existing skills and further develop those skills to provide a specialist community resource. Professional contacts in other parts of the country, particularly rheumatology nurse specialists, provided support and information on literature, study days and forums.

The local community provided an Arthritis and Rheumatism Council representative, a local hall that could be used for exercise classes, a local school pool with the potential for hydrotherapy sessions, a private physiotherapist and voluntary transport.

National organisations, such as the Arthritis and Rheumatism Council, Arthritis Care and the Ankylosing Spondylitis Association, were other valuable information resources. The business world, including drug companies and appliance centres, helped the team to keep up to date with the latest research and equipment. The local press and professional journals provided opportunities to publish articles and provided a valuable resource with which to encourage the development of similar initiatives in other practice areas.

Joint protocol

The local hospital consultant was invited to the health centre to discuss the development of a joint protocol (Fig. 16.3). Decisions were made regarding the development and format of the clinic, clinical assessment, investigation and drug monitoring guidelines. The aims of the education to be provided were also outlined along with a checklist.

Liaison with the hospital rheumatology department was through:

- Use of shared-care cards
- Letters
- Advice by telephone from the consultant, regarding complicated cases
- General practitioner accepting a clinical assistantship.

To assess its effectiveness, the team planned an audit of patient satisfaction, effectiveness of joint injections and the uptake of non-steroidal anti-inflammatory drugs.

Educational development

The general practitioner, practice and district nurse each undertook a self-appraisal to assess deficient areas of knowledge regarding the musculoskeletal disorders. The general practitioner felt that he would develop his skills through a clinical assistantship and by attending relevant study days. The district nurse spent time working in two rheumatology wards at the Royal Bath Hospital in Harrogate and alongside a rheumatology nurse practitioner in her outpatient clinic at Leeds General Infirmary. Team members were invited to sit in on the hospital outpatient clinics, attended numerous study days and became members of the Primary Care Rheumatology Society and the Royal College of Nursing Rheumatology Nursing Forum.

The cooperation of many rheumatology departments across the country enabled educational handouts for patients to be developed, on many topic areas.

Development of assessment tools

A pre-clinic questionnaire was developed to assist in the initial evaluation of patients' needs. This was based partly upon the Stanford Health Assessment Criteria

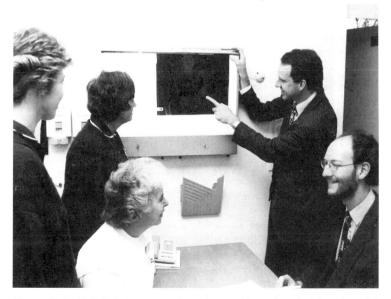

Figure 16.3 Multidisciplinary cross boundary working – the principles of good shared-care. The team includes: district nurse, practice nurse, hospital-based rheumatology nurse specialist, general practitioner, consultant rheumatologist.

(Kirwan & Reeback 1986), in combination with the depression, pain and social activity sections of the arthritis impact measurement scales (Meenan et al 1980). Using the questionnaire, a patient's physical, psychological and social needs can be assessed (see Ch. 4). It is given to patients prior to their clinic attendance, to allow them time to consider their responses at home, and it is evaluated at the clinic.

In addition to the questionnaire, a clinic assessment sheet (Fig. 16.4) and flow chart (Fig. 16.5) were designed to record baseline information and a pain and stiffness daily diary card was developed.

Advertising the clinic

All patients with RA were sent a letter of invitation to the clinic and a tutorial was given by the practice nurse, district nurse and general practitioner to encourage referrals from other members of the primary health care team. A poster was placed in the health centre reception and details printed in the health centre newsletter, to advertise the clinic. The immediate and overwhelming response gave early indications of the clinic's necessity.

Clinic format

Initially, the clinic was run twice monthly, with 30 minute appointments for new patients and 20 or 10 minute follow-up appointments. However, as a result of the demand for appointments, this was soon altered to a weekly clinic.

The clinic is open to patients with any form of musculoskeletal disorder, through referral by:

- The patient
- Fellow primary health care team members
- Hospital consultants.

Patients are initially seen by the district nurse and practice nurse who identify priority needs, in partnership with the patient. This is achieved through evaluation using the pre-clinic questionnaire, initiating the use of the pain/stiffness daily diary card where appropriate and by undertaking clinical assessment and investigations as per protocol.

Having identified a patient's educational needs, topics are selected from the education checklist and discussed and handouts provided to reinforce the information given. An opportunity is provided at the patient's next visit, to answer any subsequent queries.

The nurses are also responsible for assisting the general practitioner with appropriate treatment and undertaking referrals to other professionals as required. The general practitioner is on hand to deal with any diagnoses, poor symptom control, initiating alterations in prescriptions, undertaking joint injections and acupuncture. Patient recall depends very much on the status of their disease and is a decision that is made on an individual basis.

REFLECTIONS ON SEAMLESS CARE

The clinic has now been operating for 5 years and the experience of running it since 1992 has enabled the health centre arthritis team to reflect on some of its advantages and disadvantages. The examples described in Case Studies 1 and 2 illustrate the way in which the clinic works.

Provision of a much-needed service

The need for the clinic has been reflected in the response received from the population it serves. The initial twice a month clinic sessions were quickly increased to weekly, as the excess demand for clinic appointments became apparent. Within the first 18 months approximately 142 new patients were seen with 430 consultations. The clinic now continues weekly, serving approximately 10 patients a week.

Clinic effectiveness

A limited survey of patients' satisfaction with the clinic was undertaken in 1994, based partly upon a patient satisfaction questionnaire designed by the Rheumatism Research Unit, University of Leeds (Hill et al 1992, Hill 1997). Twenty-eight questions were sent to 20 patients who had attended the clinic. The questions were grouped into topics:

- Overall satisfaction
- Giving of information
- Empathy with the patient
- Technical quality and competence
- Attitude to patients
- Access and continuity.

The item producing the lowest score concerned the extent to which patients were asked which treatment they would prefer and that producing the highest score was 'visiting the clinic is not a stressful situation'. The survey results have enabled the team to examine ways of improving the clinic.

Evidence of increasing participation in preventing deterioration of their illness has been identified through the numbers of patients attending local initiatives involving exercise classes, local health walks

SONNING COMMON HEALTH CENTRE ARTHRITIS MANAGEMENT RECORD	Patient label
Date:	

Type of arthritis:	Date of diagnosis:
Occupation:	Lives alone yes no Dependents yes no If yes, relationship to patient:
Current medication:	

Has had the following X-rays:	Dates	Report
Height (cms):		Ideal weight:
Past arthritic medical history:		
Comments from questionnaire:		
Pain score:	Depression score:	
Sleep pattern:		

ACTIVITIES OF DAILY LIVING ASSESSMENT

ACTIVITY	COMMENTS	AIDS/DEVICES IN USE
1. Dressing/grooming		
2. Rising		
3. Eating		
4. Walking		
5. Hygiene		
6. Reach		
7. Grip		
8. Activities		

Figure 16.4 Arthritis management record sheet (with permission from L. Dargie, J. Proctor and W. Bird; skeleton illustrations adapted from Black's Medical Dictionary, 3rd edn, p. 83, with permission from A. & C. Black).

Education checklist	LFT given	Discussion/date
Disease process		
Drug therapy		
Investigations		
Exercise		
Pain control		
Pain diary		
Managing a flare		
Joint protection		
Rest, positioning, splinting		
Diet		
Feet and footwear		
Roles of multi-disciplinary team		
Joint injections/operations		
Aids/appliances		
Financial benefits		
Coping strategies		
Co-op card needed		
? Depression		
Alternative medicine		

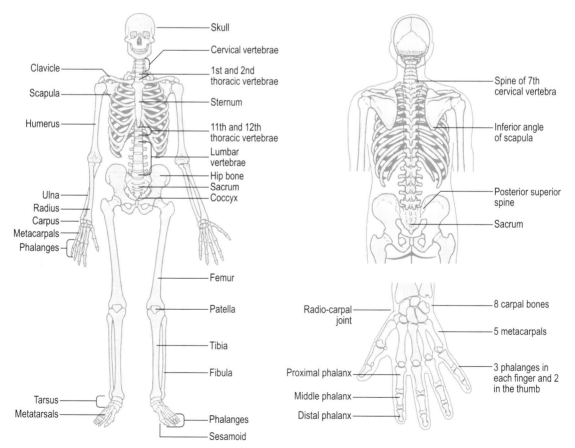

Figure 16.4 Cont'd.

JOINT PAIN FUNCTION LEVELS

Date	Weight Kgs	BP	PPS	DMS	Daily analgesic	Hb	RAHA	ESR	CRP	A	B	C	D	Comments/medication

Joint pain 1–5

DMS : Duration of morning stiffness	Daily analgesics
PPS : Present pain score (Max = 35)	Total number needed in last week

Joint pain : 1=No pain 5=Severe pain

Figure 16.5   Assessment flow chart (with permission from L. Dargie, J. Proctor and W. Bird).

Case Study 16.1 Osteoarthritis of the knees

Jean is a 62-year-old overweight woman with a 5-year history of painful knees. A diagnosis of OA had been made several years earlier and since diagnosis her pain had been reasonably well-controlled with regular paracetamol. Recently her pain had increased and she was able to walk only short distances and stairs had become a considerable challenge. She made an appointment at the health centre arthritis clinic because of her increasing pain and disability. She completed a pre-clinic questionnaire and from this it was identified that she required more information regarding OA and her treatment options. She was advised to lose weight and to wear soft insoles or trainers to reduce the stress on her knee joints. On examination, her knees were tender to touch but showed no effusions. She was commenced on distalgesic and advised of the possible side effects of these drugs. Jean was reviewed frequently and during this time her education was continued with simple home exercises, advice and information sheets on pain control and joint protection. Referral was made to the dietician and the occupational therapist and she was advised to attend local exercise classes that run alongside the arthritis clinic.

For several months Jean's pain appeared to be well-controlled, but following a holiday that required her to walk longer distances than she usually managed, there was a rapid deterioration of her right knee. The knee became unstable and gave way frequently. X-rays at this time showed extreme OA changes to the joint. When seen in the clinic her pain was improved with patella–femoral strapping that also made the joint feel more stable. A saline washout of the joint followed by a steroid injection gave her short-term relief.

She was referred to the local hospital for surgical opinion. Whilst waiting for her hospital appointment, a six week course of acupuncture was arranged which also offered temporary relief. After a wait of several months, Jean had a right knee replacement from which she recovered well and was delighted to be pain free almost immediately following surgery.

Following physiotherapy in hospital, she was discharged to the care of her husband and the district nurse, but she continued to attend the hospital physiotherapy department. She was visited by the district nurse involved in the arthritis clinic and continued to make good progress. Once mobile, she was followed up in the clinic and continued to see the dietician. The pain in her left knee was well-controlled on paracetamol. Jean's previous education had enabled her to be aware of self-management techniques, which should help to prevent future problems and to minimise the support needed from the arthritis clinic.

Case Study 16.2 Rheumatoid arthritis under control

Peter is a 28-year-old furniture restorer recently registered at the health centre, having moved from an inner city area. He is married with one child. Two years earlier, Peter had been diagnosed as having RA by his former general practitioner, following an episode of painful swollen hands. The rheumatoid factor at that time had been strongly positive. Since diagnosis, Peter's pain had been controlled with non-steroidal anti-inflammatory drugs. As his symptoms had settled down he had continued working, attended his surgery for occasional check-ups. Peter had read about RA and was well-informed about the disease process and treatment options.

Soon after moving to the area, he recognised a 'flare' of his disease and made an appointment at the health centre arthritis clinic. On examination, his hands were painful and carpometacarpal joints were red and swollen. He felt generally unwell and was also complaining of pain in his right shoulder. His erythrocyte sedimentation rate, taken at the surgery was 65. It was decided to refer him to the local consultant rheumatologist, with a view to being commenced on disease modifying drugs. He was given depomedrone 120 mg intramuscularly to settle his 'flare' until he could be seen at the hospital. Peter's condition improved over the next few days and his pain was controlled with non-steroidal anti-inflammatory drugs. When seen by the consultant rheumatologist, he was commenced on methotrexate. Baseline liver function tests and a chest X-ray were carried out at the hospital and he was transferred back to the health centre arthritis clinic for monitoring. Peter had been seen by the rheumatology nurse specialist at the hospital who had counselled him on the side effects of methotrexate and informed the arthritis clinic of his treatment. Continuity of care was to be maintained through the recording of blood test results and investigations on a shared-care card. In this way, the hospital were able to advise clinic staff of any alterations to his management.

Since Peter commenced methotrexate, his RA has been well-controlled. Regular blood test results have remained satisfactory and having experienced no further flares, he was able to return to work.

designed by the general practitioner and supported by the Countryside Commission (Bird 1995) and local health cycling. Patients also contribute towards a practice scrapbook of interesting articles and have expressed their appreciation of the accessible advice and support provided by the nurses. Often they have suggested that just to talk about their problems offers an enormous relief of stress, a factor that has been shown to increase pain levels and affect a person's ability to cope with their illness.

The reflex prescription of non-steroidal anti-inflammatory drugs has now been replaced by a stepwise management protocol. Such a protocol has taken many patients away from the doctor and drugs and towards a self-management plan taught by the nurses.

Cost-benefit

Ill health prevention and health promotion through the management of the musculoskeletal disorders could produce significant benefits, not only to the patient, but to the health care system, through longer-term financial savings. The arthritis clinic has endeavoured to promote prevention of physical and emotional impairment through the support and education of its patients, as opposed to crisis intervention.

It has been suggested that the direct cost savings brought about by such care could pale in comparison to the indirect savings (Mazzuca 1994). However, when resources are scarce, it is the direct cost-savings that often take precedence over the longer-term benefits of the indirect savings. Studies are increasingly being undertaken into the direct cost-savings of education and support programmes for patients with arthritis and other musculoskeletal disorders (Lorig et al 1993, Weinberger et al 1993).

In 1995, the prescribing costs of the health centre, for drugs used in the rheumatic diseases and gout group, and which included non-steroidal, anti-inflammatory drugs, was 17% below the Family Health Services Association average (PACT 1995). Figure 16.6 illustrates the significant reduction in the expenditure on such drugs compared to 1993, when non-steroidal anti-inflammatory drugs accounted for approximately 81% of the musculoskeletal group. This was prior to the practice becoming a fundholding practice in 1994. As well as financial savings, there are indirect advantages such as a reduced incidence of drug related side effects.

The arthritis clinic has demonstrated that by utilising the skills of nurses fully, it is possible to reduce hospital consultants' waiting lists, save general practitioner time and start the community on the path to self management whilst simultaneously offering a

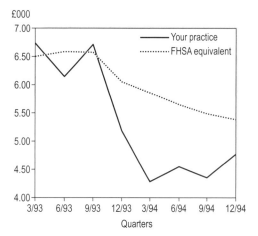

Figure 16.6 Sonning Common Health Centre Practice prescribing costs comparing 1994 with 1993 (musculoskeletal and joint disease). (Reproduced by kind permission of the Prescription Pricing Authority.)

more individual and appropriate service to patients. However, this is only on a small scale, and the full benefits of long-term prevention of some musculoskeletal disorders and accompanying cost-savings are unlikely to be achieved unless there is a radical reconsideration of the way in which services are provided locally and nationally (Horbury 1995).

Raising awareness of needs

The experience of setting up a community-based arthritis clinic prompted the team to educate other health professionals as to the benefits of such an initiative. Lectures have been given to groups of general practitioners, practice and district nurses across England and the clinic has played host to many interested health professionals.

Practice nurses in particular have been keen to initiate similar ventures. However very few have succeeded, mainly due to a lack of human and financial resources. This lack of response was reflected in a project aimed at initiating the education of practice nurses by rheumatology nurse specialists, in which there was only a 2% participation rate by practices approached. Although closer cooperation between hospital clinic and primary care was seen as desirable, patient education was considered as being the exclusive province of the hospital clinic. Practice nurses who were eager to learn and general practitioners who were keen to improve standards were encountered, but the acceptance of additional demands on time and reorganisation, without financial reimbursement, were impositions that few general practitioners felt able to bear in the present climate (Grahame & West 1996).

District nurses have also exhibited a keen response. However, many are restricted to working their traditional domain outside the health centre/surgery setting. A common response by district nurses to the team lectures, was amazement that a health manager should allow their district nurse to spend a morning a week working in the surgery. There is no doubt that initially the commitment produced an increased workload, but it allowed the district nurse to develop rheumatology skills that could be utilised in the community, which ultimately reduced the burden on the general practice.

THE FUTURE

In their quality guidelines, Arthritis Care (1994) supported the view that 'adequate and appropriate health care of all kinds should be readily available to all people with arthritis who need it'. The recognition of the existing problems and the adoption of the principles of good shared-care by primary and secondary health care teams can make a major contribution to meeting such a goal. Arthritis Care suggests that District Health Authorities should encourage and support joint initiatives and strategies by health providers. Additional investment will be required if this is to happen, but only then can the concept of a seamless service be realised in practice.

Action points for practice:

- Briefly outline what effects the projected future demand for musculoskeletal services may have on hospital in/outpatient care.
- Make a list of outcomes that could be achieved if primary and secondary health professionals were to adopt the principles of good shared-care in rheumatology.
- Mr Roberts is a 68-year-old man exhibiting symptoms of early OA of the hands and knees. His present condition does not warrant a referral to the hospital rheumatology department. What support could the primary health care team at his local surgery give?
- A community nurse would like to set up a shared-care initiative in rheumatology at their surgery. What difficulties may be encountered in her endeavours?
- Having read this chapter take time out to reflect upon the following questions:
- Could links be improved between primary and secondary rheumatology care in your area of practice?
- Do you envisage any difficulties in implementing shared-care schemes?
- What could you do to influence the support of such initiatives?

RERERENCES

Arthritis Care 1994 Quality guidelines number three. Community health care for people with arthritis
Barrett C W, Tomes J 1992 Shared care – the way forward. Hospital Update Plus 18(4): 7–10
Bird H 1985 Nurses: an underused resource. British Medical Journal 290: 1589
Bird W 1995 Health walks. Sonning Common Health Centre
Blaaw A, Schuwirth I, Van Der Vleuten C, Smits F, Van Der Linden S 1995 Assessing clinical competence: recognition of case descriptions of rheumatic diseases by general practitioners. British Journal of Rheumatology 34: 375–379
Branch W 1994 Primary care practice and training in rheumatology. Arthritis and Rheumatism 37(3): 305–306
Charlton C, Fleming D, McCormick A 1995 Morbidity statistics from general practice. HMSO, London
Consumer Association 1992 GPs, your verdict. Which? April 1992: 202–205
Dargie L, Proctor J 1993 Arthritis clinics in practice. Practice Nurse 1–14 June: 144–148
Dargie L, Proctor J 1994 Setting up an arthritis clinic. Community Outlook 4(7): 14–17
Davis P, Suarez-Almazor M 1995 An assessment of the needs of family physicians for a rheumatology continuing medical education programme: results of a pilot project. Journal of Rheumatology 22(9): 1762–1765
Freeman G K, Richards S C 1993 Is personal continuity of

care compatible with free choice of doctor? Patients' views on seeing the same doctor. British Journal of General Practitioners, 43: 493–497
Grahame R, West J 1996 The role of the rheumatology nurse practitioner in primary care: an experiment in the further education of the practice nurse. British Journal of Rheumatology 35: 581–588
Hasler J 1994 The primary health care team. John Fry Trust Fellowship. Royal Society of Medicine Press, London , ch 3, p 21–30: ch 6, p 79
Haslock I 1987 The practising rheumatologist's view. In: Baillière's Clinical Rheumatology: epidemiological, sociological and environmental aspects of rheumatology. Baillière Tindall, London, ch 11, p 645–663
Helliwell P, O'Hara M 1995 Shared care between hospital and general practice: an audit of disease-modifying drug monitoring in rheumatoid arthritis. British Journal of Rheumatology 34: 673–676
Hickman M, Drummond N, Grimshaw J 1994 A taxonomy of shared care for chronic disease. Journal of Public Health Medicine 16,4: 447–454
Hill J 1986 Arthritis at home. Journal of District Nursing October: 4–11
Hill J 1991 Caring and curing. Nursing Times 87(45): 29–31
Hill J, Bird H A, Hopkins R, Lawton C, Wright V 1992 Survey of satisfaction with care in a rheumatology

out-patient clinic. Annals of Rheumatic Diseases 51: 195–197

Hill J, Bird H A, Harmer R, Wright V, Lawton C 1994 An evaluation of the effectiveness, safety and acceptability of a nurse practitioner in a rheumatology out-patient clinic. British Journal of Rheumatology 33: 283–288

Hill J 1997 Patient satisfaction in a nurse-led rheumatology clinic. Journal of Advanced Nursing 25: 347–354

Hjortdahl P, Laerum E 1992 Continuity of care in general practice: effect on patient satisfaction. British Medical Journal 304: 1287–1290

Horbury J 1995 Bone and joint disorders. In: Bradlow J, Bennet V, Breton S et al (eds) A health strategy for Oxfordshire 1995–2000. Oxfordshire Health

Hyde V 1995 Community nursing: a unified discipline? In: Cain P, Hyde V, Howkins E (eds) Community nursing: dimensions and dilemmas. Arnold, London, ch 1, p 8

Kirwan J R, Reeback J S 1986 Stanford health assessment questionnaire, modified to assess British patients with rheumatoid arthritis. British Journal of Rheumatology 25: 206–209

Kirwan J R 1994 Effect of national health service reforms on outpatient rheumatology workload. British Journal of Rheumatology 33: 1181–1183

Knox J D E 1987 Rheumatic diseases: a general practitioners view. In: Clinical rheumatology: epidemiological, sociological and environmental aspects of rheumatology. Baillière Tindall, London, ch9, p601–622

Liebman J, Hull A, Blauner M, Barkey J, Vignos P, Moskowitz R 1986 Identifying needs and community resources in arthritis care. Public Health Nursing 3(3): 158–170

Lorig K, Mazonson P, Holman H 1993 Evidence suggesting that health education for self-management in patients with chronic arthritis has sustained health benefits while reducing health care costs. Arthritis and Rheumatism 36: 439–446

Mansfield C 1995 Attitudes and behaviours towards clinical guidelines: the clinician's perspective. Quality in Health Care 4(4): 250–255

Maycock J 1990 Primary health care: a catalyst for better rheumatology care. Nursing Standard 4(50): 54–55

Mazzuca S 1994 Education and behavioural and social research in rheumatology. Current Opinion in Rheumatology 6: 147–152

Meenan R F, Gertman P M, Mason J H 1980 Measuring health status in arthritis: the arthritis impact measurement scales. Arthritis and Rheumatism 23: 146–153

NHS Management Executive 1991 Integrating primary and secondary care. Department of Health, London

Nottingham Health Authority 1990 In: District nurse learner pack 1994. Nottingham Community Health NHS Trust

Orton P 1994 Shared care. The Lancet 344: 1413–1415

PACT 1995 Analysis and prescribing review for Sonning Common Health Centre Pharmaforce

Prescription Pricing Authority 1995 Analysis of Sonning Common Health Centre prescribing costs

Tinson S 1995 Assessing health need: a community perspective. In: Cain P, Hyde V, Howkins E (eds) Community nursing: dimensions and dilemmas. Arnold, London, ch 7, p 144

Vetter N, Charny M, Lewis P, Farrow S 1990 Prevalence and treatment of symptoms of rheumatism and arthritis among over 65 year olds: a community profile. British Journal of General Practice 40: 69–71

Weinberger M. Tierney W, Cowper P, Katz B, Booher B 1993 Cost-effectiveness of increased telephone contact for patients with osteoarthritis. Arthritis and Rheumatism 36: 243–246

FURTHER READING

Mowbray House Surgery, Northallerton, North Yorkshire 1993 How others do it (Rheumatoid arthritis management in primary care) Mims Magazine Weekly 2 February

Sonning Common Health Centre, Reading, Berkshire 1993 How others do it (Osteoarthritis management in primary care) Mims Magazine Weekly 22 June

Appendices

CONTENTS

Appendix 1

Health assessment questionnaire

Reproduced with permission from British Journal of Rheumatology 1986(25): 206–209

Health Assessment Questionaire

Name `...------------------------------------------------` Date `.----------------------------------`

Age `.----------------------------------`

To the patient: Please complete this record and give it to the doctor seeing you today.
Tick the one response which best describes your usual abilities over <u>the past week.</u>

	Without *any* difficulty (0)	Without *some* difficulty (1)	Without *much* difficulty (2)	Unable to do (3)	
1 Dressing and grooming Are you able to: –Dress yourself, including tying shoelaces and doing buttons? –Shampoo your hair?	`------` `------`	`------` `------`	`------` `------`	`------` `------`	*□
2 Rising Are you able to: –Stand up from an armless chair? –Get in and out of bed?	`------` `------`	`------` `------`	`------` `------`	`------` `------`	□
3 Eating Are you able to: –Cut your meat? –Lift up a full cup or glass to your mouth? –Open a new carton of milk (or soap powder)?	`------` `------` `------`	`------` `------` `------`	`------` `------` `------`	`------` `------` `------`	□
4 Walking Are you able to: –Walk outdoors on flat ground? –Climb up 5 steps?	`------` `------`	`------` `------`	`------` `------`	`------` `------`	□

Please tick any <u>aids or devices</u> that you usually use for any of these activities

`----` Walking stick
`----` Walking frame
`----` Crutches
`----` Wheelchair

`----` Devices used for dressing (button hook, zipper pull long-handled shoe horn)
`----` Built-up or special utensils
`----` Special or built-up chair

Other (specify): `-------------------------------------------------------------------`

Please tick any categories for which you usually <u>need help from another person</u>

`----` Dressing and grooming
`----` Rising

`----` Eating
`----` Walking

PTO

*Enter highest score for each section in box

To the patient: Please complete this record and give it to the doctor seeing you today
Tick the one response which best describes your usual abilities over <u>the past week</u>

	Without *any* difficulty (0)	Without *some* difficulty (1)	Without *much* difficulty (2)	Unable to do (3)	
5 Hygiene Are you able to: –Wash and dry your entire body? –Take a bath? –Get on and off the toilet?	------ ------ ------	------ ------ ------	------ ------ ------	------ ------ ------	☐
6 Reach Are you able to: –Reach and get down a 5lb object (e.g. bag of potatoes) from just above your head? –Bend down to pick up clothing from the floor?	------ ------	------ ------	------ ------	------ ------	☐
7 Grip Are you able to: –Open car doors? –Open jars which have been previously opened? –Turn taps on and off?	------ ------ ------	------ ------ ------	------ ------ ------	------ ------ ------	☐
8 Activities Are you able to: –Run errands and shop? –Get in and out of a car? –Do chores such as vacuuming, housework or light gardening?	------ ------ ------	------ ------ ------	------ ------ ------	------ ------ ------	☐

Please tick any <u>aids or devices</u> that you usually use for any of these activities

_ _ _ _ _ Raised toilet seat   _ _ _ _ _ Bath rail
_ _ _ _ _ Bath seat   _ _ _ _ _ Long-handled appliances for reach
_ _ _ _ _ Jar opener (for jars previously opened)

Other (specify): ---

Please tick any categories for which you usually <u>need help from other persons</u>

_ _ _ _ _ Hygiene   _ _ _ _ _ Gripping and opening things
_ _ _ _ _ Reach   _ _ _ _ _ Errands and housework

We are also interested in learning whether or not you are affected by pain because of your illness
How much pain have you had because of your illness in the past week?
Place a mark on the line to indicate the severity of the pain

No pain _____ Very severe pain   ☐

$$\text{Final score} = \frac{\text{Total score}}{\text{No. of categories}} = \quad \boxed{}$$

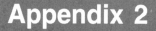

Appendix 2

Patient information – pain in rheumatoid arthritis (RA)

What causes pain in RA?

Pain is the first thing that most people notice when they get RA. It can start in just one joint or in a number of joints. One of the causes of this pain is inflammation. When there is little inflammation, you often feel less pain. However, this is not the whole story. Other things such as anxiety, depression and fatigue (tiredness) can make the pain feel worse or become harder to control.

Does pain have a purpose?

Yes, it does. It stops us from hurting ourselves. For instance, a child will drop a hot object before it is badly burnt. Pain is also the way our body tells us that there is something wrong with it. If we are in a lot of pain, or the pain carries on for some time, we usually go to the doctor who puts a name to the problem. However, the pain from RA is different. It seems to forget what it came for! The pain tends to become 'chronic'. Chronic pain is pain that lasts longer than 6 months. This kind of pain can be harder to control than short-term pain.

How much pain should I feel?

Pain is a very personal experience. People with the same disease may have different levels and types of pain. This means that someone with very bad RA may feel less pain than another person with mild RA.

The amount of pain you feel does not only depend on how active your RA is. It can also change when you become interested in what you are doing or what is going on around you. Many people find that their pain is worse when they are sitting alone doing nothing, or are in bed in the dark where there is nothing to take their minds off it. People often feel less pain when they are doing something that they enjoy. Pain can also change from day to day. Doing too much can cause this. For example, overdoing the housework or rushing around at work. Very often it seems to change for no reason at all.

Will I get rid of my pain?

Most people with chronic pain never get rid of it altogether but that does not mean that it cannot be kept at a reasonable level. Of course what is 'reasonable' is different for each person. For example, someone with a high pain tolerance may not wish to take painkilling tablets, even if their pain is severe. Those who do not like taking drugs may prefer to take less painkiller but put up with more pain.

At the end of the day the pain belongs to the person who feels it. It is for you to decide what you can live with. The doctors and health carers are there to advise you about the kinds of pain relief there are. It is for you to choose what you would like to try.

What kinds of drugs will help?

There are several kinds of drugs that can help to control pain. These include:

- Analgesics
- Non-steroidal anti-inflammatory drugs (NSAIDs)
- Steroids
- Antidepressants

What else will help my pain?

- Massage
- Relaxation
- Distraction
- Splinting
- Heat.

Heat

Heat will not cure pain, but many people find it very comforting. There are two types of heat, **Dry** and **Moist**.

Examples of **Dry** heat include:

- **Electric pads**

These are used if you have just one or two painful joints.

- **Electric blankets**

These are good if you have pain all over.

- **Hot water bottles**

Good for just one or two painful joints. Some people prefer to use a hot water bottle rather than a pad as they feel the weight of the bottle on their joint helps.

- **Hot/cold pack**

These are easy to use. They can be heated in a microwave oven or in hot water. They mould to the joint and are easy to keep in place with a towel.

Examples of **Moist** heat include:

- **Hot shower or bath**

Very good at relieving 'all over' pain. Make sure that the bathroom and your towels are warm. This will help to prolong the good effects of the moist heat.

- **Wash basin or bowl of hot water**

A good method of helping to reduce pain in the hands or feet.

You can use any of these methods of dry or moist heat to ease the pain but do follow a few simple safety rules.

- **Always** protect the skin with a towel or cloth before applying a hot water bottle.
- **Never** use boiling water in a hot water bottle.
- **Always** follow the safety guide, which comes with electrical appliances.

Cold

Some people find that they get better pain relief by using cold therapy. The most common methods are:

- **Bag of frozen peas**

Useful for larger joints such as knees or elbows. They mould well to the joint when kept in place by a towel.

- **Hot/cold pack**

Useful for larger joints. Can be kept in the freezer.

To use the above methods, cover the joint with a cloth or towel. This will stop you getting an ice burn. Place the peas or the pack over the joint and then wrap a towel around it to keep it in place. Leave it in place for about 10–15 minutes.

- **Never** use ice on your hands or feet if you have poor circulation.

Massage

Massage can be a very potent painkiller. lt can be done for you by your partner or a friend, or if the joint is easy to reach, you can do it for yourself. Always use massage oil as you can break or stretch the skin. This can be bought quite cheaply from a chemist or stores such as Body Shop. Some people prefer to use aromatherapy oils, but these should be used with caution. Some essential oils can have a bad effect if you are taking blood pressure tablets or are pregnant. If you are not sure, ask your doctor, nurse or chemist.

Relaxation

Relaxation really can help you to overcome pain. There are very good scientific reasons for this. Unfortunately, it is not easy to learn how to relax and it is even more difficult to relax when you are in pain! You usually learn from audio cassettes and many hospitals will either give you one or record one for you. You can only learn these methods by practice and it may take a number of months before you are really good at it.

Distraction

Some people who have chronic pain are able to use this method for a few hours each day. Others can only do it for short periods. The idea is to take your mind off the pain by concentrating deeply on something. This can be hard to do when you are in pain.

Methods of distraction are:

• Visual distraction

Look through a magazine and choose a picture that you like. Look at it closely and then start to describe it out loud in detail. When you have done this, close your eyes and try to describe it again from memory. Let your mind run free and try to think if the picture reminds you of a place or holiday that you have had. Go over this in your mind. As you get better at it, you will find that you can distract your mind away from your pain.

• Hearing distraction

Many people find this method of taking their mind off their pain very useful. It works best if you can use a personal cassette player and listen through earphones. Choose a piece of music that you like and try to concentrate on it. When the pain gets worse, increase the volume. If the music makes you think of any images such as waves breaking on a beach, follow them through. If you don't like music, choose a talking book or a funny tape, humour is a great way to distract your mind from your pain. This is a very good way of helping when you are in bed in the dark.

• Social distraction

Good company can divert your mind from your pain so do try to get out as much as possible or invite your friends to visit you. Make it clear that you may have to ask them to leave if it gets too much. This isn't a slur on their company, it is just one of the difficulties you have with your RA. You need to help them to understand your problems.

Rest

Pain can make you feel more tired than usual. If you are always in pain, or if the pain has woken you in the night then you're going to feel pretty tired! When you feel more tired you will find it more difficult to control the pain. The best way to control your pain is to take more rest. Don't feel guilty, you're not being lazy. You have good cause to feel tired. Try to pace yourself and take periods of rest after each spate of activity. It is a good idea to make yourself lie down on a settee or bed for set periods of time each day. Try adding one of the other pain relief methods, such as relaxation or distraction. Try to spoil yourself a little – after all it's all part of the treatment.

Splinting

It's a good idea to rest any joint that is very painful. A good way to rest a single joint is to wear a splint. A splint will stop you making movements that cause pain. They can also prevent the pain from starting. If you are wearing splints all day, you should remove them every 2 hours and do some gentle range of movement exercises. This will help to stop the joint becoming stiff.

Combining different methods

As you can see, there are many different ways of reducing your pain. Most people find that they get the best relief by not just staying with one method. They get better results by using a number of different methods at the same time. A good example is to take non-steroidal anti-inflammatory tablets and analgesics, but also to use relaxation and heat. There are many things you can try so if one combination does not help, try another.

Take control of your pain – don't let it control you

Remember

- Pain is a personal experience; it belongs to the person who feels it
- No two people have the same pain and it is for you to decide what you can stand
- Use more than one method of pain control. If it doesn't work, try another

- Take your anti-inflammatory drugs regularly
- Take analgesics before the pain gets severe. They work better this way
- If you are in lots of pain take your analgesics regularly and don't be frightened to take the maximum amount if you need to
- Rest if you feel tired. This will help you to control the pain
- Do not give up. If one method does not help, always try something else.

Appendix 3

Guidelines for nurses on the use and administration of intra-articular injections, sodium aurothiomalate and intra-muscular methotrexate in rheumatoid arthritis

APPENDIX 3.1 GUIDELINES FOR NURSES ON THE USE AND ADMINISTRATION OF INTRA-ARTICULAR INJECTIONS (by kind permission of the RCN Rheumatology Nursing Forum)

1. What is an expanded role?

Role extension refers to nurses carrying out tasks not included in their normal training for registration. Most of these tasks related to medical technical interventions are usually carried out by doctors (Wright 1995).

2. Accountability

The scope of professional practice (UKCC 1992) acknowledges that nurses are involved in negotiating the boundaries of practice and should be responsive to the needs of patients and clients. The onus is on each individual nurse to recognise their own level of competence and decline any duties or responsibilities unless they are able to perform them in a safe and skilled manner. Each nurse is also accountable for maintaining and improving their knowledge and should be familiar with the contents of the following documents.

- UKCC Exercising Accountability 1989
- UKCC Scope of Professional Practice 1992
- UKCC Code of Professional Practice 1992
- UKCC Standards for the Administration of Medicine 1992

3. What are intra-articular injections?

These are injections into the synovial joints. Long acting steroids are generally used for joint injections and hydrocortisone is used for soft tissue injections.

4. Indications for joint injections

(a) Relief of pain from localised inflammation of the joint (e.g. rheumatoid arthritis)
(b) Relief of pain from soft tissue discomfort
(c) To aid mobilisation
(d) To assist with rehabilitation (e.g. physiotherapy)
(e) To improve function.

5. Contraindications of joint injections

(a) Local infection
(b) Intra-articular fracture
(c) Anti-coagulant therapy
(d) Bleeding disorders.

6. Preparation the nurse must undertake prior to the administration of intra-articular injections

The nurse must be able to demonstrate evidence of competency in the administration of intra-articular injections in accordance with the Scope of Professional Practice (UKCC 1992).

Evidence of competency should indicate that the nurse has knowledge of:

- Anatomy and physiology of the joints and soft tissues
- Drugs used and their effects and side effects
- Indications and contraindications for intra-articular injections
- Potential complications
- Aspiration and injection technique.

Evidence of assessment of competency should be available.

The employer must have precise knowledge of the employee's activities, and agree to them being undertaken by the employee; in accordance with vicarious liability.

7. The nurse's responsibility when giving intra-articular injections

(a) Obtain written instructions from the prescribing doctor detailing the drug, dosage and site of administration.
(b) Ensure the patient has given informed consent.
(c) Use an aseptic or no touch technique.
(d) Aspirate the joint if swollen.
(e) Send a sample of synovial fluid for culture if it is very opaque, green or foul-smelling.
(f) If no obvious signs of infection or contra-indications are present, administer the prescribed drug into the site stated.

(g) Document the drug, dosage and site of administration in the care records.
(h) Provide the patient with after care advice.

8. After care advice

The nurse must advise patients that:

(a) The joint may be painful for 24 hours after the injection. Take analgesia if necessary.
(b) It may take several days before benefit is felt.
(c) The injected joint should be rested as much as possible 24–48 hours after the injection.
(d) Short term facial flushing may be experienced.
(e) Localised skin atrophy may occasionally occur.
(f) To contact the Rheumatology Department if the patient has any concerns.

9. Potential complications following the administration of intra-articular injections

(a) Infections
(b) Damage to the articular cartilage
(c) Tendon rupture
(d) Skin atrophy.

REFERENCES

Wright S (1995) The role of the nurse: extended or expanded? Nursing Standard, May, 10 9(33): 25–29

BIBLIOGRAPHY

Dixon A, St J Emery P 1992 Local Injection Therapy in Rheumatic Diseases. Eular Publishers.
Dieppe P et al 1991 Arthritis and rheumatism in practice. Gower Medical Publishing.
Doherty M et al 1992 Rheumatology Examination and Injection Techniques. WB Saunders Co. Ltd

APPENDIX 3.2 GUIDELINES FOR NURSES ON THE USE OF AND ADMINISTRATION OF SODIUM AUROTHIOMALATE IN RHEUMATOID ARTHRITIS (by kind permission of the RCN Rheumatology Nursing Forum)

1. What is sodium aurothiomalate?

Sodium aurothiomalate (intramuscular gold) belongs to the group of drugs known as slow-acting anti-rheumatic drugs (SAARDs). These drugs suppress clinical and laboratory markers of disease activity and are thought to slow the progression of the disease but the precise mode of action is unknown. Unlike non-steroidal anti-inflammatory drugs (NSAIDs) which produce an immediate therapeutic effect, SAARDs are unlikely to produce any benefit before 12 weeks and often take as long as 24 weeks before improvement is attained.

2. Indications for using sodium aurothiomalate

Sodium aurothiomalate is used in cases of active rheumatoid arthritis.

3. Contraindications

Females who are pregnant or are breast feeding should not be given intramuscular gold.

Likewise those who have gross renal or hepatic disease, history of blood dyscrasias, exfoliative dermatitis or systematic lupus erythematosus.

4. Administration and dosage of sodium aurothiomalate

The drug is given by deep intramuscular injection, followed by gentle massage of the area.

An initial test dose of 5–10 mg is usually given and if there are no adverse reactions (skin rash or hyper-sensitivity), weekly injections of 20–50 mg are administered until a response occurs. Most patients will feel no benefit until they have received a total dose of between 500–800 mg. Once in remission and providing they do not experience any side effects, patients are usually maintained on a dose of 50 mg administered monthly, but the physician may vary the dose according to the activity of the disease. If no major improvement has occurred after reaching a total dose of 1000 mg (excluding the test dose) the treatment is usually discontinued, although sometimes weekly injections of 100 mg for 5 weeks are given.

5. Adverse reactions

Side effects occur in approximately 30% of patients and can appear at any time during the course of the treatment, even after the patient has been successfully treated with sodium aurothiomalate for many years. They are mostly mild, but up to 5% experience severe reactions which are potentially fatal.

Skin. Skin reactions are perhaps the most common of the side effects to intramuscular gold and are usually mild. However, if they do develop, the injection should be withheld and their presence should always be reported to the physician as they may be the fore-runners to severe gold toxicity. This side effect occurs most commonly after a total cumulative dose of 300–400 mg.

Rashes may be localised or general and range from minor reactions to major skin lesions. They can mimic almost any skin eruption.

Pruritus or 'itching' is quite common and is often first felt between the fingers.

Mucous membranes. Stomatitis and mouth ulcers can develop in some patients. Pharyngitis should raise the question of leucopenia. Patients sometimes complain of a metallic taste in the mouth which although unpleasant is not a permanent side-effect.

Blood. Thrombocytopenia, neutropenia, agranulo-cytosis and fatal marrow suppression can develop but the latter is rare. Bruising, particularly around the shins, can be the first indication of thrombocytopenia. A fever and sore throat can indicate the presence of agranulocytosis.

Eosinophilia may be an indication of developing toxicity but does not always necessitate stopping gold.

The drug manufacturer recommends that a full blood and platelet count is taken before each injection is given and this should be meticulously adhered to. These results should be recorded sequentially. A sudden fall in platelet or white cell count outside normal limits may be reason for the physician to suspend treatment. A fall on three consecutive occasions, even if within normal limits, should also be reported as he/she may wish to suspend or modify the treatment.

Blood dyscrasias are most likely to happen when between 400 mg and 1000 mg of intramuscular gold has been given but can occur at anytime during treatment.

Kidney. Proteinuria develops in about 10% of patients but is severe in less than 2%.

A gradual increase in protein concentration is more significant than a single result and so if protein is detected, do not give the gold but ask the patient to return a few days later for a retest. If the protein persists, consult the physician as it may be necessary to estimate the amount of protein excreted in 24 hours by a more accurate measure than use of dipstix.

If blood and protein are present, eliminate the possibility of a urinary tract infection by collecting a midstream urine specimen; if the MSU is negative, the physician may decide to stop the gold.

Rarer side effects. Rarer side effects include, peripheral neuritis, alopecia and colitis.

A small number of patients may experience flushing, nausea or vertigo after an injection.

The nurse's responsibility when giving sodium aurothiomalate

Before beginning the gold injections, you should discuss the treatment with the patient. This should include an explanation of what the treatment is for, how it is to be given, how the treatment will help and what side-effects may occur. It is also important to make sure that the patient knows where the treatment and monitoring will take place, and who they should contact if they are unable to attend or if they experience any problems. It is always helpful to provide written information to the patient as a backup to this verbal explanation.

Before each injection

1. Inspect the skin for rashes and ask if any pruritus has been experienced.
2. Ask the patient if they have experienced any soreness of the throat, developed mouth ulcers or loss of taste.
3. Ascertain that blood has been taken for a full blood count.
4. Check that the prescribing doctor has seen and approved the results of the previous blood tests.
5. Inspect the skin for bruising.
6. Inquire if the patient has experienced any undue bleeding such as epistaxis or bleeding gums.
7. Ask the patient if they are experiencing any 'flu' like symptoms.
8. Test that the urine is free of protein and blood.
9. Record the dose given, haematology and urinalysis results, the presence of any unwanted effects and any action taken on the patient's gold card.

If the monitoring reveals any adverse effects, withhold the gold and report the symptoms to the doctor. These guidelines should be read in conjunction with the national guidelines for the monitoring of second line drugs, produced by the British Society for Rheumatology.

APPENDIX 3.3 GUIDELINES FOR NURSES ON THE USE OF AND ADMINISTRATION OF INTRA-MUSCULAR METHOTREXATE IN RHEUMATOID ARTHRITIS (by kind permission of the RCN Rheumatology Nursing Forum)

1. What is methotrexate?

Methotraxate is an anti-metabolite cytotoxic agent. It can be administered via the oral, subcutaneous and intra-muscular route. It suppresses clinical and laboratory markers of disease activity and is used to slow the progression of the disease, but the precise mode of action is unknown. Unlike non-steroidal anti-inflammatory drugs (NSAIDs) which produce an immediate therapeutic effect, methotrexate is unlikely to produce any benefit before 4–6 weeks and often takes as long as 2–4 months before improvement is evident.

2. Indications for using intra-muscular methotrexate

Methotrexate is used in cases of:

(a) Active rheumatoid arthritis
(b) Psoriatic arthropathy
(c) Polymyositis
(d) Inability to tolerate oral methotrexate.

3. Contraindications

Relative contraindications:

(a) Abnormal liver function
(b) Alcohol (increases the risk of liver damage)
(c) Smoking (increases the risk of pneumonitis).

Absolute contraindications:

(a) Pregnancy and breast feeding
(b) Chronic viral hepatitis.

4. Administration and dosage of intra-muscular methotrexate

Deep intra-muscular methotrexate is given weekly in doses between 5–25 mg according to disease severity and individual response.

5. Adverse reactions

Side effects may occur any time during the course of treatment.

Gastrointestinal. Patients may still experience nausea even when the intra-muscular route is used. Anti-emetics and / or drug reduction may be considered.

Skin.

- Stomatitis and mouth ulcers can develop in some patients
- Some patients may experience hair loss
- Herpes zoster and systemic fungal infections can occur
- Patients may notice accelerated nodules whilst taking this drug.

Most rheumatologists routinely prescribe folic acid on a daily or weekly basis to try and minimise the risk of the above side effects.

Respiratory. Acute pneumonitis is rare but can be life-threatening and should be considered if the patient has a dry cough or has experienced recent breathlessness. A sputum specimen must be collected and sent for culture in the event of a productive cough.

Incidences of opportunistic infections, such as *Pneumocystis carinii* pneumonia have occurred in patients taking methotrexate.

Blood. Thrombocytopenia, neutropenia, agranulocytosis and fatal marrow suppression can develop but the latter is rare. Regular monitoring of the blood is required.

Liver. Methotrexate can cause abnormal liver function and hepatic fibrosis. The liver enzyme AST, when persistently elevated is the best guide to toxicity. (N.B.: Alkaline phosphatase and gamma – CT may be elevated in acute rheumatoid arthritis).

6. Drug interactions

TRIMETHOPRIM and PHENYTOIN must be avoided because they increase the risk of bone marrow suppression. Be aware that aspirin, acidic NSAIDs and probenecid may increase the effects of methotrexate.

7. The nurse's responsibility when giving methotrexate

Before administrating intra-muscular methotrexate each nurse must be aware of the local policy regarding the handling, administration and disposal of cytotoxic agents.

Prior to commencing methotrexate the nurse must check and document that the patient has had:

(a) A chest X-ray within the last 6 months (lung function tests may be requested by some rheumatologists).
(b) Females have received contraceptive advice to avoid pregnancy whilst on, and for 6 months after taking methotrexate.
(c) Fertility – males are advised that reduced spermatogenesis may occur but is reversible.
(d) Alcohol – advised to avoid all alcohol.
(e) Smoking – advised to reduce or stop.

Before beginning the injections the nurse should discuss the treatment with the patient. Explanation should be given of what methotrexate is for, how it is to be given, how it will help and potential side effects. It is also important to make sure that the patient knows where the treatment and monitoring will take place

and who they should contact if they are unable to attend or if they experience any problems. It is always helpful to provide written information to the patient to support the verbal explanation.

Before the injection

1. Ask the patient if they have experienced breathlessness, a dry productive cough, mouth ulcers, nausea or any overt signs of infection. The injection should be witheld if any of these have occurred.
2. Ascertain that blood has been taken for FBC, ESR or PV and LFTs. A blood test should be avoided up to 3 days after administration of methotrexate as it can reduce the WBC and platelet count. Danger signs include a progressive fall in the haemoglobin, white cells, neutrophils or platelets and abnormal liver function.
3. Check that the prescribing doctor has seen and approved the results of the previous blood test. (Some units may have nurse-led protocols to take the responsibility for carrying this out).
4. Record the dose given, blood results and the presence of any unwanted effects and any action taken in the patient's monitoring booklet.

If the monitoring reveals any adverse effects, withhold the methotrexate and report the symptoms to the doctor. These guidelines should be read in conjunction with the national guidelines for the monitoring of second line drugs, produced by the British Society of Rheumatology.

Administration and disposal of methotrexate

1. Administration.

(a) Aseptic technique is essential at all stages.
(b) Contact between the nurse and the methotrexate should be avoided by the use of:
   (i) Thick latex or PVC gloves
   (ii) Plastic apron and water repellent armlets
   (iii) Safety goggles/mask.

2. Disposal. Potentially hazardous equipment includes:

(a) Sharps (vials, ampoules and needles) which should be discarded in the appropriate sharps container according to local policy.
(b) All other disposable equipment including protective clothing which should be treated as dry clinical waste and placed in the designated bag according to local policy.

REFERENCES

Carroll G et al 1994 Incidence, prevalence and possible risk factors for pneumonitis in patients with rheumatoid arthritis receiving methotrexate. J Rheumatology 21: 51–4

Furst et al 1990 Adverse experience with methotrexate during 176 weeks of a long term prospective trial in patients with rheumatoid arthritis. J Rheumatology 17: 1628–35

Groendal H et al 1990 Methotrexate and trimethoprim-sulphamethoxazole – a potentially hazardous combination. Clinical and Experimental Dermatology 15: 358–60

Kremer J M et al 1994 Methotrexate for rheumatoid arthritis: suggested guidelines for monitoring liver toxicity. Arthritis Rheum 37: 316–28

RCN 1989 Safe practice with cytotoxics. Royal College of Nursing Oncology Society – RCN, London

Shiroky J B et al 1991 Complications of immunosuppression associated with weekly low dose methotrexate. J Rheumatology 18: 1172–5

Stewart K A et al 1991 Folate supplementation in methotrexate-treated rheumatoid arthritis patients. Semin Arthritis Rheum 20: 332–8

Multiprofessional care and discharge planning list

Reproduced with permission of the Nuffield Orthopaedic
    Centre NHS Trust

NUFFIELD ORTHOPAEDIC CENTRE NHS TRUST

<u>MULTI-PROFESSIONAL CARE & DISCHARGE PLANNING CHECKLIST</u>

Ward:

Admission Date:

Diagnosis/Operation:

SECTION I

All patients will be asked these questions which are to help us ensure that your stay in hospital and return home are as well planned as possible.

This section must be completed for every patient coming into hospital at the following stages where relevant.

SCREENING QUESTIONS [please delete yes or no as appropriate]	OUT PATIENTS	PAC	WARD
1. Do you have someone who is willing and able to care for you at home if necessary?	YES/NO	YES/NO	YES/NO
2. Are you able to wash, dress, walk, get to the toilet, make and eat your meals without assistance?[1] [2]	YES/NO	YES/NO	YES/NO
3. Do you already receive any services? eg District Nurse, Meals on Wheels, Home Help	YES/NO	YES/NO	YES/NO
4. Are you worried about anyone or anything at home whilst you are in hospital?	YES/NO	YES/NO	YES/NO
5. Are you worried about managing when you go home from hospital?	YES/NO	YES/NO	YES/NO
Signed (Nurse): Signed PATIENT/CARER: Date:			

NOTES:

1 If supervision is required, the patient is **not** independent. 2 If equipment is used but no help is required the patient is independent.

Does the patient have any communication problems eg hearing, language?

Are there any other reasons why further assessment is necessary?

ACTION: Please consider if as a result of information gained you need to make an **early referral** for specialist assessment or liaison with Occupational Therapist, Social Worker, Physiotherapist, District Nurse etc.

HOME SITUATION [delete as appropriate]
LIVES: ALONE/WITH (including pets):
ACCOMMODATION
FLAT/HOUSE/BUNGALOW   WARDEN CONTROLLED/RESIDENTIAL CARE/OTHER:
Toilet UPSTAIRS/DOWNSTAIRS   Bedroom UPSTAIRS/DOWNSTAIRS   Bathroom UPSTAIRS/DOWNSTAIRS
Steps to house YES/NO
COMMENTS

CURRENT COMMUNITY SERVICES	CURRENT PRIVATE SERVICES
Home Care:	Private Nursing/Care:
Meals on Wheels:	Chiropody:
Day Services:	Cleaning Services:
Community Nurse:	Other:
Named Care Manager: (including SW/Community OT)	
Community/Out Patient Physio:	

SECTION II PATIENT NEEDS AND SERVICES REQUIRED ON DISCHARGE

PHYSIOTHERAPY				REFERRED TO: FIRST SEEN DATE:		DATE:
NEEDS IDENTIFIED	**ARRANGEMENTS MADE**					
To be independent:	YES	NO	N/A	COMMENTS		DATE & SIG.
on transfers from bed and chair						
walking with appropriate aid FWB PWB NWB						
climbing a single step						
climbing stairs						
Out Patient Physio arranged						
Other:						
				ARRANGEMENTS COMPLETED	PHYSIO SIG: DATE:	

OCCUPATIONAL THERAPY	REFERRED TO: FIRST SEEN DATE:			DATE:	
NEEDS IDENTIFIED	**ARRANGEMENTS MADE**				
To be independent & safe:	Home Checked	Activity Completed	Equipment Required	Equipment Delivered	DATE & SIG.
Transfers bed					
chair					
toilet					
bath/shower					
car					
Personal Care/Dressing					
Domestic ADL					
Education/Advice given	YES / NO / N/A				
Assessment of Home Environment (Home Visit)	YES / NO / N/A THOSE INVOLVED	DATE:		TIME:	
Referral for Community Equipment	DATE:				
Other:					
	ARRANGEMENTS COMPLETED		OT SIG: DATE:		

TO BE COMPLETED BY THE APPROPRIATE PROFESSIONAL PRIOR TO DISCHARGE

NURSING	
NEEDS IDENTIFIED AND ARRANGEMENTS MADE	DATE & SIG.

Community/Nursing Home bed required on discharge YES/NO		
Bed requested at:	Request accepted YES/NO Booking date: For:	
Transfer details of Community Hospital/ Nursing Home:	Date of transfer:	
GP Letter Written: GIVEN/POSTED:	**TTO's** Ordered: Given: Patient's own drugs to be returned YES/NO Patient's own drugs returned YES/NO	
Out Patient Appointment Date: GIVEN/POSTED:	**Transport** OWN/HOSPITAL Booking date: For: Booking No:	
Patient's Personal Property/Valuables Checked by: and: Recorded in Property Book YES/NO Property returned to patient:	Date: In HOSPITAL/WARD safe YES/NO Patient's own walking aids returned YES/NO Property taken home:	
District Nurse/Practice Nurse Required for: Date asked to see patient: Booked by:		
Knowledge/Skills/Information 1. Knowledge of wound care 2. Understands Drug Therapy 3. Knows who to contact for advice/help 4. Other 5. TED stockings 6. Learning check carried out	 GP Tel No: Consultant's Secretary Tel No: To be worn for: following discharge	
COMMENTS	

TO BE COMPLETED BY THE NURSE PRIOR TO DISCHARGE

PATIENTS NEEDS AND SERVICES REQUIRED ON DISCHARGE

SOCIAL SERVICES AND OTHER PROFESSIONALS	REFERRED TO: FIRST SEEN DATE:	DATE: TIME:
NEEDS IDENTIFIED	ARRANGEMENTS MADE	DATE & SIG.
Comments	ARRANGEMENTS COMPLETED	SW SIG: DATE:
	Continuation Sheet YES/NO	

DISCHARGE PLAN (NAMED NURSE/PRIMARY Nurse to complete this section)

Proposed Discharge Date: ....

NAMED/PRIMARY Nurse: ....

Change of Nurse: ....

Patient	( )	Community Nurse	( )
Carer	( )	Warden	( )
Nurse	( )	Head of Home	( )
Physiotherapist	( )	Care Manager (SW/Community OT)	( )
Occupational Therapist	( )	Community Physiotherapist	( )
Doctor	( )	Community Hospital Nurse	( )
Social Worker/Care Manager	( )	Day Care Services	( )
Other Professional	( )	Others	( )
		GP	( )
Going Home Package Completed	( )		
Going Home Package Given to Patient/Carer	( )		

Discharge Destination: ....

to check arrangements on discharge where appropriate with:

```
GP Sticky
```

Signature of Patient: ....

Signature of NAMED/PRIMARY Nurse: ....

Actual Discharge Date:

COMMENTS (including Doctor's comments)

THIS CHECKLIST TO BE FILED IN MEDICAL NOTES ON DISCHARGE

CARE & DISCHARGE PLANNING 93/NOC (2)

Appendix 5

Drug treatment for rheumatoid arthritis

There is no cure for rheumatid arthritis (RA), but drugs can help to control the pain and stiffness and some can put it into remission.

Four types of drugs are usually used. They are **anti-inflammatory**, **analgesic**, **slow acting anti-rheumatic** and **steroids**. Each one is given for a different reason and at a different stage of the disease. It is usual for you to be taking more than one type of drug at the same time. This is not a problem as most drugs given for arthritis mix with each other.

How should I take them?

It is better to take most types of tablets for arthritis with or after a meal as this makes them less likely to upset your stomach. Some drugs, such as D-penicillamine, should be taken on an empty stomach so please read the label on the bottle and your drug information sheet.

What drugs will I take?

Remember that each person is different and what suits one person may not suit another. Finding the right drugs for you could take a little time. If you try one drug and it doesn't help or it upsets you, it doesn't mean that this will happen with all drugs. Many tablets come in bottles with childproof tops and this can be a real problem for people with painful hands. If you can't open your tablet bottle, ask the chemist for a bottle with an ordinary screw cap. Please remember that if you have small children in or visiting your home that they get into everything.

Do keep all drugs out of their reach.

Analgesics

Analgesics are pain killing tablets. There are a number

of different kinds of analgesics. You can buy some drugs 'over the counter' like **paracetamol** but others such as **distalgesic** are only on prescription.

Commonly used analgesics

Paracetamol, distalgesic, co-codamol, co-dydramol, benoral, aspirin.

There are quite a few more but remember, most drugs have more than one name.

What do they do?

Analgesics are also known as painkillers. Although they can stop pain for some people, they usually lessen rather than stop it altogether.

What do they look like?

They are usually in tablet form, but they can also come as a liquid. Sometimes they are given as injections.

How quickly do they work?

They start to work very quickly, often within half an hour of taking them.

How should I take them?

You may take analgesics at any time of day and the number you take will vary. To be safe, you need to know the most you can take in 24 hours. For instance, the most **paracetamol** or **distalgesic** that you can take each day is two tablets four times a day but the number that you take from this dose is up to you. Some days you may need to take eight tablets whilst on others only four or six.

Some people worry about taking analgesics and tend to wait until they are in a lot of pain before they take them. In fact the tablets work much better if you take them as soon as your pain starts to build up.

Another good time to take them is as a way of preventing your pain from starting. If you are going to do something that you know causes you pain, like doing the shopping, take a couple of painkillers **before** you start.

If you are having a 'flare' it's a very good idea to take your analgesics on a regular basis until the arthritis has calmed down.

One good thing about analgesics is that you don't have to wait until you eat a meal to take them. They work more quickly if you take them just with a glass of water or juice. Aspirin is an exception to this rule as it can irritate the stomach and so should be taken with food.

Can I take them with my other tablets?

Yes, they mix well with all your tablets for your RA, but it is better to avoid alcohol with **some** analgesics. Check your tablet bottle label.

If you are taking tablets for some other condition, check with your doctor, nurse or chemist that they mix.

Are there any side effects?

Side effects are rare. Some analgesics can cause dizziness, sickness and occasionally headaches. Paracetamol can cause constipation.

Non-steroidal anti-inflammatory drugs

There are many different types or 'families' of anti-inflammatory drugs. They are all similar, but some will suit you better than others. If you try one and it doesn't work, don't worry too much because you can try another one that might help.

Commonly used anti-inflammatory drugs

Brufen, voltarol, naprosyn, indocid, froben, feldene, ponstan, oruvail.

Most of these drugs are only on prescription, but **Brufen** can be bought 'over the counter'. If you buy drugs without a prescription, do check that they are safe to take with your other tablets.

What do they do?

These drugs lessen the pain, stiffness and swelling which inflammation causes. They are not a cure for RA but they do help the 'symptoms'.

What do they look like?

They are usually tablets but sometimes they can be suppositories. There are also some anti-inflammatory gels that you can apply to your muscles or joints.

How quickly will they work?

They usually work quite quickly. Some people notice a difference within hours of taking them but it usually takes a few days before you feel the best effect.

How should I take them?

There are over 30 different kinds of anti-inflammatory drugs and you take each one in a different way. You take some as often as four times a day and others only once a day. The number of times that you need to take the drugs depends on how quickly it gets out of your body. With some tablets only half the amount of drug is left in the body after 2 hours. For these to be effective they will need to be taken about four times a day. Other drugs leave the body more slowly so you do not have to take them so often. You will get the best effect from the tablets by taking them regularly so that you keep the proper amount in the body.

You should always take anti-inflammatory tablets with or after food **never on an empty stomach**. If you can't manage to take them with a meal each time, take them with a drink of milk and a biscuit.

Are there any side effects?

The most common side effect is indigestion or an upset stomach. This sometimes makes people feel sick. A few people get stomach ulcers and any drug can cause a rash. Luckily these side effects are quite rare. Some anti-inflammatory drugs such as indocid can cause headaches or dizziness.

Anti-inflammatory drugs are usually quite safe, but they can sometimes cause a problem for some people if they already have a stomach ulcer or are on drugs that thin the blood.

Slow Acting Anti-Inflammatory Drugs (SAARDS)

This type of drug is taken if the arthritis is very active and is likely to destroy the joint. We can tell that this may happen by a blood test called Plasma Viscosity or PV. When the disease is active this blood result is higher than normal. Anti-rheumatic drugs bring the plasma viscosity down to more normal levels. This is quite different from the other drugs used in your treatment. You can take analgesics and anti-inflammatory drugs endlessly and they will not alter the plasma viscosity. Only slow acting anti-rheumatic drugs can do this.

Commonly used slow acting anti-rheumatic drugs

Sulphasalazine, hydroxychloroquine, gold, D-penicillamine, methotrexate.
This is not a full list, but these are the ones used most often.

What do they do?

These drugs are also known as **long-term drugs**. They slow the arthritis down and stop the disease from getting worse. This does not mean that the arthritis just stays the same as it was when you began the drugs. People start to feel much better. For instance there is less pain and stiffness and the tiredness that many people feel starts to lift. Walking up and down stairs or getting in and out of bed can become easier. Anti-rheumatic drugs really can improve the quality of your life.

What do they look like?

They are usually tablets, but one type of gold comes as an injection.

How long will they take to work?

Most of these drugs are slow to start working. It usually takes 10–12 weeks before you start to feel better and for some people it may take as long as 6 months. Methotrexate can start working a bit earlier, usually after about 4 weeks.

How do I take them?

You take all the anti-rheumatic drugs in a different way. Sulphasalazine and D-penicillamine start as a small daily dose that is slowly built up. Hydroxychloroquine is taken once a day and methotrexate is only taken once a week. Gold injections are also given once a week until you start to feel better and then about once a month. Not all of these tablets are taken with food; you should take D-penicillamine and methotrexate on an empty stomach.

You can take all of these drugs for as long as they are helping and are not causing any side effects.

Can I take them with my other tablets?

You can take anti-rheumatic drugs with both anti-inflammatory drugs and analgesics. Avoid taking D-penicillamine at the same time of day as iron or indigestion tablets. Methotrexate does not mix with aspirin, water tablets and some antibiotics.

Remember, if you need to take one of these drugs you will be given an information sheet that tells you all about it.

Are there any side effects?

A few people do get side effects. This usually happens at the start of treatment, but it can happen even if you have been on the drugs for many years. Each drug may have a different side effect and with most anti-rheumatic drugs you need to have regular blood and urine tests.

STEROIDS

Steroids are only taken when other drugs are not helping your rheumatoid arthritis. This is because they can have side effects if they are given in high doses over a long period of time. Steroids can be taken either as a tablet or as an injection.

Commonly used steroids

Prednisolone is the most commonly used steroid tablet for RA.

What do they do?

They dampen down the inflammation and that helps to lessen the pain, swelling and stiffness.

What do they look like?

They come either as tablets or as an injection into a joint or muscle. The 2.5 mg and 5 mg tablets are usually 'enteric coated'. This means they have a coating around them to help to stop stomach irritation.

How long will they take to work?

They usually start to work within a day or two, especially when given by injection.

How do I take them?

You usually take tablets just once a day but some people need to split the dose. They are best taken in the morning with or just after eating food. If they are given by injection into a joint you will be given an information sheet about the injection.

Can I take them with my other tablets?

Yes, they are safe to take with anti-inflammatory drugs, analgesics and slow acting anti-rheumatic drugs.

Are there any side effects?

Steroids can have side effects, but in small doses or when given into a joint, they are not a great problem to most people.

When taking steroid tablets some people put on weight or get a swelling of the face. More serious effects occur if they are taken in high doses. These include stomach ulcers, high blood pressure, thinning of the skin and bones and even diabetes.

The body can become addicted to steroids making it very hard to come off them.

Special information

You should never stop taking steroids suddenly as this could make you very ill. When you come off steroids the dose that you take is lowered gradually.

People who take steroids by mouth should always carry a special '**steroid card**'. This is in case you are in an accident and need an operation or treatment quickly. If this happens you will need to be given steroid by injection.

Appendix 6

Useful addresses

Arthritis Care
18 Stephenson Way
London NW1 2HD

Arthritis and Rheumatism Council
Copeman House
St Mary's Gate
Chesterfield
Derbyshire S41 7TD

British Acupuncture Council
Park House
206-208 Latimer Road
London W10 6RE
Phone: 0181 9640222

British Association for Counselling (BAC)
1, Regent Place
Rugby
Warwick CV21 82PJ
Phone: 01788 578328

Bristol Cancer Help Centre
Grove House
Cornwallis Grove
Clifton
Bristol BS8 4PG
Phone: 01272 743216

British Complementary Medicine Association (BCMA)
St Charles Hospital
Exmoor Street
London W10 6DZ
Phone: 0181 9641205

British Holistic Medical Association
179 Gloucester Place
London NW1 6DX
Phone: 0171 2625299

British Reflexology Association
12 Pond Road
London SE3 9SL
Phone: 0171 8526062

British School of Reflexology
92 Steering Road

Old Harlow CM17 0JW
Phone: 01279 429060

Family Planning Association
(see under Family Planning in telephone book)

International Society of Professional Aromatherapists
ISPA House
82 Ashby Road
Hinkley
Leics. LE10 1SN
Phone 01455 637987

National Federation of Spiritual Healers
Old Manor Farm Studio

Sudbury on Thames
Middlesex TW16 6RJ
Phone: 01932 783164/5

Reiki Association
2 Manor Cottages
Stokley Hill
Peterchurch
Hereford HR2 0SS

S.P.O.D.
(The Association to Aid the Sexual and Personal
Relationships of People with a Disability)
286 Camden Road
London N7 0BJ

Index

About the
PROFESSIONAL DEVELOPMENT RECORD

The United Kingdom Central Council (UKCC) PREP regulations require you to maintain a personal professional portfolio, in which you record evidence of your professional development.

This book provides you with excellent educational material to assist your study and develop your practice. Reading all or parts of it can contribute to your professional development.

The *Professional Development Record* (overleaf) is designed to help you record your study activity in your portfolio and show how it has enhanced your practice. To use the Record, you can do either of the following:

• photocopy the Record and place it directly into your portfolio, or

• use it as a basis for your own individual entry.

The aim of the Record is to help you plan how this book assists your professional development, to the benefit of yourself, your colleagues and your patients/clients.

Further information:

• If you do not have a portfolio and would like to purchase one, please contact your local bookseller or, in case of difficulty, phone our Customer Services Department on 0181 300 3322.

• If you need further information about PREP, you should contact the UKCC on: 0171 333 6550.

PROFESSIONAL DEVELOPMENT RECORD

Book (fill in author, title, year of publication, publisher):

Date of completion of book (or selections from book):

Duration of study time:

Reason for reading the book:

Intended learning outcomes:

Evaluation of material read:

Planned influence on practice:

Evaluation of influence on practice:

Learning outcomes achieved: